Praise for *Our Bodies, Ourselves: Menopause*

"I highly recommend this wonderful book to any woman navigating the changes of midlife. The mix of sound information, inspiring stories, and insight into the social context of menopause is unique and invaluable. Any midlife woman can use it to find information and affirmation to make health decisions that are right for her."

—Karen Carlson, M.D., Deputy Director, Center of Excellence in Women's Health, Harvard Medical School

"To the great good fortune of women entering the mid-life years, the legendary *Our Bodies, Ourselves* women have produced a book distilling the multiple complexities of our current understanding of that very normal transit in every woman's life, the menopause. So much has been learned about menopause in the last twenty-five years—what a challenge it had to be to treat the subject in a comprehensive, comprehensible manner, which this book admirably does. The information is responsibly up to date, the explanations reader friendly, the advice coolly wise, the mood sympathetically upbeat. *Our Bodies, Ourselves: Menopause* is a worthy companion to the classic pathfinder book by the same organization."

—Isaac Schiff, M.D., Chief of Obstetrics and Gynecology Service at Massachusetts General Hospital

"*Our Bodies, Ourselves: Menopause* is more than just another health reference book. Through accurate medical information and illustrative stories that value women's lives, it gives women the power to be advocates for their own health and well-being. Not only are women able to become more informed consumers, they are inspired to become involved socially and politically in creating a better future for women's health and health care."

—Mary Hayashi, Founder of the National Asian Women's Health Organization

"Once again, the Boston Women's Health Book Collective has provided us with a book all women can trust."

—Byllye Avery, Founder of the National Black Women's Health Project

"There's so much bad information about menopause. Here finally is great information, coupled with a clear-headed guide around the myths, misinformation, and vested interests that have made information-seeking so difficult."

—Janine O'Leary Cobb, Founder of "A Friend Indeed"; Author of *Understanding Menopause*

"A first choice for women seeking trustworthy information about menopause. Sound medical information enhanced with personal experiences and insightful social commentary. Many thanks to the dedicated women of the Boston Women's Health Book Collective for once again advancing women's health care!"

—Margery Gass, M.D., Former President, North American Menopause Society

"For those who want to navigate, understand, even celebrate menopause, this new book is an essential companion. Packed with words of wisdom for every woman, and with ideas about how to pro-

mote a healthy, nonmedicalized menopause, this is sure to be treasured—and referred to—as much as *Our Bodies, Ourselves* was when we were a bit younger.
—Abby Lippman, Chair of the Canadian Women's Health Network

"*Our Bodies, Ourselves* taught me about my body thirty years ago. I used it to transform my relations with my doctors and become a fierce advocate for my rights and my life. Now I am a great-grandmother and Our Bodies Ourselves is providing a book on menopause, which could not be more timely! This is visionary work that lasts a lifetime."
—Loretta J. Ross, National Coordinator of SisterSong Women of Color Reproductive Health Collective

"Enlightening, well-researched, and candid, *Our Bodies, Ourselves: Menopause* offers a complete range of medical and scientific information and advice plus wonderfully reassuring and inspiring personal anecdotes, photos, and sketches. If you're a woman over fifty, this is *the* book to keep on your bedside table."
—Nancy Thayer, Author of *Hot Flash Club*

"Who's afraid of menopause? Not the authors of this book, who offer practical health information and the wisdom of experience to help other women through this life transition."
—Kathleen Turner, Actor

"*Our Bodies, Ourselves: Menopause* allows us to enter this stage of our lives fully armed with the vital information we need to address any physical, mental, and spiritual challenges that arise. And it empowers us to make the change a true celebration!"
—Jeanie Linders, Writer/Producer of *Menopause The Musical®*

"Our Bodies Ourselves has done it again! After raising us from girlhood to womanhood and never shying from 'taboo' topics, our beloved guides to our own bodies are now here to lead us through menopause with this detailed, inclusive, and woman-centered book– a must-read for every woman in her middle years."
—Helen Zia, Author of *Asian American Dreams: The Emergence of an American People*

"*Our Bodies, Ourselves: Menopause* is a must-read for women of all ages. It clearly and accurately presents valid, research-based findings for women to use to make truly informed decisions about the value of treatments such as hormone replacement therapy, as well as alternative/nonmedical modalities. Whether you are a health care practitioner or a health care consumer, you will want this book in your library."
—Ann M. Voda, Ph.D., R.N., past President of the North American Menopause Society and the Society for Menstrual Cycle Research; author of "Menopause Me and You: the Sound of Women Pausing"

Other Major Books by Members of the Boston Women's Health Book Collective

Our Bodies, Ourselves: A New Edition for a New Era

Changing Bodies, Changing Lives

Ourselves and Our Children

The New Ourselves, Growing Older

OUR BODIES, OURSELVES:
Menopause

THE BOSTON WOMEN'S HEALTH BOOK COLLECTIVE

With a preface by
Vivian Pinn, M.D.

A TOUCHSTONE BOOK
Published by Simon & Schuster
New York London Toronto Sydney

This publication contains the opinions and ideas of its authors. It is intended to provide helpful and informative material on the subjects addressed in the publication. It is sold with the understanding that the authors and publisher are not engaged in rendering medical, health, or any other kind of personal professional services in the book. The reader should consult his or her medical, health, or other competent professional before adopting any of the suggestions in this book or drawing inferences from it.

The authors and publisher specifically disclaim all responsibility for any liability, loss, or risk, personal or otherwise, which is incurred as a consequence, directly or indirectly, of the use and application of any of the contents of this book.

TOUCHSTONE
Rockefeller Center
1230 Avenue of the Americas
New York, NY 10020

Copyright © 2006 by The Boston Women's Health Book Collective

TOUCHSTONE and colophon are registered trademarks
of Simon & Schuster, Inc.

For information regarding special discounts for bulk purchases,
please contact Simon & Schuster Special Sales at 1-800-456-6798
or business@simonandschuster.com.

Designed by Katy Riegel

Manufactured in the United States of America

10   9   8   7   6   5   4   3   2   1

Library of Congress Cataloging-in-Publication Data
Our bodies, ourselves : menopause / The Boston Women's Health Book Collective ;
with a preface by Vivian Pinn.
      p.   cm.
    Includes bibliographical references and index.
    1. Menopause—Popular works.   2. Middle-aged women—Health and hygiene.
3. Middle-aged women—Attitudes.   I. Boston Women's Health Book Collective.
RG186.O97   2006
618.1'75—dc22   2006044362

ISBN-13: 978-0-7432-7487-6
ISBN-10:   0-7432-7487-3

Contents

HEALTH CONCERNS

KNOWLEDGE IS POWER

Preface

Our Bodies, Ourselves: Menopause serves an important role in translating the latest scientific findings about the menopause transition into information that women can understand and use. A valuable theme throughout this book is the need for each woman to make good personal health care decisions. Good decisions involve gathering and evaluating information, weighing what is important at a personal level, finding the necessary resources for the type and quality of care required, and managing the associated costs. *Our Bodies, Ourselves: Menopause* presents an invaluable discussion of the most up-to-date information about menopause and a comprehensive view of health care alternatives for addressing symptoms associated with it. The authors discuss menopause in the larger context of a woman's overall physical, mental, and social well-being. Each chapter will help readers analyze information and apply it to themselves.

Menopause is a natural process that unfolds over years as women age (except when it occurs as a result of surgery or chemical treatments). Many women experience few or no problems associated with it and do not need medical treatment. This fact demonstrates the importance of understanding menopause as a natural occurrence in the lives of women as they age rather than considering it a disease. Women who do experience problems, and the health care providers who advise them, need to know the safest and most effective medical and nonmedical treatments.

To address this need, the National Institute on Aging and the Office of Medical Applications of Research of the National Institutes of Health sponsored a state-of-the-science conference in 2005: The Management of Menopause-Related Symptoms. Experts presented information on the biology of the menopausal transition, the nature of the symptoms women experience, strategies for relieving the common problems associated with the menopausal transition, and the risks associated with some treatments. This included information from the Women's Health Initiative (WHI), a large clinical trial that included a study of the long-term effects of estrogen with or without progestin in preventing chronic conditions such as heart disease, bone fractures due to osteoporosis, stroke, and breast and colon cancer. The WHI studies were stopped early because they demonstrated that risks outweighed benefits when women were taking the most commonly used hormonal preparations and dosages. After weighing all of the scientific evidence, including research conducted since the end of the WHI, an independent panel prepared a state-of-the-science statement regarding key issues surrounding the science of menopause. (This statement may be found at http://orwh.od.nih.gov/pubs/pubs_reports.html.)

In spite of advances from research and continuing scientific studies of menopause, there are still many aspects of menopause that must be further investigated. The panel stated that much more research is needed to clearly define the natural history of menopause, associated symptoms, and effective and safe treatments for bothersome symptoms. Best practices for preventing postmenopausal health problems must be further explored. Research studies on menopause must be expanded to more inclusively address the diversity of women for whom the results will influence decisions about medical care. Many continuing and new studies of menopause are already under way, and more will be supported to answer emerging questions about menopause and women's total body health and longevity. As these studies are completed and their results reported, the scientific community should reassess the state of knowledge about menopausal symptoms and treatments and about how to navigate the menopause transition.

Women and health care providers need trustworthy information in order to make responsible, informed decisions regarding health and well-being. *Our Bodies, Ourselves: Menopause,* written in language that can be understood by diverse populations of women, provides just such information.

Vivian W. Pinn, M.D.
Director, Office of Research
on Women's Health
National Institutes of Health
Department of Health and Human Services
Bethesda, Maryland

Introduction

The first newsprint version of *Our Bodies, Ourselves*—the groundbreaking book about women's health—did not even mention menopause. Back in 1970, sexuality, birth control, and childbearing were the main concerns of the book's authors, most of whom were in their twenties. When the Boston Women's Health Book Collective did decide to include menopause, in the 1973 edition, the mother of one collective member helped write the new section. Since then, *Our Bodies, Ourselves* has evolved into a comprehensive book for women at every stage of life, covering issues such as body image, relationships, and violence against women.

While producing the thirty-fifth anniversary edition of *Our Bodies, Ourselves,* the editorial team realized that several topics covered in a chapter or two in the "mother book" were ripe for more in-depth treatment. One of these was menopause. We decided to create a new book devoted entirely to the health concerns of women going through this transition. The result is the book in your hands now.

Like *Our Bodies, Ourselves,* this book features women speaking from our own experience. It also combines trustworthy medical information based on the best available evidence and thoughtful analysis of the social, cultural, and political forces affecting our health, just as *Our Bodies, Ourselves* does.

Our Bodies, Ourselves: Menopause is distinctive among current books on menopause in its rejection of the medicalization of women's natural life transitions; its evenhanded consideration of all treatment options, whether "conventional" or "alternative"; and its focus on understanding individual women's health in social and political context. While emphasizing that menopause is a natural process, not a disease to be treated, and that most women have a relatively easy time with the transition, this book does not deny the real challenges that some women face. Rather, it sifts through the evidence, offers illustrative personal narratives, and provides the best information available to help women make educated health care decisions.

BEYOND SELF-HELP

This book gives individual women tools to take care of ourselves during the menopause transition, from tips on eating well and becoming more physically active to strategies to cope better with stress. It provides helpful, clear information about signs of menopause that women may experience, such as hot flashes and vaginal dryness. Because most women experience menopause at midlife, and menopause is often associated with other health concerns of midlife and aging, this book covers those issues, from heart disease, osteoporosis, and cancer to problems of memory and mood.

But *Our Bodies, Ourselves: Menopause* is about more than self-help. It puts our individual choices in social context. Many factors, from pharmaceutical companies' influence on medical research and training to society's ageism and sexism, are beyond an individual's control. We can change these conditions only by advocating with others for policies and programs that protect the health of our families and communities.

FROM "I" TO "WE"

Throughout this book, women share their menopause experiences. Some of these first-person stories are told anonymously, set off in italicized passages in the text. Longer stories are set apart from the main text in boxes, with the name and photograph of the woman telling her story.

The inclusion of diverse voices is also embodied in the all-embracing "we" of this book.

The "we" refers to all women, whatever our racial, ethnic, and class backgrounds, countries of origin, sexual orientations, or gender identities. The choice to refer to women as "we" rather than "they" reflects the early decision of the Boston Women's Health Book Collective to change the title of its book (initially *Women and Their Bodies*) to *Our Bodies, Ourselves.* By speaking about women's bodies with the voice of personal experience, referring to "our bodies" rather than "their bodies," the book rejects the distancing voice of some medical texts. It celebrates that this is a book written for and about women—and primarily by us.

A COLLABORATIVE EFFORT

With the publication of *Our Bodies, Ourselves: Menopause,* we are launching a series of books that consider specific topics in women's health in greater detail than it is possible to do in *Our Bodies, Ourselves.* Our next project will be a book on childbearing, an issue that has been central to our advocacy for women's health from the very beginning. We hope that the titles in this new series will complement and expand on the work of our original book, which has been translated into twenty languages and has sold more than 4 million copies over the decades.

In preparing this book, we have collaborated with a wide-ranging group of contributors, who wrote and reviewed sections based on their expertise. We offer our thanks to them for their dedication and hard work. We also owe a great debt of gratitude to everyone who has contributed over the years to *Our Bodies, Ourselves* and to the organization that produces it, particularly the founders, staff, and volunteer board members. In addition, we want to acknowledge the trailblazing work of founder Paula Doress-Worters and Diana Laskin Siegal on *Ourselves, Growing Older,* a comprehensive guide to women's health after age forty that was first published in 1987.

Women of all ages now have greater access to information about our bodies, health, and medical care than was imaginable back in 1970, thanks in large part to the efforts of these pio-

neering advocates of women's health. We are proud to carry their mission forward with this new project.

Judy Norsigian, executive director, and Heather Stephenson, editor, for the Boston Women's Health Book Collective

Approaching Menopause

CHAPTER 1

Understanding Our Menopause Experiences

When I was fifty-two, my youngest son had just started college, my mother had relocated to a continuing care community close to me, my husband was stressed at work, and I was trying to define my next career steps. In the midst of my life, my body took over and signs of menopause began: very heavy irregular bleeding due to fibroids, occasional night sweats, and some vaginal dryness. . . . I had to acknowledge I was aging and couldn't take my body for granted. I needed to take care of it.

When I stopped having my periods, I was really happy about that. I realized that I could relax. I didn't have to worry about getting pregnant. I'm looking forward to the times ahead. I have vaginal dryness, but I use a range of lubricants so it is not a huge problem. Sex has changed but not in a negative way. Sometimes I feel great joy, other times less joy. But that's the way life is, isn't it?

The younger women I knew all thought it was never going to happen to them (ha!). And all my older women friends insisted, "Oh, it's nothing." So I had no one to talk to. That was very hard on me. Late in the process I found an excellent online support group, but by then, I realized that I was in a better position to give advice than to receive it. I think more women need to talk about this.

Those of us who are approaching menopause may wonder how it will affect us physically, emotionally, and socially. Most of us have questions, whether we anticipate the end of our periods with excitement, anxiety, or a combination of the two. While talking about menopause used to be considered taboo, women today are sharing our experiences more openly, through discussions with friends and family, in support groups and online chat rooms, and in the media. Women's health advocates have long pushed for better research on midlife and menopause and worked to raise awareness of the biological, social, and political factors that influence our menopause experiences. This book offers the information, resources, and support we need to make informed decisions and take care of ourselves as we approach and experience the menopause transition. When we learn more about menopause, we can proceed with increased confidence, the knowledge that we are not alone, and a critical perspective on the cultural messages that surround us.

For most women, menopause is a natural biological change that occurs at midlife. For others, menopause is the consequence of a health condition, medical treatment, or surgery, or it

KEY TERMS

SUDDEN AND EARLY MENOPAUSE

Sudden or early menopause can be induced by surgery involving the removal of both ovaries and by other medical treatments and health conditions. The term early menopause also refers to women who experience menopause naturally but earlier than usual (generally before the age of forty). (For more information, see Chapter 4, "Sudden and Early Menopause.")

MENOPAUSE TRANSITION

The transition to menopause, sometimes called *perimenopause,* is often a gradual process, involving the fluctuation of hormonal levels and some physical changes before the last menstrual cycle. It spans a period of one to six years or more. For most women, the menopause transition begins in our mid-forties and is completed in our early fifties.

MENOPAUSE

Menopause is defined as the end of menstruation. However, because our periods can be sporadic as we approach menopause, a woman is said to have reached menopause only after she has not had a menstrual period for twelve months. At menopause, we no longer ovulate and our ovaries produce significantly less estrogen. Menopause either occurs naturally or is induced by surgical removal of the ovaries or other medical treatments. Often people use the term menopause to refer to the entire menopause transition.

POSTMENOPAUSE

Postmenopause refers to the time following menopause.

occurs naturally but earlier than usual. Because such a transition is earlier or more abrupt, it may pose different challenges. Our experiences as we go through the menopause transition vary greatly. For some women, the transition is quite rapid; for others, it is slow or intermittent. It is impossible to predict with certainty what changes our bodies will go through or precisely how they will affect us.

Most of us, if we have not already experienced sudden or early menopause, begin to undergo a number of physical changes when we are in our forties. We may wonder if these changes are normal and if they are associated with menopause. A forty-eight-year-old says,

I think I'm in the beginning of my menopause. I've noticed a change in my menstrual cycle. In the last two or three months my periods have been a bit irregular and my flow is a lot heavier than it used to be. I'm normally just like clockwork.

In addition to changes in our menstrual cycles, we may experience other signals of the menopause transition, including hot flashes, night sweats, vaginal dryness, and insomnia. Some of us also experience problems such as memory loss, mood swings, and reduced sexual desire, although evidence suggests that these problems are more likely correlated with the aging process, other medical conditions, or life stressors than with menopause. The only changes that are scientifically recognized as associated with menopause are the end of menstrual bleeding, hot flashes, night sweats, insomnia, and vaginal dryness.[1]

Menopause is not a disease that needs to be "fixed" or "cured" by physicians and drugs. For the majority of us, in fact, the transition to the postmenopausal years involves relatively minor discomforts that do not require medical intervention or treatment. Most signs of menopause are temporary. For example, the hot flashes and

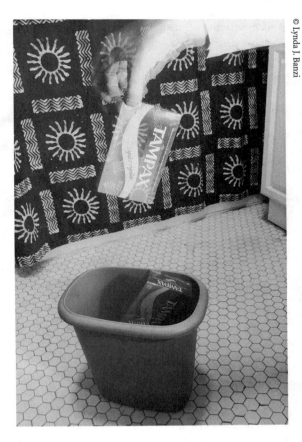

night sweats some of us experience are a response to changing hormone levels; when our hormone levels stabilize, the hot flashes usually stop within a few years. Knowing that these signs will end on their own may make them easier to tolerate or manage.

A minority of women experience problems associated with menopause that are severe enough to interfere with daily life.

I began having night sweats (I think I had them for a long time before I was really aware that it was night sweats and not just restless sleep). At work I would have sudden onsets of profuse sweating to the point of drenched hair and soaked shoes. . . . I am a registered nurse and always thought that I would sail right through meno-

pause because I understood the physiological changes and did not fear it. Ha! . . . I know that few people have as severe a reaction to the hormonal changes of menopause as I did, but I think women and men should be more aware of the things that can happen.[2]

The Massachusetts Women's Health Study, one of the largest and most comprehensive studies of midlife women and menopause, showed that the vast majority of women have positive or neutral attitudes toward menopause.[3] Many of us find that the experience and symbolism of the menopause transition motivate us to take stock of our lives, think about what's most important to us, become more attentive to our health needs, and make changes in how we take care of ourselves. In a 1998 Gallup survey sponsored by the North American Menopause Society, a majority of postmenopausal women said they were happier and more fulfilled than when they were younger. They reported improvements in their family and home lives, partner relationships, and friendships. In addition, approximately three-quarters of the women, who lived in the United States and ranged in age from fifty to sixty-five, said they had made some type of health-related lifestyle change, such as stopping smoking, at menopause/midlife.[4]

As we approach menopause, we may feel fearful because we have heard more about the small percentage of women who have very difficult menopausal transitions than we have about the majority, who have a relatively easy time of it.

It scared me at first because I felt I had no control. I sometimes went through three months of hot flashes and then I wouldn't have anything for six months. Things were happening to me that I didn't know if they were right or not. I couldn't understand what was happening. . . . It was hard to talk to anybody, including my mother.

In popular media, menopause is often presented as a time of physical and mental degeneration that women dread. Women going through the transition are frequently portrayed as emotionally unstable and irrational—people who may break into tears for no reason, become angry without provocation, and seem "out of control" (all because of our hormones). In reality, studies have shown that emotional changes are *not* inevitably part of the menopause transition.[5] The mood symptoms some women experience during the menopause transition do not appear to be caused by hormonal changes; they are far more likely to be linked to life stress, a history of depression, and health status at midlife.

Fears and anxieties about menopause can be created, exaggerated, or manipulated by drug companies, media pundits, and self-help gurus who focus attention on the potential problems associated with menopause (and the supposed solutions they are selling) rather than providing a balanced and accurate picture of women's real experiences. As *Aged by Culture* author Margaret Morganroth Gullette puts it, "Women have less to fear from menopause than from menopause *discourse*."[6] When we have little information and few positive role models, we are left vulnerable to believing all the negative things we hear about menopause. Learning to recognize and resist these sometimes damaging influences can prepare us to better understand and cope with the menopause transition.

For most American women, the context within which we experience menopause includes **ageism** (negative stereotypes and institutionalized discrimination against older people), **sexism** (prejudice and discrimination against women), and **medicalization** (the notion that natural biological processes need medical supervision or intervention). These societal attitudes can undermine our confidence and encourage unnecessary reliance on hormone treatment, other medical interventions, or "expert" advice.

Our menopause experiences are also often affected by our cultural, racial, and ethnic heritage, our socioeconomic class, and our individual life histories and life circumstances. There is no single path that all women take to and through menopause.

AGEISM AND SEXISM

I had my first hot flash at age fifty-two, the same age my mother was when she started menopause. But she told me she remembered feeling old. I don't. I feel like a younger older woman. I had my youngest daughter when I was forty-two. My sense of the life span has increased, with the expectation that I will have many active years, until my eighties, hopefully. There is so much I want to do.

Both women and men are living longer than we did in the past, for a wide variety of reasons: better sanitation, vaccinations, more control over reproduction, better understanding of the link between lifestyle and poor health, and better medical treatments and technology. A woman in the United States who reaches menopause today can expect to live approximately thirty more years, making her postmenopausal stage of life nearly as long as her reproductive years.[7] In 2002, the 33 million women in the United States who were fifty-five or older made up nearly 23 percent of the female population.[8] As more women reach midlife and change the demographics in our country, we have an opportunity to reframe the issues and construct a vision that will improve the health, well-being, and social status of women at midlife.

Unfortunately, entrenched negative stereotypes about "being old" can make it difficult for us to accept our natural aging process. We feel pressure, in overt and subtle ways, to live up to impossible ideals of eternal youth and beauty. Although society has changed somewhat, sexist attitudes linger and affect women as we age. A woman in her early forties says,

I don't like the word "menopause." . . . Whenever I heard that word when I was younger, I felt like it didn't relate to me. And now when I hear other women talk about menopause, it's all negative. . . . You're viewed as getting old and you're deteriorating.

In cultures where age is particularly venerated and respected, menopause is perceived very differently. In contexts where women look at aging in a positive light and are seen by others as sources of wisdom, menopause is likely to be less stressful.

We also may feel resistant to the idea that aging may bring with it a certain amount of discomfort, pain, and limitations to mobility. Such resistance is supported by our consumer culture, which promises us quick fixes for everything from menstrual cramps to acne, usually for a price.

Aging is separate from menopause, but it is part of it. I don't feel old, but I'm getting aging spots on

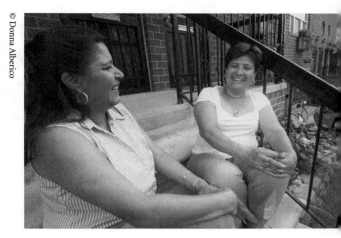

© Donna Alberico

my hands and my face. My hair is turning white. I'm starting to get that "boxy" shape. I look at other women my age, and I think, Gee, they look old. They act "old." But then, it's like, Oh my God. Am I that old? Maybe I'm just deceiving myself. Maybe I'm old, too, but I just can't see it. Maybe I need to go out and dye my hair and paint my toenails to feel good about myself. I don't like the way it makes me view myself.

Aging is a natural part of life. We can resist the cultural messages that devalue older women by joining advocacy groups for midlife and older women and by reaching out and appreciating one another. Building friendships with older women can offer us alternative role models. A forty-four-year-old woman says,

I went to a women's brunch where most of the women ranged from the mid-thirties to the mid-fifties. I was curious about one much older woman who turned out to be a sculptor in her seventies. She invited me to visit her at her studio near the shore. I drove down with a photographer friend, bringing a picnic lunch, and enjoyed a delightful afternoon viewing her recent work, each of us sharing her experiences as a woman trying to do creative work at different times in the life cycle.[9]

MEDICALIZATION

When I entered midlife, I experienced some of the same kinds of frustrations that I did as a woman giving birth. Once again, I found myself regarded by the medical profession as a patient in need of treatment. I was encouraged to view the natural process of menopause as a negative change that, if left untreated, would jeopardize my health. Thanks to the women's health movement, I found my voice. My own hormones are keeping me a healthy, active sixty-six-year-old.

In our culture, major biological transitions that women experience, such as childbirth and menopause, are often medicalized. The term *medicalization* refers to treating a natural process as if it were a medical condition requiring intervention. The normal physical changes associated with menopause in particular tend to be perceived as pathologies requiring both medical and cosmetic "help," perhaps because aging itself is so medicalized.

Some medical researchers, health care providers, and drug companies have defined menopause as a hormone "deficiency" condition due to ovarian "failure." According to this view, menopause is a condition like thyroid deficiency or diabetes: If it is left untreated, we will be at greater risk for many chronic diseases, a lower quality of life, and premature death.

This view was the rationale for the widespread use of long-term hormone treatment for postmenopausal women from the 1960s to early in this century.[10] After all, if our ovaries had failed us and we had become deficient, it made sense to replace our hormones, hence the term "hormone replacement therapy." For decades, many doctors and women were convinced that boosting estrogen levels would treat all signs of menopause, make women feel younger, and ward off diseases of aging. This belief persisted even though no well-designed long-term clinical trial of hormone treatment had been conducted. We now know that hormone treatment is likely to carry more risks than benefits for most women. (For more information, see Chapter 7, "Hormone Treatment.")

Several factors may help to explain why menopause has been perceived as a deficiency. One is the long history of attributing ill health and characteristics considered undesirable for women to our reproductive organs and hormones. For example, terms like *hysteria* (derived from the Greek word *hustera*, which means "womb") reflect the former belief that

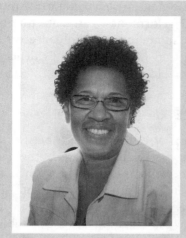

"I decided that I needed to care for myself."

YVONNE ATWELL

I knew very little about what the menopausal experience would be like or how it might influence one's mind and body. Information was sketchy at best and none specific to Black women. I gained weight almost overnight and my eating habits also changed. I wanted sweet foods, yet sugar made me tired and lazy.

There were times I thought, What is wrong with me? I felt so confused. The day I put the iron in the fridge and the milk in the linen closet was the day I sat down and cried, thinking I must be losing my mind. I remember speaking to my sister about this. She laughed and said the same thing had happened to her early in her menopause experience. Talking to my sister helped ease some of the stress I was feeling. I was on my own, working three part-time jobs and trying to raise a teenage daughter. I didn't have time to worry about what was happening to my mind and body.

I knew that I had to somehow find a way to care for myself, because as a Black woman I didn't trust the system to know about me or my race. My doctor suggested that I go on HRT [hormone replacement therapy] because the hot flashes kept me awake at night. I knew enough about HRT not to trust that this was the best solution for me. Besides, my doctor had no information on the effects of HRT on Black women.

At some point I made a concerted effort to design and develop my own health plan. I decided that I needed to care for myself and spend as little time with a doctor as possible. My plan consisted of meditation, reading everything I could find on menopause and Black women, changing my eating habits, joining a fitness club, and finding a program that would help me develop my inner strength through positive thinking and awareness.

It has been ten years since I entered menopause and I have no regrets about my decisions to take care of my own physical and mental health. I still attend the doctor on a regular basis. I still weigh the pros and cons of her advice and decide if the information she is giving me is what I need or if I should consider other options.

Presently I feel that I'm in better physical and mental health than at any other time of my life. I still get night hot flashes, but they are no longer severe. Most of the time I feel happy and blessed to be well, to enjoy my three daughters and my two grandchildren. I feel I am experiencing a place of empowerment and self-control unlike any other time in my life.

behaviors considered inappropriate for a woman were somehow caused by her uterus. Some women in the nineteenth century had hysterectomies in attempts to treat a wide variety of problems. Similarly, some doctors believed that the ovaries were the source of ill health and advocated their removal. During the same era, higher education for adolescent girls was discouraged for fear that taxing girls' brains would ruin their reproductive organs.

Another reason that so many doctors have viewed menopause as a deficiency condition is that they are more likely to see in their offices women who are experiencing distress than those who aren't. Women who have a relatively easy time during and after the menopause transition simply don't visit doctors as often. This makes it seem to doctors (and others) that menopause is more stressful for most women than it actually is.

Doctors are also more likely to see women who have severe distress immediately after their ovaries are removed (a procedure that often accompanies hysterectomies). The sudden change in hormone levels caused by surgical removal of both ovaries usually results in more distress than natural menopause does. (For more information, see Chapter 4, "Sudden and Early Menopause.")

Finally, the pharmaceutical industry must be recognized as a driving force in the medicalization of menopause. Many studies on hormones have been sponsored by pharmaceutical companies, which influence both the way the studies are done and how the results are interpreted. These studies are then published in prestigious medical journals and become accepted as scientifically valid; legitimate criticisms of these studies often do not reach the lay public. The pharmaceutical industry also sponsors "continuing education" seminars for physicians, reinforcing the use of hormones either as a treatment for menopause or as a preventive measure for chronic diseases. Research has shown that doctors' prescribing practices are often strongly influenced by promotional messages rather than by scientific evidence.[11]

The story of the widespread prescribing of hormone treatment before long-term clinical trials had confirmed their safety is a dramatic example of the power of the pharmaceutical industry and inadequate research to influence women, doctors, and government agencies.

(For more information on hormone treatment, see Chapter 7, "Hormone Treatment"; for more information about industry influence on research, see "Can We Trust the Evidence in Evidence-Based Medicine?" page 24.)

THE ROLE OF HORMONES

The reduction of estrogen levels that women experience at menopause represents the natural state for women; our ovaries have not "failed" us and we are not "deficient." The higher levels produced when women are younger allow for ovulation and the possibility of pregnancy; beyond our reproductive-age years, these higher levels are no longer necessary. (For more information about how hormone levels change during the menopause transition, see Chapter 3, "What's Happening in Our Bodies.")

Reduced estrogen production can be health-enhancing in some ways. Decreased estrogen can reduce our risk for certain hormone-related health problems. For example, estrogen is strongly linked with the risk of breast cancer. Almost all studies show that women who took hormones long-term after menopause had a higher risk of breast cancer than women who did not. Other hormone-related disorders, such as fibroids (benign tumors) and endometriosis (a condition in which tissue like that of the uterine lining grows outside the uterus, causing pain, infertility, and other problems), are greatly decreased after menopause.

Any premenstrual syndrome or painful menstruation a woman might experience will likely stop when menstruation stops. For this reason, menopause may be especially welcomed by those of us who have painful monthly cramps, as well as by women who experience heavy bleeding during the menopause transition. A thirty-nine-year-old woman says,

I've always had a lot of problems with my periods, so I look forward to no periods. Ever since I was a teenager, I've had to go to bed for the first day when I first get my period because I feel so sick. I thought I would outgrow this problem after I had babies. But no. It just kept on. So that's one good thing to look forward to.

The end of our fertility, while not always welcome, is also health-enhancing in some ways, because multiple pregnancies can strain our bodies.

This does not mean that all of the physical changes related to menopause are experienced as positive. For example, lower estrogen levels tend to be associated with vaginal dryness, a sensation that many of us find unpleasant. Still, knowing that this is the normal way that our bodies experience the movement through the natural human life course allows us to identify which changes we feel we can embrace, which we can tolerate, and which we wish to find ways to alleviate.

Going through perimenopause, I wanted to do everything naturally. I tried the progesterone cream, went to a homeopathic doctor, talked to my friends who were in menopause. My hot flashes were so bad, I was waking up about every two hours, and they got bad during the day. My period stopped altogether and I was fine with that. But then sex, which had been wonderful, hurt. I was dry and sore and felt like I was getting infections. . . . I was so miserable, I decided to try hormones. I am so glad I did! I'm on the combination [of estrogen and progestogen] and it's a lifesaver. . . . My friends have been pretty surprised. They thought I'd be the Soy Bean Queen and avoid HR [hormone replacement], but I've never felt better.

One doctor suggested I go on hormone replacement pills but I said no. I don't like taking med-ication unless I feel it's absolutely necessary. I'd rather jump into the shower to cool down than take a pill. I would prefer to ride it out without hormones.

(For more information about the risks and benefits of hormone treatment, see Chapter 7, "Hormone Treatment.")

The medical myths surrounding menopause need to be dismantled. We must become informed consumers and develop critical perspectives on treatments available to us and research being conducted. Government, the medical establishment, and women's health groups need to work together in order to ensure that this will happen. Individual women also need to take care of ourselves and one another. Women's health depends on it.

RACIAL AND ETHNIC DIFFERENCES

Our experiences of the menopause transition are shaped by our particular cultural or ethnic background, class, and sexual orientation, as well as other social and genetic determinants. For example, the traditional role of black women as the pillars of our families and communities can result in black women's jeopardizing our health by "overdoing it." An African-Canadian woman says she cannot show her feelings openly even when she feels vulnerable because she is expected to be the "strong" one:

I think menopause is hard for Black women. We tend to downplay emotional things. We're like the M&M's with the hard shell up to survive racism, but the soft part inside that is love and tenderness. That shell is our survival key. I think, being strong Black women, a lot of us are worn down. We go into menopause emotionally, physically

IS MENOPAUSE THE SAME AROUND THE GLOBE?

The majority of the world's languages do not include a word for menopause. Women in many parts of the world understand the end of menstruation as part of an aging process in which, more often than not, biological changes are less important than social changes, such as enjoying improved status in the community and becoming a grandmother.

Anthropological research suggests that both the biology of aging and the cultural meanings associated with it vary around the world, and that biology and culture may affect each other. For example, the signs of the menopausal transition that are often noted in North America and Europe, in particular hot flashes and night sweats, do not occur equally among all populations of perimenopausal and postmenopausal women. Research in India, Indonesia, Taiwan, Hong Kong, Japan, Singapore, China, Korea, Thailand, Malaysia, and the Yucatan, Mexico, all reveal low reporting of hot flashes and night sweats. In parts of Africa and the Middle East, research indicates that hot flashes are, on average, experienced more often than among North American and European women.

Similarly, older women around the globe are not equally at increased risk for heart disease, bone fractures, or other conditions. White women in the United States have an almost seven times greater risk of dying from heart disease than Japanese women[12] and a more than seven times greater risk of experiencing a hip fracture than women in Beijing.[13] African women have significantly lower rates of hip fractures than African-American women, even allowing for the possibility of substantial underreporting.[14]

Many factors affect our experiences of menopause and our development of diseases. Biological, nutritional, lifestyle, psychological, and social variables all need to be considered, as well as cultural and language differences and individual variation.

drained. We have the tendency to think, This is not going to happen to me.

Mexican-American women may be confronted with issues at menopause that result from bicultural life experiences. In Mexico, as in many other Latin American countries, women are unlikely to discuss menopause with others, including with their daughters, so the sensations and changes associated with menopause may come as a surprise to many women.

Pudor or modesty is an important value in many Latina communities. Therefore, for midlife Latina women, consulting a medical practitioner, especially to discuss personal or sexual matters, may be uncomfortable. Pudor may also be part of the reason that some Latinas do not use the terms for our sexual anatomy, referring instead to the area "de abajo" ("down there"). In the United States, however, one routinely is expected to answer questions about menstrual status and other intimate issues at medical appointments.

Making matters even more difficult, those of us who are Latina immigrants in the United States may be confronted with a set of cultural values regarding aging that is different from the values we grew up with. In many Latin American communities, the status of women, and our power within the family, grows as we grow older. In the United States, midlife women, and especially immigrant women, may find that our status declines.

For many Latina immigrants, who are disproportionately poor, financial and social responsibilities often take priority over the experience of menopause. The menopause transition may be perceived as a normal part of life that does not require medical attention. One Mexican-American woman said, in Spanish,

Menopause? No, I didn't go to a doctor for that. We [do not] go to a doctor for every cut we get. We just take care of things ourselves.

A number of studies have documented cultural differences in our perceptions of menopause. For example, African-American women seem more likely to view the cessation of menstruation as a relief and look forward to not worrying about pregnancy after menopause. By contrast, white women perceive menopause as more of a medical problem and more readily seek prescription therapy and written resources for information.[15]

A large-scale study with the acronym SWAN—Study of Women's Health Across the Nation—has allowed researchers to analyze the impact of ethnicity on menopause. A multiethnic sample of 16,065 African-, Chinese-, European-, Hispanic-, and Japanese-American women between the ages of forty and fifty-five confirms that manifestations of menopause vary by race/ethnicity, lifestyle, and socioeconomic status. The SWAN analysis highlighted a substantial amount of ethnic variation. For example, more African-American women reported hot flushes, more Latinas reported vaginal dryness and an earlier menopause, more white women reported difficulty in sleeping, and Asian-American women reported fewer symptoms despite having lower estrogen levels compared with the averages in the study group.

Socioeconomic disparities were also found in the SWAN analysis. The majority of symptoms were more frequently reported among women who had difficulty "paying for basics," as well as women who smoked and those who rated themselves less physically active than other women their age. This diversity in the physical sensations associated with menopause suggests that our cultural expectations regarding our bodies as well as differences in health practices such as diet, and economic patterns such as access to healthy food and safe places to exercise, strongly shape our experiences of menopause.[16]

Spiritual and religious beliefs provide some women with an important source of strength. An African-American woman explains how her faith is central to coping with the menopause transition:

There are times when I'm sitting in a meeting or something, and I have such bad hot flashes, and, oh my goodness, and I'm just so hot . . . and all the emotional things that I don't understand. So I just go right to my spirituality. I pray. And because of that, it makes me feel less overwhelmed, more at peace. Afterwards, I feel more refreshed, rejuvenated.

MIDLIFE TRANSITIONS

For many of us, it is not the hormonal or physical transitions of menopause so much as the social transitions associated with midlife that are the tipping point for emotional or lifestyle changes. For some women, menopause and midlife are a time of transition toward a new phase in life or a trigger for adopting a new life

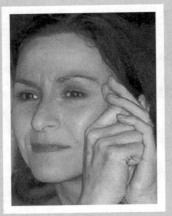

"I was sweating with the big girls now."

CHARLOTTE LOPPIE

My experience of menopause has been largely shaped by my bicultural (Aboriginal/European) background. Many indigenous cultures view health as holistic and approach experiences like menopause from a naturalistic perspective. Yet Western culture takes a somewhat more disease/deficiency view of this life change. I entered perimenopause straddling these two worldviews, and keeping my balance was not always easy.

It began during the winter of 2002; after almost six years of reading and research about the menopausal transition, I awoke one frigid, December night in a blistering sweat. Quite suddenly it seemed like some internal register had jacked up the temperature in my pajama top. I quickly removed the offending garment and lay there feeling an odd sense of elation. I had arrived—my first hot flash. I was sweating with the big girls now; I was a crone, on my journey toward the wisdom and maturity of elderhood—corny, to be sure, but very fulfilling.

More than two years has passed since my first "trial by fire." I have finally arrived. The journey, I fear, was not always as serene and joyful as I previously had imagined. The lack of sleep almost did me in and the loss of control left me feeling quite weary. I am still among the ranks of countless flashing, sweating, tired middle-aged women. Yet I can easily flip that coin and tell you about the clarity of my vision these days; about the big changes I have made in my most intimate relationships; of the self-love and self-worth I finally found, somewhere in my tired eyes, my aging face, and my tormented body.

philosophy. Some of us go back to school, while others may decide to use our life experiences and increased confidence to make changes in our community. This may be a time in which we develop a stronger sense of identification with our mothers. Or it may be a time of sadness in which we grieve for opportunities we missed earlier in life—for children we did not bear or raise, or other paths we did not take. For many of us, menopause is simply a non-event.

I was a stay-at-home mom of sorts. While raising my kids, I went to school one class at a time. It took me about twenty years to finish my bachelor's and then my master's degree. I was never quite sure what I was going to do with these degrees, but I kept going. And then, all of a sudden, it became quite clear to me. Not only was I going for a Ph.D. but I knew I would have to somehow leave home to do it. Where did I get the confidence to think that I was smart enough to earn a Ph.D.? What made me think I could possibly go away and expect my husband to take care of himself and our three college-age kids and manage the household? It couldn't be just because my oldest son applied and was accepted into a Ph.D. program. It couldn't be just because my youngest, twins, were reaching eighteen, the magic age when they legally become adults. I knew I was just entering my midlife. That's it! It must be the hormones!

Many of us reach menopause while also experiencing the "dependency squeeze." At midlife we are often caught between the responsibilities of raising children or grandchildren and caring for aging parents or other relatives. Or we may be coping with an "empty nest." At the same time, we may be working in demanding jobs. Balancing these roles can cause us stress and may be the source of problems that we mistakenly think are signs of the menopause transition. The opposite also may be true; the physical signs of menopause may erode coping skills.

Menopause happened when there were a lot of other things happening in my life. I was leaving my job, my house, and I was moving to another city. So at first I thought I was just under a lot of stress.

It's important to be in tune to our body because it's often trying to tell us something. Unfortunately, I think by the time we finally get the message, our body has already been trying to tell us something for a long time, and we suffer the consequences of not having listened. But it's more than what is happening to our bodies, it's also our minds. Our state of mind is tied up with our bodies. Like sometimes I feel kind of lethargic, but I think, OK, this is physical, but it has something to do with my emotions, too.

(For more information about family and social changes, emotional well-being, and stress reduction, see Chapters 10 and 11, "Family Life and the Workplace" and "Emotional Well-Being and Managing Stress.")

FINDING OUR BALANCE

The point for many of us is to find the right balance between acknowledging the very real changes in our bodies at menopause and also understanding that our life experiences at any age are affected by many social, political, economic, and cultural factors that have little to do with hormones and that cannot be "treated" with either medication or pop psychology. By honestly looking at our life situation, our relationships, our families, and our society, we may be better able to resist the ageism, sexism, and medicalization that are so central to the American way of experiencing menopause.

Menopause can provide an opportunity to know ourselves and our bodies better. A fifty-two-year-old woman says,

It's another stage of life. . . . Your body is going through another journey. It's part of a woman's natural life cycle. It's not something to be frightened of. When you reach this stage, you're more aware of who you are as a person. You learn to feel more comfortable within yourself.

Menopause can result in our feeling satisfaction at having successfully come through a long journey. In Germaine Greer's terms, the older woman is one who climbs her own mountains, "in search of her own horizon, after years of being absorbed in the struggles of others."[17] While we may stumble at times, we find the strength to continue. At the end of this transition, we can look forward to a new phase of life that can be liberating and empowering.

The change of life means that you change. . . . Priorities change. Needs change. Emotions change. I think it sometimes scares people because they are afraid of change.

The menopause transition can inspire us to be more attentive to our health needs, eat well, and exercise. Many of us are motivated to quit smoking or cut back on our drinking.

When we understand menopause, we can become more comfortable and accepting of the changes it will bring. Having gone through menopause, a fifty-eight-year-old woman says she looks on life very differently now:

A few years ago I would have said, "Oh my gosh, menopause? That's old!" But now that I'm at that stage, I feel differently. I feel like I don't have to apologize for things I feel. I look at things differently and I'm more relaxed. It's just like—I don't know how to explain it—I just feel happier. Things don't bother me the way they used to. If I can't get things done today, then there's always tomorrow. I've matured. I've become wiser. My outlook on life is different. Now I tell younger women, these are the most wonderful years. I think that's where my menopause has brought me. I'm feeling very good about that.

NOTES

1. National Institutes of Health, "NIH State-of-the-Science Conference Statement on Management of Menopause-Related Symptoms," March 21–23, 2005, accessed online at consensus.nih.gov/2005/2005 MenopausalSymptomsSOS025.html.htm on October 25, 2005.

2. Excerpted from the website A Fine Kettle of Fish: Menopause, at www.queendom.com/kettle/meno pause/k_menopaus2.html, accessed on October 27, 2005.

3. Nancy E. Avis and Sonja M. McKinlay, "The Massachusetts Women's Health Study: An Epidemiologic Investigation of the Menopause," *Journal of the American Medical Women's Association* 50, no. 2 (March–April 1995): 45–9, 63.

4. W. H. Utian and P. P. Boggs, "The North American Menopause Society 1998 Menopause Survey, Part I: Postmenopausal Women's Perceptions about Menopause and Midlife," *Menopause* 6, no. 2 (Summer 1999): 122–28, available online at www.ncbi.nlm.nih.gov/entrez/query.fcgi?CMD=search&DB=pubmed.

5. National Institutes of Health, "NIH State-of-the-Science Conference Statement on Management of Menopause Related Symptoms."

6. Margaret Morganroth Gullette, "What to Do When Being Aged by Culture: Brief Annals of the Twentieth-Century Hormone Wars," *Tikkun* 18, no. 4 (July/August 2003): 64.

7. Avis and McKinlay, "The Massachusetts Women's Health Study: An Epidemiologic Investigation of the Menopause."

8. U.S. Census Bureau, "Women and Men in the United States: March 2002" and "The Older Population in the United States: March 2002," accessed at www.census.gov/prod/2003pubs/p20-544.pdf. and www.census.gov/prod/2003pubs/p20-546.pdf on October 20, 2005.

9. Paula B. Doress-Worters and Diana Laskin Siegal, in cooperation with the Boston Women's Health Book Collective, *The New Ourselves, Growing Older: Women Aging with Knowledge and Power* (New York: Simon & Schuster, 1994), xxiii.

10. Nancy Krieger et al., "Hormone Replacement Therapy, Cancer, Controversies, and Women's Health: Historical, Epidemiological, Biological, Clinical, and Advocacy Perspectives," *Journal of Epidemiology and Community Health* 59, no. 9 (September 2005): 740–48.

11. Testimony of Michael Wilkes, M.D., Ph.D., before the U.S. House Committee on Government Reform, May 4, 2005, accessed at reform.house.gov/UploadedFiles/UC%20Davis%20-%20Wilkes%20Testimony.pdf on October 26, 2005.

12. World Health Organization, *World Health Statistics Annual 1995*, Geneva, 1996.

13. L. Xu et al., "Very Low Rates of Hip Fractures in Beijing, People's Republic of China," *American Journal of Epidemiology* 144 (1996): 901–7.

14. C. W. Slemenda and C. C. Johnston, "Epidemiology of Osteoporosis," in *Treatment of the Postmenopausal Woman: Basic and Clinical Aspects,* edited by R. A. Lobo (New York: Raven Press, Ltd., 1994).

15. K. T. Pham, J. A. Grisso, and E. W. Freeman, "Ovarian Aging and Hormone Replacement Therapy: Hormonal Levels, Symptoms, and Attitudes of African-American and White Women," *Journal of General Internal Medicine* 12 (1997): 230–36.

16. E. B. Gold, B. Sternfeld, J. L. Kelsey, et al., "Relation of Demographic and Lifestyle Factors to Symptoms in a Multi-racial/Ethnic Population of Women 40–55 Years of Age," *American Journal of Epidemiology* 152 (2000): 463–73.

17. Germaine Greer, *The Change: Women, Aging and the Menopause* (Toronto: Knopf Canada, 1991), 67.

CHAPTER 2

Making Health
Care Decisions

Making good health care decisions can be challenging. A good decision involves gathering and evaluating information, weighing what's important to us, finding the resources we need to maximize the quality of care we receive, and dealing with the associated costs. Each phase of this process can be complex as we clarify our values, our fears, and our resources. We may ask ourselves whether we place a priority on avoiding any interventions that might increase future cancer risk, however slightly. Or is it more important to us to achieve immediate relief of symptoms so that we can function better here and now? Are the effects on our sexuality of choosing or refusing particular interventions extremely important to us or of relatively minor importance? Are we comfortable accumulating financial debt in order to pursue treatments, or is worry over finances likely to cause us more distress than the condition for which we seek treatment?

While we struggle to clarify our needs and make our decisions, we also realize that many of the factors that affect our health—from toxins in our food and air to the influence of pharmaceutical and insurance lobbies—are not in our individual control. They are largely determined by social policies, government regulations, and economic realities. Much of our power to shape our experience of menopause is limited by the access we have to appropriate economic and medical resources. Our country's failure to provide a comprehensive, integrated health care system that ensures access to all means that we spend enormous energy, time, and resources trying to navigate the existing system. To create change at the systematic level, we must work together to advocate for our health and the health of our communities. (For more information, see Chapter 20, "The Politics of Women's Health," and Chapter 21, "Finding Our Power, Organizing for Change.") This chapter focuses on what we can do as individuals to navigate the current health care system, educate ourselves, and improve our own care.

We make decisions that affect our health constantly. For example, we may decide to have fresh fruit for a snack instead of getting french fries at the drive-through. We may decide to walk to the movies instead of drive. We may decide to quit smoking—or to continue smoking. Such decisions add up. Our lifestyles can have profound effects on our well-being and reduce (or increase) our need for medical care. Regular exercise, healthy eating, and stress reduction may reduce some problems associated with the menopause transition.

When I began experiencing a number of menopausal signs, I decided to use herbal remedies, to exercise regularly, and to pay more attention to what I ate. I belong to a women's group, which helped me a lot. We shared information, gave each other suggestions, and supported each other's decisions.

As I was approaching my fiftieth birthday, my daughter gave birth to twins. I was totally delighted and knew I would take an active part in their lives. However, I also realized that if I didn't take care of myself, I would not have the energy to take care of them. I started walking every day, made sure I was eating more nutritious meals, and best of all, I was finally able to quit smoking. Four years later, I am in the best shape of my life and I can keep up with my grandchildren. I am having the time of my life!

Our ability to make healthy choices and carry them through is often limited by eco-nomic and social realities, and it is important that we avoid blaming ourselves for not living the "perfect" lifestyle.

FACING MENOPAUSE

MENOPAUSE AS A NORMAL LIFE EVENT

Women in the United States often think of menopause as requiring medical treatment, but menopause is not a disease. It is a normal, natural part of a woman's life. Occasionally it involves problems for which we may explore self-help techniques, complementary or alternative treatments, or conventional health care.

It is important to remember that many signs and complaints of menopause are temporary. They usually last a few years. Enduring two years of hot flashes is different from experiencing them for the rest of our lives. Mood swings may seem less problematic if we remember that they will fade. Times of transition are often rocky, but as we move through them, we may gain a sense of balance and equilibrium.

When I began to have hot flashes, I felt grateful. I thought of [the times] when I would miss work because of severe menstrual cramps and of all the money I had spent for menstrual supplies. I knew the hot flashes would end and there would be no more cramps!

We may make different decisions at different times, depending on our values and the severity of our menopause-related complaints.

A couple of years [after menopause], I started to experience hot flashes in earnest. They almost took on a life of their own. And they certainly took over mine. I'd start my morning with a shower and would be sweating before I finished dressing. I'd sit at my computer at work and that unpleas-

ant, overwhelming feeling would flare. Many days I'd have to go into the ladies' washroom, strip down to my bra and fan myself before I could return to my desk. I endured the symptoms since I didn't want to go back on the [hormone treatment] drugs.

[But eventually I decided] to go back on hormone therapy. . . . I'm now taking hormone therapy once every five days. Am I getting hot flashes again? Yes, but only first thing in the morning, even before I get out of bed and before my shower. I can live with this.

IT MAY NOT BE MENOPAUSE

Knowing whether a health concern we are experiencing is related to menopause or not can be difficult. Sometimes our health care providers, and we ourselves, assume that all our health problems are related to menopause just because we are going through the menopausal transition. Sometimes a provider may suggest a treatment without understanding the true cause of the problem. Hot flashes, night sweats, insomnia, and vaginal dryness are the only physical problems clearly and consistently shown by research to be related to menopause.

AGEISM AND MEDICALIZATION

Ageism is the systematic devaluation of a person because of her or his age. In the youth-oriented culture of the United States, getting older is equated with loss of power, loss of status, and disease. Medicalization may cause health care providers and others to think of menopause in terms of disease and medical intervention. (For more information on medicalization, see page 8.)

We may internalize anti-aging attitudes, which make us vulnerable to market pressures pitching cosmetic surgery and medications that claim to prolong youth.

To resist commercial manipulation that plays into our insecurities about the normal physical changes we experience as we go through the menopause transition, we need to be able to distinguish the signs of normal aging from disease, as well as understand the impact of internalized and institutionalized ageist attitudes.

INTERVENTIONS AND THEIR CONSEQUENCES

Medical interventions often affect us in ways that go beyond the specific therapeutic goal we may have had in mind. In fact, many of us have learned that medical interventions often lead to further interventions. This particularly seems to be the case for two of the interventions most often offered menopausal women: hormone treatment and hysterectomies.

When I was in my early forties, I was having complications before the Change. The doctor did a hysterectomy and gave me hormones. . . . they don't tell you that by taking replacement hormones, you can develop gallbladder disease. I ended up losing my gallbladder, and then that sets you into a different lifestyle because all your food is passed through you, so you end up having to go to the bathroom all the time. I kept telling my girlfriend that I know where all the bathrooms are at.

GATHERING INFORMATION

Gathering and evaluating information are crucial to making good decisions about health care during the menopause transition. Our knowledge of our body, our life history, and information about possible remedies and their effects help us to make wise decisions for ourselves.

As in other situations, a good place to start is with our friends and family members. With menopause, as with our periods, pregnancy, and childbirth, the range of "normal" experiences is very wide. Many women find formal and informal support groups to be helpful in providing a sense of what the experience has been like for a variety of women. Such groups help us feel that we are not alone, give us support for our decisions, and offer additional ways of thinking about our situations.

When we speak to friends, relatives, and other women, we come to understand that while health care professionals have expertise regarding diagnosis and interventions, only we can figure out what's important to us. As we listen to opinions, some of which are contradictory and some of which are similar to ours, we realize that we have the right to act in ways consistent with our values and priorities. This is true even if our decisions are contrary to the mainstream medical position, differ from the decisions our friends made, or fly in the face of the advice given by the menopause pundits we see in the mass media.

Health care providers can be an important source of health information. However, they often are constrained by limited time; bureaucratic rules; financial incentives from employers to restrict services (particularly in managed care settings); personal biases about treatments or prejudices about certain groups of people; lack of knowledge about prevention, self-care, and alternative treatments; and concerns about liability. Therefore it is important to seek information from additional sources, including family and friends, support groups, libraries, and medical and health information websites.

Health care providers today operate within a medical environment that requires what is called "informed consent" from patients; that is, unlike in the past, providers are required to tell us about the risks and benefits of proposed treatments. However, given the time constraints of office visits and the complexities of modern medicine, we often find that the choices doctors give us are confusing. When our providers quickly cite statistics or use jargon that we don't understand, we may feel frustrated. It is important to remember that it is our right to ask for clearer explanations. We can ask the provider to write down the numbers so that we can think about them at home, and we can ask the provider to explain terms that we are not familiar with.

We may feel particularly upset when the

provider presents us with a major decision that we simply do not feel competent to make. No choice seems quite right, and we feel that weighing the alternatives actually adds to our burdens rather than lightens them. At these times, we may find ourselves wishing for an old-fashioned doctor who would tell us what to do rather than present us with difficult choices. When that happens, it's good to remember that the old-time paternalistic doctor did not always make good decisions. It also may be helpful to tell ourselves that in many cases there is no "perfect" decision; we must weigh which decision is right for us.

EVALUATING INFORMATION

As a parish nurse, the most popular guidance I have given to midlife women is "Go to [a bookstore] or the library and read the introductions to books and articles. Check the author and sources. Be sure to note if the book or article was published by a drug company that might be selling a product. Then read through the books that appeal to you and check the sources again. Then let's talk through your questions."

We may find that gathering information from libraries, websites, or other sources is relatively easy, but evaluating it is harder. An abundance of health information is available, but its quality varies greatly. Some materials push dubious medicine, both conventional and alternative; some are concerned only with selling you their products; and some may be biased by the drug companies, professional societies, and other advertisers that support them. Studies conducted through 2002 found that between 20 and 90 percent of health information on the Internet was incomplete or inaccurate.[1] Separating questionable or misleading information from accurate and reliable material can be daunting.

Below are some questions to ask yourself to help evaluate the quality of any material you find.

- *Who wrote or created the material?* Any health information, whether in a brochure, in a book, or online, should have the author or persons responsible for the material clearly identified. You may have to look hard to find this information for sources other than books: On brochures it is often in fine print at the bottom of the last page; on websites it can often be found on the "About Us" pages.
- *Who is paying for the research, article, ad, or website? What is the person or group's motivation?* The source of funding can affect what information is presented and how it's presented. For example, drug company–sponsored information tends to downgrade or ignore nonmedical or nonpharmacological approaches and is slow to present innovative alternatives or preventive treatments. Try to determine if the author(s) or site owner(s) have a financial interest or anything else to gain from proposing one particular point of view over another. Paid ads in magazines and newspapers and websites touting the products they sell should also be questioned.
- *What is the basis of the information presented?* In addition to the authorship of the material you are reading, the evidence that material is based on should be provided. Medical facts and figures should have references, and opinions or advice should be clearly labeled as such and set apart from information that is evidence-based (that is, based on research results).
- *What research was done, and what did it prove?* Check pages 23–27 for information on evaluating a research study.
- *When was the material written or compiled?* All content should have a date on it, so you can tell when the material was written or last

revised. Information on safety can change. Material on treatments for life-threatening diseases and invasive procedures may be out-dated in months, while information about self-care and day-to-day health concerns is likely to be accurate for somewhat longer.

- *Does the information sound too good to be true?* Be wary of "cures" for incurable diseases or remedies that cover too many conditions (cramps, depression, and obesity all in one pill, for example). Question materials that credit themselves as the sole source of infor-mation on a topic as well as materials that dis-parage other sources of knowledge.

Some good sources for health information include:

- Consumer guides, such as *Consumer Reports* on medications and its website, www.con sumerreports.org/mg/home.htm, that evalu-ate medical care and specific medications.
- Government guides, such as Medline Plus (http://medlineplus.gov), the Centers for Disease Control and Prevention (www.cdc. gov), and the National Institutes of Health website (www.nih.gov). Government re-sources tend to be reliable, although in some instances they reflect the influences of politi-cal organizations and/or the pharmaceutical industry.
- Medical databases such as PubMed, which provides articles from published medical journals for free at www.ncbi.nlm.nih.gov/ entrez/query.fcgi; and the Cochrane Collabo-ration, which produces systematic reviews summarizing the best evidence on health topics and interventions (www.cochrane. org/reviews/en/topics/index.html).
- The National Women's Health Network and its newsletter, *The Women's Health Activist,* and website, www.nwhn.org.
- The Center for Medical Consumers and its

newsletter *Health Facts for Informed Decision Making,* and website, www.medicalcon sumers.org.
- Public Citizen Health Research Group and its newsletter, *Worst Pills Best Pills News,* and website, www.citizen.org/hrg.
- The Our Bodies Ourselves website, www.our bodiesourselves.org.

UNDERSTANDING RESEARCH RESULTS

As we learn more about menopause, we may read and hear many competing claims and sta-tistics. Understanding the different types of re-search studies behind these numbers can help

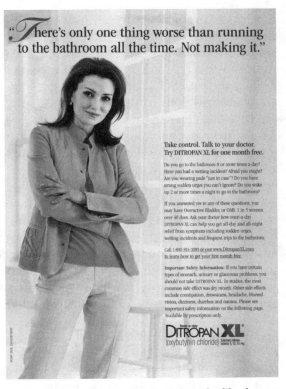

Drug companies exploit our fears about bodily changes during the menopause transition, with ads that imply their products are the best solution.

CAN WE TRUST THE EVIDENCE IN EVIDENCE-BASED MEDICINE?

When we and our providers seek solutions to our health problems, we depend on medical research to tell us which treatments work best, how likely it is that a particular treatment will help us, and what kind of risks the treatment entails. We expect this *evidence-based medicine* to bring us the best possible care.

Health professionals' trusted sources of scientific evidence include research published in respected medical journals, continuing education courses presented by experts, and clinical practice guidelines. Clinical practice guidelines are established by expert review committees charged with reviewing the best of medical research to define standards of good care.

What few of us know is that medical research has undergone a quiet but radical transformation over the past two or three decades.

Before 1970, the vast majority of clinical research was funded from government sources.[2] This has changed dramatically. Three out of four of the clinical trials published in the top medical journals (*The Lancet,* the *New England Journal of Medicine*, and the *Journal of the American Medical Association*) are now funded by pharmaceutical companies.[3] In 1991, about 80 percent of drug company–sponsored research was still being done in universities, where academic checks and balances supported the independence of researchers. But by 2000, only 34 percent of this research was still being done in academic medical centers. The rest had been transferred to for-profit research companies.

When drug companies fund research directly through private contracts, they are able to influence the results in many ways. Drug companies are not required to compare their products to other known treatments. They can select the age and gender of the people included in a study to highlight the benefits of the drug and minimize the risks. (For example, they can choose to study their product on healthy younger people who take few other medications and are therefore less likely to have adverse effects, despite the fact that the drug is more likely to be taken by older people taking multiple medications.) The drug companies can end studies if the results don't appear favorable and choose not to publish studies that don't come out the way they had hoped. And many of the authors of the research articles published in even the most respected medical journals don't have access to all of the data from their own studies—only the data the drug companies choose to let them see. By controlling the design of the research, the criteria by which patients are selected, the analysis of the data, and the selection of results to be published, drug companies shape medical knowledge.

Research funded by the pharmaceutical and biotech industries is far more likely to produce results that support the sponsors' interests. Two studies published in 2003, one in the *Journal of the American Medical Association (JAMA)* and the other in the *British Medical Journal,* showed that commercially funded studies were 3.6 to 4 times more likely than noncommercially funded studies to show positive results for the sponsor's product.[4] Another *JAMA* study that looked only at highest-quality studies found even stronger bias: The odds that commercially funded research found the sponsor's product the treatment of choice were 5.3 times greater than for studies funded by nonprofits.[5]

The agencies we count on to protect the interests of health consumers are increasingly compromised. More than half of the funding for the Center for Drug Evaluation and Research, the division of the U.S. Food and Drug Administration that approves new drugs and oversees drug safety, comes from user fees paid by drug companies.[6] The medical journals we trust to independently evaluate the articles they publish are also being influenced by the biomedical industries, as they depend on money from pharmaceutical advertising and from selling reprints of published articles to corporate sponsors, who then distribute them to physicians. The committees that produce clinical practice guidelines, which inform and direct health care professionals, are now dominated by experts with active financial ties to one or more companies that make the drugs under consideration.[7] And about 70 percent of continuing medical education courses for doctors are now paid for by the drug and other medical industries. Since doctors must participate in continuing medical education to maintain their medical licenses, it becomes increasingly difficult for any of them to avoid being exposed to industry-sponsored messages.

As commercial interests gain an increasing role in determining our "medical knowledge," it is important to understand that the fundamental reason that companies help create and distribute this information is to promote their products and improve their corporate bottom lines. Our health is relegated to, at best, a secondary consideration. We need to question whether doctors should be given financial incentives to follow clinical practice guidelines, as some now are, when those guidelines may be based on incomplete or biased research. Already we have evidence that such "pay for performance" incentives can lead to inappropriate care for older people with multiple chronic diseases.[8]

We need to demand that the public know when medical experts receive research funding or advising fees from drug and biomedical companies. And we need to advocate for stricter standards in the regulatory agencies that evaluate research results and oversee clinical guidelines. As individuals we can ask our health care providers if they practice under "pay for performance" programs and then consider this fact when making decisions about their recommendations for diagnostic tests and prescription medications.

The commercial takeover of our medical knowledge is, at its core, not a scientific problem but a political one. The solution will require an engaged and active citizenry. For more information, see *Overdosed America: The Broken Promise of American Medicine*.[9]

us evaluate their results and make informed health care decisions.

There are three major types of research studies:[10]

1. In a **cohort study,** researchers follow a group, or cohort, of women for a period of time. The researchers determine whether the women experience a particular exposure, such as whether they take a drug or supplement, exercise, smoke, or eat certain foods. The researchers follow all women in the cohort (both those who do and those who do not experience the exposure of interest) to see whether the women experience a particular outcome (for example, development of a certain disease). The researchers then calculate the risk of developing the outcome (called the *incidence rate*).

Cohort studies can detect relationships between exposure and outcome but they cannot definitively claim that the exposure or treatment *causes* the outcome.

2. In a **case-control study,** researchers investigate two groups, one group of women who have a certain outcome, such as a disease, and one group of women who do not. The group of women with the disease is called the *case group,* and the others are known as the *control or comparison group.* Researchers determine whether or not the women experienced specific exposures of interest (such as diet or exercise). Identifying case and control groups based on outcome is the hallmark of case-control studies, which are common when the outcome of interest is rare (such as certain cancers) or when it is not possible for practical or ethical reasons to assign different groups to different treatments (such as smoking or experiencing abuse). Like cohort studies, case-control studies show a relationship between treatment and outcome but they cannot definitively claim that the relationship is causal.

3. In a **randomized controlled trial,** researchers recruit women to participate in a study. Once the women agree to participate, they are assigned randomly to receive either the treatment being tested or a *placebo* (such as a sugar pill). The study is called *randomized* because there is no rhyme or reason to whether a woman ends up getting the treatment or the placebo. If neither the women participating in the study nor the health professionals working with them know which group each woman is in, the study is called *double-blind.* The placebo helps with the blinding, so that the woman and her doctor can't tell by looking at the pill she's taking whether it's an active treatment or a sugar pill. Randomized, double-blind placebo-controlled trials are thought of as the "gold standard" in research. They attempt to test whether treatment X causes outcome Y, and they can come the closest to claiming *causation* because of the blinding, the randomization, and the use of a placebo. The idea is that everything is held constant, except whether women are taking the placebo or the actual treatment.

Understanding Relative versus Absolute Risk

Statistics about health can be confusing because risk can be measured in different ways. **Risk** indicates whether or not a treatment or behavior (an exposure) is associated with an increased likelihood of developing a disease or condition (an outcome).

Relative risk is an indicator of the strength of the association between exposure and outcome. It is used to assess the importance of a particular factor or treatment in the development of a disease or condition. Relative risk is often expressed as a percentage. For example, a study might conclude that women who took a specific medicine had, on average, a 25 percent decreased risk of developing a particular disease than women who did not take the drug. Relative risk is always an average for a group.

Absolute risk describes the effect of an exposure on an outcome in the general population (as opposed to comparing specific groups). In the population overall, how harmful is an exposure? What is the likelihood of developing a particular condition? Absolute risk provides answers to these questions. For example, women in a certain country or city might have a one in ten chance of developing a certain condition during their lifetimes. (This would be the same as a risk of 10 percent.) Like relative risk, absolute risk estimates represent averages for a population, not the proscribed fate of any individual.

Sometimes studies report what sound like dramatic changes, for example a 50 percent decrease in risk for developing a certain disease. But if this is a decrease in the relative risk, and the absolute risk of developing the disease is small, the number of women affected will be low. For example, if the relative risk of developing a disease is cut in half by taking a certain drug, but only one in 100,000 women who do not take the medicine develop that disease each year, only one in 200,000 women per year would avoid developing the disease if the whole group took the medicine—and all of the other women would be at risk of experiencing its unwanted "side" effects.

Understanding what research results tell us about our risk of developing a certain disease or condition is an important part of making health care decisions. It's also important to remember that there is enormous variation among individuals and that our decisions are informed by our values and preferences as well as scientific evidence.

MAKING DECISIONS

EVALUATING DRUGS

Pharmaceutical companies and the corporate media advertise drugs targeting women who may have vague complaints to encourage us to ask our doctors for the drugs advertised. These advertisements are misleading and can cause harm.

No drug is completely safe. We each have to determine the risks and benefits of a prescribed medicine. Some adverse effects occur so rarely that they become apparent only when millions of people have taken a drug. Since every year the number of drugs on the market increases, it is important to ask your provider to explain why she or he has selected a particular drug for you. Your provider may have been given information about the drug from a company promoting its use; consider doing some independent research yourself, too. Related questions to consider are

1. Will this drug address my primary health concern? Will it cure the underlying problem or only alleviate symptoms?
2. What are my chances of developing a condition if I take the drug (for prevention), or if I don't?
3. How significant is the drug's benefit?
4. What are the most worrisome risks?

EVALUATING TREATMENTS

To learn more about a proposed treatment, whether conventional or alternative, ask your provider and do some research on your own. Questions to consider include

1. What is the treatment's success rate and how do we know it?
2. Is the treatment permanent (such as surgery)?
3. Is it systemic (affecting the whole body, as in chemotherapy or hormonal therapy)?
4. Is it cumulative (staying in the body and increasing with each treatment, as in radiation)?
5. Can the effects be harmful, and how?
6. Are there less drastic treatments available?
7. What will happen if the recommended treatment is not followed, and how is this known?

What's the worst thing that could happen from taking this drug? What are the chances of that happening? What will happen if I stop taking the drug?

5. How long has this drug been studied?

The example of hormone therapy for menopause shows how drugs are often used before their effects are fully known. Since 1923, when estrogen was first isolated, drug products for menopause have never undergone rigorous studies until health risks and/or deaths were documented. In 1996, the National Institutes of Health, at the urging of feminist groups, began what was supposed to be a ten-year study of the effects of hormone therapy on women. In 2002, the study was stopped because the risk of breast cancer and heart disease was found to be higher than any measurable benefit. (For more information, see Chapter 7, "Hormone Treatment.")

It is essential for all of us to evaluate any studies that physicians or others use to assure us a drug is safe, and to advocate for increased and unbiased research.

BARRIERS TO RECEIVING MEDICAL CARE

Because the U.S. medical system is so expensive, many of us face barriers to receiving the best possible care. In addition, because there is a tremendous imbalance of power between most health care consumers and many health care providers, institutionalized discrimination exists for those of us in less powerful sectors of the population. Making health care decisions can be especially difficult for women who are treated as second-class citizens by medical institutions. This group includes women as a whole; low-income women and uninsured women (who may find that very few

---

EVALUATING RESEARCH RESULTS

If you are trying to understand the results of a research study, consider these questions:

1. For how long was the study carried out? Sometimes it takes a generation (twenty years) to know the effects of a drug. An example was diethylstilbestrol (DES): Children born to mothers who took DES during pregnancy did not develop cancer until they were teenagers.
2. How many subjects were in the study? (A study that has only fifty people, rather than thousands, cannot be generalized to an entire population of potential users of the drug.)
3. Were the people studied similar enough to you (in characteristics such as age, race/ethnicity, and number and types of conditions) that the findings may be most helpful for your situation?
4. Who sponsored the study?
5. Did the study ask people to remember a behavior in the past? (Many times these studies are inaccurate because people do not always remember a past behavior or they answer in a way that will "help" the researcher.)
6. How were so-called side effects (all effects) considered?

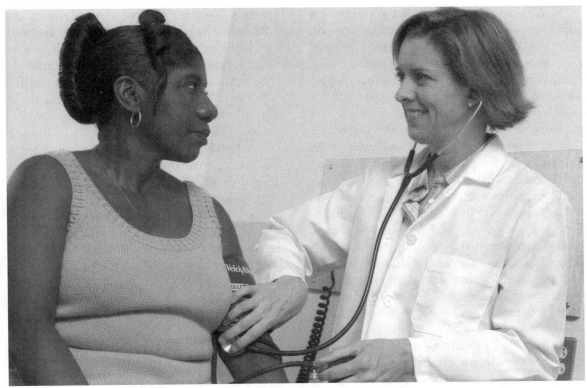

choices of providers or treatments are available to us); women of color and older women (whose concerns may be dismissed as "unimportant" or "whining"); women with disabilities (who may face mobility or communication issues); lesbian, bisexual, and transgender people; and immigrant women, especially those of us who are not fluent in English. Ultimately, changing current practices will require significant changes in public policy. In the meantime, being aware of how the medical system reflects society as a whole can help us deal with this system and improve the way we are treated.

COSTS AND INSURANCE COVERAGE

The costs of medical care present one of the largest barriers that many of us face when we try to obtain information and care. The single most common way of paying for appointments with health care providers, hospital visits, and prescription drugs in this country is medical insurance. Managed care is a type of medical insurance in which the insurance company "manages" medical services with rules, such as allotting certain numbers of visits to physical therapists, allowing certain numbers of days of hospitalization for particular procedures, and requiring participating providers to work in accordance with the guidelines set out by the managed care company. Medical insurance is often linked to our employment or that of a household member. Other common ways of paying for medical care are various government programs, such as Medicaid, Medicare, disability programs, military benefits, or their state equivalents, and individual out-of-pocket payments.

Medical insurance involves payments to a company, whether we need medical care or not, and the acceptance of that company's rules of how we receive medical care. Medical insurance companies make huge profits because people (collectively) pay more for insurance overall than it costs to provide the care.

Some of us, for a number of reasons, have a type of very limited medical insurance often known as catastrophic insurance. It "kicks in" only after we have paid some baseline sum (often $5,000 per year) out of pocket on medical expenses. Another kind of limited insurance may cover medical expenses up to a certain amount or only for a given period of time. Some insurance plans include dental care and prescription drugs (and sometimes devices) and some do not. In general, medical insurance is expensive. There are more than 45 million people in the United States—over 15 percent of the population—who are not covered by any medical insurance.[11]

Some people may choose health care providers who are rarely covered by medical insurance plans, such as herbalists, massage therapists, or Reiki masters. Or we may want more treatments by providers such as psychotherapists or physical therapists than are covered by our plan. To accept the requirements of a managed care insurance plan, which often includes limitations on our choice of health care providers, is an important health care decision that is often not consciously examined. Some of us drop out of such plans because of their limitations and requirements.

If your insurance plan doesn't cover less conventional care, such as acupuncture, you can sometimes find less expensive options. For example, supervised care by students, especially at massage and acupuncture schools, is often cheaper than going to private practitioners. Many "alternative" practitioners have different fee scales for regular, long-term, or older patients than for first-timers or one-timers. As with trying to get the best price for other goods and services, it can help to ask. You may also want to ask providers how many treatments they think you will need, so you can determine whether you want to make such a financial commitment.

Many of us participate in medical insurance plans despite the limitations and requirements, because of their apparent comprehensive nature, their wide acceptance, and our awareness that, with just a bit of bad luck, our medical needs or those of our families could easily bankrupt us. Since insurance companies often will pay for medications but not for complementary or alternative treatments, having insurance coverage can strongly influence a woman's decision to take drugs for menopause-related complaints.

I have medical insurance; when I turned fifty, my doctor urged me to begin hormone replacement therapy, assuring me that it would protect me from osteoporosis, heart disease, and a number of other ailments. My insurance would pay for the drugs—with a small copay.

Those of us who do not have medical insurance often face additional challenges in getting the information that we need in order to make health care decisions that are right for us. Because we may not have a family doctor or steady health care provider, we need to make even greater efforts to keep track of our health histories, previous tests and screenings, and past treatments. We also need to keep track of the bills that we are sent: Double-billing or billing for services that we were told we would not have to pay for happens far too often.

People who don't have medical insurance may be charged more for medical services than people who have insurance. That is because insurance companies negotiate "bulk" rates with hospitals, labs, and others. It is perfectly appropriate for you to ask in the billing department what rate is paid by a large insurer in your area for your treatment and then send a letter to the head of the billing department offering to pay that rate. Many medical facilities are willing to negotiate a lower rate if that means that they will receive at least some of the money they are owed. Offering to pay a lower amount does not always lead to an agreement, but it does work surprisingly often. It is worth asking to speak to someone in the billing department who has experience in working with uninsured patients. Many times you can arrange to pay a small amount of your bill each month.

Hospital social workers can be great resources both in terms of helping advocate for you within the hospital, and in terms of helping you sign up for municipal, county, state, and federal programs that pay bills for people with lower incomes. We often need to ask to see a social worker; this service may not be offered to us without our asking.

For many of us, the cost of medication is more than we can handle, and we find ourselves skipping doses or taking medication in less than optimal ways. You can order medication online from other countries where prices are lower for the same medication that you would buy in the United States. Also, pharmaceutical companies have patient assistance programs (PAPs) to distribute a limited amount of free and discounted medication. The downside is that the application is too complex for most people. However, in many communities, charitable organizations (such as Catholic Charities) employ someone to help people fill out and submit this kind of application. You also should be sure to tell your provider if you cannot afford the drugs she or he has prescribed.

If your provider gives you a prescription, you should ask how much it will cost to fill it. Even if the doctor does not know, your question reminds your provider that handing out a prescription that you cannot possibly fill is not a "best practice" of medicine. And by asking, you may prompt your provider to prescribe a different drug that costs less or come up with a more appropriate treatment for your circumstances. At the very least, we can ask the provider, "What will happen if I take half the dose?" or "What will happen if I take this medicine for two weeks rather than for a month like you prescribed?" Getting this information will allow us to make informed decisions and understand the risks we take, even in situations in which no decision is truly optimal.

RACISM AND DISCRIMINATION

Racism and other forms of bias create barriers to obtaining appropriate health care and health information with which to make decisions. Some providers stereotype women, offering different diagnoses and treatment to women of color and low-income women, even when our symptoms are identical to those of middle-class white women. Many of us find that providers treat those of us who are lower income and/or women of color as if we are not able to absorb information about current health issues. Therefore, those providers do not take the time to explain treatment options. And we ourselves may feel uncomfortable telling the provider that we do not understand what she or he has said. Providers may not be sensitive to or aware of our needs if we do not share their socioeconomic or ethnic background. Having access to caregivers with backgrounds similar to our own often makes a positive difference.

Those of us who have physical and mental disabilities and chronic illnesses may need to consider other potential barriers, such as the accessibility of transportation and providers' offices, when making health care decisions. Providers are not always knowledgeable about particular disabilities or conditions. Because of their lack of experience with people with disabilities and social stigma about disabilities, they may be uncomfortable interacting with us. Local agencies for people with disabilities can help with referrals to appropriate providers who are knowledgeable about people with disabilities. When gathering information, those of us with impaired hearing need to ask for written material. If we have impaired vision, we may need large-print material. Those of us with multiple chronic conditions or disabilities need to make sure that the provider understands how these conditions or disabilities are affected by other conditions or treatments.

Some lesbian, bisexual, or transgender (LBT) people do not seek health care because we believe or are told that certain services are not necessary. For example, we may incorrectly think that if we have sex with women, we are not vulnerable to sexually transmitted infections or do not need regular preventive care. We also may have had bad experiences with providers in the past, which affect our decisions about current health care. In addition, those of us who have partners are often unable to get health insurance through them, because many employers and insurance companies will not provide spousal benefits to unmarried couples. Fortunately, this is changing. When seeking a provider, those of us who are lesbian, bisexual, or transgender may want to ask other LBT friends and acquaintances for recommendations, look for a local LBT health clinic or community center for referrals, or search for a doctor on the Gay and Lesbian Medical Association's website (www.glma.org).

LANGUAGE BARRIERS

Those of us who do not speak English fluently find it more difficult to gather the information that we need in order to weigh our decisions and advocate for ourselves. It can be helpful to call health care providers ahead of time to see if they speak our first language or have an interpreter available. Large medical centers usually have medical interpreters, at least for the languages commonly spoken by the hospitals' clientele, and all hospitals can (for a fee) call into a telephone service that provides interpreters over the phone.* Interpreting over the phone can involve difficulties, such as lack of eye contact and the challenges of sharing one phone receiver if a phone with two receivers is not available. But it also can provide anonymity in small communities where the only people available to interpret locally may be family members or others with whom we are not comfortable sharing private medical information.

If a provider does not offer services in your language, ask if you can bring your own interpreter. When selecting someone to serve as interpreter, choose carefully. Ideally, this person should be an adult. You may also prefer to bring someone of your gender. She or he should be fluent and comfortable with both the language and the subject matter. Ask the person to take notes, so afterward the two of you can go over what the provider said to make sure you understand it.

If there is no appropriate relative or close friend to bring with you, consider asking schools, churches, or community centers for possible interpreters. Some medical centers may have a brochure with numbers to call for an interpreter and descriptions of services you have a right to have.

CHOOSING A PROVIDER

The medical care system as it is currently organized in this country places many limitations

---

* Language Line Services is one provider of this service. To learn more about it, visit www.languageline.com or call 1-877-886-3885.

on how we can choose health care providers. Providers must fulfill a number of requirements, which may or may not increase the quality of the care they give. For example, some doctors accept Medicaid and some do not. Some have sliding scale fees, and many do not. Some belong to certain managed care companies and not to others. The location and physical accessibility of care providers is also an issue for many of us. In some places, community-based health centers provide a wide range of responsive caregivers, who emphasize prevention and primary care approaches. Paperwork requirements and the behavior of support staff can be issues. Asking for relevant information ahead of time and being accompanied by someone you trust who can witness and advocate for you can improve the care you receive.

The selection of a provider or health care facility for treatment or information is an important one. If you have insurance and your insurance company requires you to select a provider from its list, you can investigate those available before you find yourself in an acute situation. One way to learn more about providers is to check the website for your state's board of registration in medicine. Many boards' websites offer information on physicians' training and specialties. Some websites may have information of past complaints or problems with the board.

You also can ask people you know about providers—such as doctors, nurses, nurse practitioners, and physician assistants—whom they have tried. You may find that the nurse practitioner or physician assistant (PA) in a doctor's office is more accessible and comfortable to deal with in a number of situations than the doctor. You can sometimes make appointments just to interview a provider, either in person or on the phone. It is unlikely that insurance will cover the costs of such an appointment.

Those of us who are covered by Medicaid typically find that we have fewer options in choosing a provider. In fact, in some parts of the country, only a small number of providers are willing to accept Medicaid patients at all.

In general, we have a better chance of being able to choose a provider if we live in an urban area than in a rural area. Thus, rural women may want to consider (if at all possible financially) phoning providers in the nearest metropolitan area. Local public assistance offices may be able to help with transportation.

Some low- and moderate-income women enroll in medical studies to access free medical care. However, it is important to find out in advance what screenings or treatments the study will actually provide. Moreover, because medical studies typically involve a control group (people who get no treatment), even though you enroll in a study, you may find that you do not receive meaningful care. One woman who enrolled in a medical study that has since ended explains,

When I enrolled in the Women's Health Initiative, it was the only way I knew to get help. They do it all; they do physicals, they do all blood work, they send you for [screenings]. They do the Pap smear, the X-ray. They do all those things for you. But they do not treat you if they find you have any problems. If you're in a certain program [within the study], then the nutritionists and dietitians work with you on eating and what you need to do, [but] I am not in that program. I'm in the one where they just ask you questions. Different people are assigned to different programs. It's just at random. [For me] it just gives you screenings, but I thought, well, to me that was a big help in itself, . . . because at least I can have it done, you know, 'cause my grandmother died from cervical cancer. Both grandmothers died from cancer. One of my aunts and one of my cousins. So I thought, well, at least they check you here.

CONSIDERATIONS IN CHOOSING A PROVIDER OR CLINIC

In choosing a provider or clinic, make a list of information that you want to have. Then you or your advocate can call and ask for that information. Your questions may include:

1. How long must I wait to get an appointment?
2. What determines how long an appointment is?
3. How long is the usual wait in the office before seeing the provider? (Getting the first appointment of the day or the first appointment after lunch may shorten your waiting time.)
4. How many patients does the practitioner usually see in a day? How many days each week does the provider see patients? Does the provider accept phone calls or have a "phone-in" hour? How long does it take providers to return phone calls?
5. Who covers for the provider on her or his days off? What about nights and weekends?
6. What hospital is the provider associated with?

GROUP VISITS

Some health care providers offer group visits for women who are going through the menopause transition. These group meetings can be a helpful supplement to individual office visits, offering more time than traditional appointments for women to get detailed information, ask questions, and share experiences. From the health care provider's perspective, the group visit is a cost-saving method for providing quality information to many women in a limited amount of time.

In a group visit, which often is one to three hours long, women can talk with the health care provider, expert guest speaker, or other meeting facilitator about emotional and physical changes that may accompany the menopause transition. Topics may include physiologic changes; self-care strategies such as relaxation, paced breathing, physical activity, and good nutrition; herbal products; alternative care treatments; hormone treatment for symptom relief; sexuality; counseling; and healthy aging in general. The facilitator may also provide a list of informational and community resources. Ideally, sessions are structured so that there is adequate time for group discussion and sharing of feelings and personal stories.

Health care providers may conduct the group visit in a comfortable place in a medical clinic. It may be a single session or multiple sessions. Many women find that multiple sessions with the same participants are more useful. Sometimes women pay a flat fee to attend each session or, in a health maintenance organization, a woman may be charged one office copayment for the group visit.

The group visit borrows in many ways from the model of women's self-help support groups. These groups are often held in community centers, libraries, or other neighborhood spaces and offer a chance for women to share information and experiences. Some midlife women's groups have multiple sessions, each session being facilitated by a woman who is an expert in the topic area.

7. How much will my visit cost? Is Medicaid, Medicare, or other insurance accepted? Is there a discount for paying in cash? Can one pay in installments? Are screening and lab tests included in the cost of the visit?
8. What kinds of medical history does the provider request? Should it be prepared ahead of the appointment time?

WHEN YOU SEE YOUR PROVIDER: WHAT TO ASK AND WHOM TO BRING

In the health care world that we live in today, providers rarely are allowed time to guide us through the many stages of health maintenance, screening, and treatment. Getting and keeping copies of medical records in general and laboratory tests in particular can save us time and money later. We can also advocate for ourselves by asking questions and bringing a friend along to our appointment.

Sometimes, during our visits to our health care providers, we don't ask questions because we feel intimidated or we think the provider is too busy to spend time with us. It is our right to ask questions and to expect a reasonable amount of time to be spent with us. We have a right to bring someone with us to take notes or to ask questions on our behalf.

As a retired nurse, I often accompany older members of my church congregation to medical appointments. I usually try to make them more comfortable by letting them know what is likely to happen next. Once, as I saw a physician get ready to examine the woman I was with, I noticed that he did not seem to be planning to wash his hands before he did the exam. So I said loudly, "And as soon as he washes his hands, he will examine you." He washed his hands.

To get the most out of your visit, spend some time beforehand thinking about what you want to get from the appointment. Write down your symptoms and when they started, and list any questions you have. You may find it useful to decide on the top three questions or problems you want to address. If this is your first visit, be prepared to discuss your health history.

Here are some questions you may want to ask:

1. What, in plain language, is the matter with me? (Keep saying, "I do not know what that means," until you have the answer you can understand.)
2. Why are you prescribing that medicine for me? What is it? How long should I take it? What are the effects of this drug on my body? What will happen if I do not take it? (Ask your provider to prescribe drugs by their generic name, if available, rather than by their brand name. This usually will save you money without affecting your treatment, as they are by law identical.)
3. What is the purpose of this test or X-ray?
4. How much will this medical care cost me?
5. Why is this operation necessary for me? What are the alternatives? (Remember that you have a right to a second opinion. If a series of expensive tests or surgery is recommended, you can tell the provider that you would like to consult another doctor before making a decision. Learning more and getting a second opinion may prevent unnecessary or harmful treatments.)

Many of us get at least some part of our medical care in clinic or training settings, where the care provider changes from appointment to appointment. Although we may not have control over who our provider will be, we can call ahead to see if it is possible to keep the same provider. If not, we need to make sure to bring the records we have with us to the appointment. At county and other public health centers, it sometimes is easier to arrange for a nurse practitioner to serve as your primary care practitioner; oftentimes, nurse practitioners work in the health center according to a more regular schedule than the physicians, and thus may be more available for follow-up and repeat visits.

CONCLUSION

Whatever we do that improves and maintains our overall health will benefit us in managing menopause. Actively making decisions, rather than passively letting things happen to us, is self-affirming and reinforcing.

Our health care decisions are strongly influenced by the particular world we live in, the opinions of those close to us, and the resources available to us. We need to know what we base our choices on and to feel that they are right for us at the time we make them. We have to practice allocating our time and energy among the many demands of our lives, including our own well-being, in a way that satisfies us and meets our own needs. We also need to find health care providers with whom we are comfortable.

Our expensive medical system makes being an alert consumer especially important. If we are informed and have support, we will have more and better choices for our health care. Still, there are limits to what each of us can do as an individual to get quality medical care. Our entire medical system needs to be reformed to ensure access to quality health care for everyone.

NOTES

1. "Expertise Online: Finding Reliable Information," *Consumer Reports* 70, no. 9 (September 2005): 48.
2. Thomas E. Andreoli, "The Undermining of Academic Medicine," *Academe* 85, no. 6 (November–December 1999): 32–37.
3. House of Commons Health Committee, The Influence of the Pharmaceutical Industry, Volume 1, April 5, 2005, 55, accessed at www.parliament.the-stationery-office.co.uk/pa/cm200405/cmselect/cmhealth/42/42.pdf on September 25, 2005.
4. Justin E. Bekelman, Yan Li, and Cary P. Gross, "Scope and Impact of Financial Conflicts of Interest in Biomedical Research: A Systematic Review," *JAMA* 289 (January 2003): 454–65; see also Joel Lexchin, Lisa A. Bero, Benjamin Djulbegovic, and Otavio Clark, "Pharmaceutical Industry Sponsorship and Research Outcome and Quality: Systematic Review," *BMJ (British Medical Journal)* 326 (May 2003): 1167–70.
5. B. Als-Nielsen, W. Chen, C. Gluud, and L. L. Kjaergard, "Association of Funding and Conclusions in Randomized Drug Trials: A Reflection of Treatment Effect or Adverse Events?" *JAMA* 290 (2003): 921–8.
6. "Effect of User Fees on Drug Approval Times, Withdrawals, and Other Agency Activities," United States General Accounting Office, September 2002, 9, accessed at www.gao.gov/new.items/d02958.pdf on September 25, 2005.
7. Rosie Taylor and Jim Giles, "Cash Interests Taint Drug Advice," *Nature* 437, no. 20 (October 2005): 1070–71; see also Patrick J. O'Connor, "Adding Value to Evidence-Based Clinical Guidelines," *JAMA* 294 (2005): 741–3.
8. Cynthia M. Boyd, Jonathan Darer, Chad Boult, Linda P. Fried, Lisa Boult, and Albert W. Wu, "Clinical Practice Guidelines and Quality of Care for Older Patients with Multiple Comorbid Diseases: Implications for Pay for Performance," *JAMA* 294 (2005): 716–24.
9. This sidebar is based on the work of John Abramson, including the 2004 book *Overdosed America: The Broken Promise of American Medicine* and the article "The Effect of Conflict of Interest on Biomedical Re-

search and Clinical Practice Guidelines: Can We Trust the Evidence in Evidence-Based Medicine?" *Journal of the American Board of Family Practice* 18 (2005): 414–18.

10. Kay Dickersin, "Behind the Numbers," *MAMM,* June 2003, accessed at www.findarticles.com/p/articles/mi _kmmam/is_200306/ai_kepm41109 on October 5, 2005, see also Charles H. Hennekens, Julie E. Buring. Sherry L. Mayrent, eds., *Epidemiology in Medicine* (Boston: Lippincott Williams & Wilkins, 1987).

11. The Center on Budget and Policy Priorities, "Economic Recovery Failed to Benefit Much of the Population in 2004," accessed at www.cbpp.org/8-30-05 pov.pdf on September 8, 2005.

A Transition and
Its Challenges

CHAPTER 3

What's Happening in Our Bodies

As the baby boomers who were born between 1946 and 1965 grow older, a greater number of women are making the transition to menopause than in past decades. Many of us in this generation want to understand our bodies in order to make informed decisions. Our large numbers have stimulated interest in menopause-related research and treatments. We are viewed by some as a market for the sale of often unnecessary and sometimes even harmful tests, services, and products. Despite this increased focus on menopause, many of us still feel uncertain about what to expect.[1] We may wonder, "What's normal?" "Does everyone else feel this way?" or even "Does *anyone* else feel this way?" We may ask, "Why can't our periods just stop, without all these other physical changes? What is going on in our bodies?"

This chapter describes the changes most women experience as we make the transition to life after menopause. It also explains how our bodies produce various hormones over the course of our lifetimes—and the effects that these hormones may have on us. The last section of the chapter provides an overview of problems—such as sleep disruption, depression, and memory and sexual concerns—that some women experience during the menopause transition.

There is a wide range of typical experiences of the menopausal transition. No two women will have the same experiences. Most research suggests that the transition occurs gradually over a decade or more and that the changes that most women notice—such as hot flashes—last for no more than about five years. Every woman who survives to midlife will experience menopause naturally if she has not already experienced it because of surgery, medical treatment, or other causes.

WHEN WILL I HAVE MY LAST PERIOD?

It is very difficult to predict when you will experience your final menstrual period. On average, U.S. women who go through natural menopause experience last periods at about age fifty-one, but the range from forty to sixty years old is considered "normal."

If you smoke or if your mother had relatively early menopause (closer to forty than fifty), you are likely to have your last period earlier than average.[2] If you are or have been poor, have relatively little formal education, or work in a blue-collar job, you are more likely to experience menopause at a younger age (for reasons that are not clear, although nutrition may be a factor). Having had your first period later than average is also associated with having an earlier menopause, as is never having been pregnant.[3]

If you drink alcohol, you are likely to have a later menopause than if you do not drink.[4] Higher income, more education, and higher job status are also associated with later menopause (perhaps because of better nutrition and other health behaviors). Women who have had one pregnancy have on average a slightly later menopause than those who have never been pregnant, and those who have been pregnant twice have a slightly later menopause on average than those who were pregnant only once, suggesting that the more pregnancies a woman has, the later her menopause.

Finally, women born later in the twentieth century are experiencing menopause later, on average, than those born earlier in the same century. This change may be because of improved nutrition.

The typical transition to natural menopause is a gradual process, with increasing irregularity of menstrual periods and eventually a final menstrual period occurring at about age fifty-one, the average for U.S. women. Smokers have their final period one to two years earlier than non-smokers, on average. (This difference may be due to decreased blood flow to the ovaries in smokers or the toxicity of tobacco to the ovaries.) The changes in our bodies that precede menopause may begin as long as a decade or more before our last menstrual period. Researchers are just beginning to understand some of these changes, as most studies of women during the menopausal transition have not included women in their late thirties and early forties.

Some of us experience a natural early menopause, with our final menstrual period occurring before we are forty years old. Some women experience induced menopause as a result of chemotherapy or radiation therapy or removal of both ovaries (bilateral oophorectomy), which often accompanies removal of the uterus (hysterectomy). (For more information, see Chapter 4, "Sudden and Early Menopause.")

THE TRANSITION YEARS

In an effort to communicate more clearly about menopause, a team of researchers and health care providers recently proposed a set of terms and definitions to describe its stages.[5]

The **reproductive stage** is the time in a

woman's life from when she starts menstruating until the menopausal transition begins.

Perimenopause is a term for the menopausal transition, which researchers divide into early and late stages.

Menopause is defined by a woman's last menstrual period. Because women's periods can be sporadic just before menopause, studies usually require that a woman have not had a period for one year in order to qualify as having experienced menopause.

Postmenopause begins after menopause (the last period). Like perimenopause, it can be divided into early and late stages. Early postmenopause includes the first five years after the final period, a time when the hormone changes that started before menopause are stabilizing. The late postmenopause extends throughout the remainder of the lifespan and is a time when ovarian hormones have reached a new, lower steady state.

MENSTRUAL CALENDARS

In addition to having irregular periods during the menopausal transition, women also frequently experience spotting (scant bloody discharge) before, after, and in between episodes of menstrual bleeding. Some of us also have longer and heavier episodes of bleeding (*men-orrhagia* or *flooding*), and some have shorter periods and less bleeding.[7] Some women have a very quick change in bleeding patterns and some experience irregular periods over more than five years.

Perimenopause was a foreign word to me when I went to my doctor. . . . I was experiencing dark blood spotting my panties with an unattractive odor. . . . It had been a few months since my regular period. It turned out that after that appointment I never had a period again, at least for about a year and a half, and then just some light bleeding.

When I was about forty-six, I started spotting between periods. Sometimes the spotting would be just enough blood to make the toilet paper pink when I wiped myself, but sometimes there were actually spots in my panties.

You may want to use a menstrual calendar to track your own bleeding (see sidebar, page 45). This may help you identify what stage of the menopause transition you are in.

The menstrual calendar on page 44 represents the experience of a woman in the early menopausal transition stage. Notice how her menstrual cycle during late July and August (July 24 to August 21) is more than seven days longer than that during July (July 3 to 24).

STAGES OF REPRODUCTIVE AGING*						
	Reproductive	Early Menopausal Transition	Late Menopausal Transition	**Final Period (Menopause)**	Early Postmenopause (the first five years after the last period)	Late Postmenopause
Menstrual Cycles	Cycles are regular for many women	Cycles may be irregular, varying by 7 or more days	Women may skip cycles, having no period for >42 days		No periods	No periods
* Adapted from the STRAW (Stages of Reproductive Aging Workshop) Criteria.[6]						

Day	1	2	3	4	5	6	7	8	9	10	11	12	13	14	15	16	17	18	19	20	21	22	23	24	25	26	27	28	29	30	31
JAN	B_2	B_1	B_1	u																			S	B_1	B_2	B_2 3	u	B_1	S	S	
FEB	S																				B_2	B_3	B_3	B_2 3	B_1 u						
MAR																	S	B_1	B_1 B_2	B_3	B_2	B_3	B_1								
APR																		B_2	B_2	B_1	B_1	S	u								
MAY													S	S	B_1	B_1	B_2	B_2													
JUN							S	S	S	B_1	B_2	B_2	B_3 u	B_1	S																
JUL				S	B_1	B_1	B_2	B_2	B_1 u															S		S		B_1	B_2 u	B_3 u	
AUG																					B_1	B_2	B_2	B_2	B_2	u	S	S			
SEP																		S	B_1	B_2	B_1	B_2 u	B_1	B_1	S	B	S	S			
OCT																													B_2	B_2 B_2	B_1
NOV	S	S	u	S														S	B_1	B_2	B_2 3	B_1	u								
DEC			B_1	B_2	B_3	B_1	S	S u																							

This record shows the bleeding patterns of a woman in the early menopausal transition stage.

The late stage of the menopausal transition occurs when a woman skips her usual period so that her cycle becomes double the length that is typical for her.

The menopausal transition may start in our early to mid-forties, although there has not been sufficient research with younger women to be certain. Estimates from studies over the past two decades suggest that women experience irregular cycles for about five to six years prior to menopause.[8] Women participating in the Seattle Midlife Women's Health Study have kept daily menstrual calendars shown here as long as fifteen years. These women's experiences suggest that the early menopausal transition stage begins at an average age of forty-six years old and lasts for an average of nearly three years. The late menopausal transition stage begins at about age forty-nine and lasts for about two years. Women in the Seattle study reached menopause at an average age of nearly fifty-two, with the earliest menopause recorded at nearly forty-four years old and the latest at fifty-nine.[9]

Even if we reach menopause at the same age, we may have very different experiences, as the following two women's descriptions show:

Menopause was fast and extremely difficult. It hit at age fifty, like a brick wall. I certainly do not miss my period. That is perhaps the only liberation.

Had my fiftieth birthday and not a period since! Signs of change: came quickly and the transition has been easy.

CHANGING HORMONES

The beginning of the menopausal transition is marked by the onset of irregular menstrual cycles in women who have had regular cycles previously. The changes in a woman's periods are a signal that changes are occurring in her ovaries.

The changes in our ovaries are orchestrated by a complex set of signals from hormones in the brain, pituitary gland, and ovaries themselves. Hormones help control the chemistry of the body. Reproductive hormones control the development of *follicles* (or egg sacs) in the ovaries. Follicles contain eggs (*ova*) that develop until it is time to release one of them

HOW DO I KNOW WHEN I AM IN THE MENOPAUSAL TRANSITION?

The most reliable way to estimate where you are in the menopause transition is to keep track of your periods on a menstrual calendar like the one on page 44 for a few months. Each day you can mark on the calendar whether you have had bleeding (B) or spotting (S).

You can identify when you are in the early menopausal transition stage when the length of your menstrual cycles differs by a week or more from one cycle to the next but you have not yet started skipping periods. Of course, some of us have irregular cycles all our lives. For us, using a menstrual calendar isn't helpful for identifying where we are in the menopausal transition. Keeping track of our cycles may be useful for other reasons, such as pregnancy planning, fertility treatment, or tracking very heavy periods before we consult our health care provider for help.

After a few months of tracking your period on a menstrual calendar, follow these steps:

1. Examining the calendar for your last few menstrual cycles, count the length of your cycle by beginning with the first day on which you have marked a B for bleeding. Then count all the days with a B marked, plus the days that have either an S (spotting) or a blank until the start of the next bleeding days (marked B). Repeat this for at least two cycles.
2. Subtract the number of days for the second cycle from the number of days for the first cycle. (It doesn't matter if you get a positive or negative number).
3. If the difference in the number of days between cycle one and cycle two is seven or more, you may be in the early stage of the menopausal transition. (Note: This will not work well if you have had irregular cycles for most of your life.)
4. If there are sixty days or more between the start of menstrual bleeding in one cycle and in the next, or if the days are about double your usual cycle length, you may be in the late menopausal transition stage. When you reach this stage, chances are that you are within two years of your last menstrual period. This is more likely to be the case if you have had a pattern that looks like the early menopausal transition earlier.

from the ovary. This happens each cycle, making fertilization and implantation possible. In addition to containing ova, the follicles produce hormones, including *estrogen,* the hormone that supports characteristics of our bodies associated with being female, such as the development of breasts and the cells lining the vagina. The ovaries also make *androgens,* hormones typically associated with support of "male" bodily characteristics such as hair distribution and muscle development.

FOLLICLE-STIMULATING HORMONE

During the reproductive stage, *follicle-stimulating hormone (FSH),* which comes from the pituitary gland in the brain, signals the ovaries at the start of every period to produce more estrogen by causing ovarian follicles to develop. FSH works something like a thermostat on a furnace, with estrogen being like the heat produced. When FSH rises, the amount of

• *After menopause, women suffer from estrogen deficiency; we either have estrogen levels that are too low or have no estrogen at all.*

Myth. Women don't stop producing estrogen altogether after menopause, but our estrogen levels do become lower. This is not a deficiency but an expected developmental change. Once ovulation and menstrual cycles stop, we still make estrone, a less active type of estrogen, by converting androgen to estrogen in fatty tissue. Estrone continues to provide our bodies with a source of estrogen after menopause.

• *If my mother had an easy time with the transition into menopause, I should.*

It is not clear if this statement is true or false. There is little evidence from studies of mothers and daughters to determine the role of genetics in menopause. There is evidence that women whose mothers had an early menopause are more likely to have an early menopause. It is uncertain whether daughters of women who had severe problems around the time of menopause are more likely to have a similar experience.[10]

estrogen the ovaries produce increases, and when estrogen levels reach a high-enough set point, FSH decreases.

As we approach our final menstrual periods, the numbers of follicles in our ovaries that are signaled by FSH to grow each cycle are much greater than they were during the reproductive stage. This leads to a rapid drop in the numbers of follicles remaining available for future development, ovulation, and pregnancy.[11] The rapid development of more follicles also can result in the production of extra-high levels of estradiol, the most active form of estrogen, for some months or years. The more rapid development of follicles is linked to rising levels of FSH.[12] FSH levels usually increase gradually until the year or two preceding the last menstrual period, when they increase rapidly.

ESTRADIOL

Estradiol is the most common type of estrogen produced by the ovaries in the reproductive stage. During the menopausal transition, as the number of remaining follicles decreases, ovulations become less regular and we begin to produce lower levels of estradiol, even though FSH continues to rise. In most women, a drop in estradiol production occurs between one and two years before the final menstrual period and for a few years after the final period, until estradiol levels reach a new, lower but steady level.

During the menopausal transition, some women experience very high levels of estradiol in response to the higher levels of FSH.[13] High levels of estradiol may cause symptoms such as breast swelling, breast tenderness, and bloating. The elevated, erratic fluctuations of estradiol may cause heavy and unpredictable vaginal bleeding in some women; if this happens to you, consult with your health care provider. High levels of estradiol may cause fibroids to grow or increase the risk of endometrial cancer (a cancer of the lining of the uterus). Vaginal bleeding is a possible sign of endometrial hyperplasia (over-development of the endometrium) and possible endometrial cancer.

When estradiol levels drop, some women may notice hot flashes. After menopause, the low estrogen levels may be associated with thinning of the vaginal tissues, which women may notice as vaginal dryness or painful intercourse. This also makes the tissues more vulnerable to infection.

INHIBINS

Inhibins are proteins in the ovaries that help control the ovulation process through their effects on FSH. Inhibin A and B keep FSH levels low during the reproductive years. Inhibin levels drop in the years prior to menopause at the same time that FSH levels rise. The drop in inhibin B levels reflects the diminishing number of follicles left for future development in the ovary.[14] As the number of follicles available to develop decreases below the level necessary for ovulation, ovulation stops.

PROGESTERONE

Progesterone is a hormone that is produced by the ovaries in the last two weeks of the menstrual cycle after ovulation occurs. It helps prepare the lining of the uterus (endometrium) so that a fertilized egg can implant. When ovulation stops, progesterone is no longer produced. Thus as the menopause transition is completed, there is a shift in the balance of hormones so that we produce much less estradiol and no further progesterone from the ovaries.

ANDROGENS

Androgens are often thought of as male hormones, but women produce androgens in our ovaries and in the adrenal cortex. The adrenal cortex is the outer layer of cells of the adrenal gland, which is located next to our kidneys. The adrenal gland secretes several hormones that our bodies can make into androgen. Some of these are called dehydroepiandrosterone sulfate (DHEAS), dehydroepiandrosterone (DHEA), and androstenedione. Our ovaries also produce the hormone testosterone.

Testosterone levels do not change dramatically during the transition to menopause, although they do decrease with aging. DHEAS levels also decrease with age in both women and men.[15] DHEAS can be metabolized to either a potent androgen or to estrogen, providing an adrenal source of androgen and estrogen for women after menopause. Androgens are responsible for male-appearing sexual characteristics, such as hair growth and distribution on the body, muscle growth, and deepening of the voice.

SEX HORMONE-BINDING GLOBULIN

Sex hormone–binding globulin (SHBG) binds to hormones in the blood, providing a way to regulate their effects. Free (or unbound) testos-

---

UNPLANNED PREGNANCY

Sometimes changes in ovulation occur in an unpredictable way. Although a woman may be having menstrual periods, she may not ovulate, or she may not have a period for several months and then ovulate. As a result, women may be at risk of an unplanned pregnancy if we assume that we have completed menopause and are no longer fertile. For this reason, **if you are having sex with a man, it is important to use a birth control method until you have not had a period for a year or longer.**

terone and estrogen are available to bind to receptors in the cells of various tissues, thus producing their effects throughout the body where these receptors are present. SHBG decreases by about 50 percent from the time a woman is in her mid-twenties until her late forties, with the greatest drop two years before menopause.[16] This drop in SHBG allows hormones like estradiol or testosterone to be more active in the body. Reduced SHBG levels occur at about the same time as the drop in estradiol levels women experience with the menopausal transition. The free androgen index, calculated as the ratio of testosterone to SHBG, rises by 80 percent during the same period, with the maximal change occurring two years before the last menstrual period.[17]

When SHBG drops, more androgen becomes available at about the same time that estradiol drops. This can result in the effects of androgen becoming more noticeable. Some of us have increased hair growth on our upper lip or face and may develop a more masculine pattern of fat distribution (fat on the belly instead of on the thighs and buttocks). Acne can resurface. Some women find these changes in our bodies troubling, but others may not experience them at all or may not be bothered by them.

ESTRONE

As the amount of estradiol produced by the ovaries decreases as women approach menopause, the adrenal gland provides an important source of another type of estrogen called *es-*

CAN HORMONE LEVELS PREDICT MENOPAUSE?

With the many hormonal changes associated with the menopausal transition, you might imagine that measuring hormone levels could help predict when you will have your last period. This is not possible, but some companies that stand to profit from testing would like you to believe that it is.

Some over-the-counter test kits have been manufactured to measure levels of follicle-stimulating hormone (FSH) in urine, but their results are unlikely to be very helpful in predicting when menopause will occur. Some laboratories will measure FSH levels in saliva, but there are no data to suggest that these levels predict when the final menstrual period will occur.

Increasing FSH levels are a useful indicator that menopause is approaching, but they are not sufficiently specific by themselves to predict that menopause will occur at a certain time in the future. In addition, no specific level of FSH clearly distinguishes women approaching menopause within a specified time period from those not approaching menopause.[18]

Measurements of FSH along with a physical exam and full medical history can be useful to women who are seeking help for infertility. They can help establish whether we have begun the menopausal transition. Since FSH levels change very quickly over the menstrual cycle, it is important to know when in the menstrual cycle a sample is obtained and to obtain a series of blood samples over a period of days or weeks to get a profile of the hormone levels over time. A single random value could represent a woman's lowest or highest level, and there is no way to be sure whether on any particular day the hormone level is low, high, or intermediate for any one woman.

trone. Women produce this kind of estrogen before and after menopause by converting androstenedione (a type of androgen) to estrone. Estrone is a much weaker estrogen than estradiol.

In effect, during the menopause transition, the body transitions from ovarian production of estrogen (estradiol) to adrenal production of estrogen (estrone). Estrone is converted from androgen in fatty tissue, so women who have more body fat produce higher levels of estrone.[19]

OTHER HORMONES

To date there is no evidence that thyroid-stimulating hormone levels change with the menopausal transition. There is also no evidence that growth hormone or other hormones change with the menopausal transition.

ETHNIC DIFFERENCES

Until recently there was little information about ethnic differences in women's experiences of the menopausal transition and beyond. As investigators for the Study of Women Across the Nation (SWAN), a study of multiple ethnic groups of women from across the United States, began to report on hormonal changes during the menopause transition, they examined whether women from different ethnic groups had different levels of hormones.

The SWAN study is following more than 2,000 women, starting at ages forty to fifty-five, over an eight-year period as they go through the menopause transition. The women are African-American, Chinese-American, Japanese-American, Hispanic-American, and Caucasian and live in various states across the country. The SWAN study is large enough to help us compare the experiences of women from different ethnic groups and take into account factors such as age and body size.

When hormone levels of women from different ethnic groups were compared, many differences were noted. But when an indicator of weight for one's height (body mass index) was also considered, most of the ethnic differences disappeared. Heavier women have higher levels of the hormones FSH, SHBG, estradiol, testosterone, and DHEAS. When body mass was taken into account, estradiol levels were not different across the ethnic groups.

However, there are some ethnic differences that can be seen even after body mass is taken into account. FSH levels are higher and testosterone levels are lower in African-American and Hispanic women than in Japanese-American, Chinese-American, and Caucasian women.[20] The effects of higher FSH and lower testosterone levels are currently unknown, but

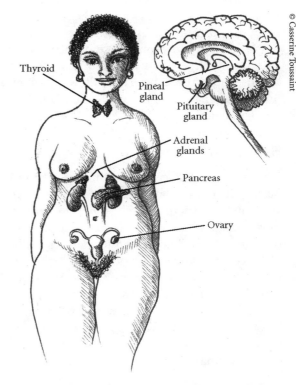

© Casserine Toussaint

Thyroid

Pineal gland

Pituitary gland

Adrenal glands

Pancreas

Ovary

Hormones are produced in many different parts of our bodies, not just our ovaries.

the SWAN study investigators will be looking at whether these differences in hormones have any effect on health, for example, heart disease or bone health.

SIGNS OF THE MENOPAUSAL TRANSITION

Problems that some women associate with changing hormones include hot flashes and night sweats; depressed mood; sleep disruption; sexual concerns; changes in cognition (thinking and judgment); vaginal dryness; urinary incontinence; and bodily aches and pain. Only a few of these become much more prevalent as women progress through the transition to menopause. Hot flashes, night sweats, vaginal dryness, and sleep disruption increase in prevalence, especially as women begin the late menopausal transition stage marked by skipping periods.[21] How long these problems persist during the postmenopause is uncertain because most studies have not followed women for more than two or three years after their final menstrual period.

HOT FLASHES

Nearly four in ten women are bothered by hot flashes during the late menopausal transition stage and postmenopause.[22] About 26 percent of women have severe hot flashes, according to one large study;[23] according to another study, 15 percent of women experience hot flashes on more than fifteen days per month and 9 percent experience them every day.[24] (For more information about hot flashes, see Chapter 5, "Hot Flashes, Night Sweats and Sleep Disturbances.")

One woman with severe hot flashes says,

Your invitation to share my story came just as I was experiencing the fourth hot flash of the day. I was, as usual, dripping with sweat and wiping my brow, under my breasts, the back of my neck, and my hands so I could continue working at the keyboard. Fortunately, I work at home, so I can strip down when necessary. Occasionally, though, I do media work, and it can be quite inconvenient to sweat away the makeup that someone has just carefully applied! Anyway, this has been going on for more than two years now but I can definitely say some days are worse than others. It's worst of all at night, and in the first year I sometimes was awakened every hour with the intensity of it. I actually get hot enough to steam up my own glasses—something that evokes unfailing sympathy from my husband, who keeps saying he can't imagine how I can cope with it. I tell him I'm not alone, there are millions of baby boomer women out there going through the same thing.

SLEEP PROBLEMS

Sleep problems seem to increase steadily across the early and late menopausal transition stages and into postmenopause, with an estimated 30 percent of women without signs of the menopausal transition reporting sleep disturbances and 45 percent reporting them three years after menopause.[25] This pattern suggests that sleep problems may worsen with progression through the menopausal transition and perhaps be related to other signs, such as night sweats. However, sleep problems increase in both women and men with age and have also been associated with the stress of poverty (for example, worry about paying for basic needs).[26] (For more information about sleep problems, see page 82.)

SEXUAL CONCERNS

Vaginal dryness becomes more prevalent during the early postmenopause, as do other sexual changes. Nearly 50 percent of women report bothersome vaginal dryness three years after menopause.[27] Some of the sexual problems women report, such as pain with intercourse, may be related to vaginal dryness.

Other changes, such as lower sexual interest and responsivity, increased in prevalence as women made the transition to menopause. Lower estrogen levels, but not lower testosterone levels, were associated with sexual problems in a large longitudinal study of women during the menopausal transition in Australia; recent reports from the SWAN study indicate that testosterone levels have minimal influence on sexual desire, a finding corroborated by another study of Australian women.[28] Our prior sexual experiences and factors related to our partners, our relationships, and other aspects of our lives influence our sexuality as well as the biological changes associated with menopause. (For more information about sexuality, see Chapter 9, "Sexuality." For more information about vaginal dryness, see Chapter 6, "Vulvovaginal Changes." For more information about testosterone and low sexual desire, see page 110.)

DEPRESSION

It is unclear if problems with depressed mood, urinary control, cognitive functioning, and joint and muscle aches and pains change because of the menopause transition. Depressed mood is common in women across the lifespan, with about 30 percent of women of all ages in a recent study noticing symptoms.[29] Women with depressed mood may have slightly lower estradiol levels, but research has found that having severe hot flashes and disrupted sleep is more frequently associated with depression than low estradiol is.[30] In addition, women who experience depressed mood during the menopause transition are more likely to have been depressed earlier in the lifespan and to have faced major stressors such as abuse.[31] (For more information, see Chapter 15, "Memory and Mood.")

MEMORY

Many women going through the menopause transition and after menopause describe problems with memory, such as difficulty recalling names, but few women rate these as serious. Women attribute memory problems to increased responsibilities and stress, advancing age, physical health problems, inadequate concentration, and emotional changes.[32] To date only one study has tracked changes in cognitive function across the menopause transition; it found there was no change in the prevalence of memory problems. In that study, memory actually improved as women progressed to the early menopausal transition stage. The only memory change noted was a modest decrease in perceptual speed after women became postmenopausal, a change usually associated with age in both women and men.[33] (For more information, see Chapter 15, "Memory and Mood.")

OTHER CONCERNS

Urinary problems, such as leaking urine, are prevalent in women during midlife, with about half of women reporting varying levels of severity of leakage. These symptoms do not seem to change with the progression to menopause. They are more prevalent in heavier women.[34] (For more information, see Chapter 14, "Uterine and Bladder Health.") Likewise, 40 to 60 percent of women across the menopausal transition experience stiffness or soreness in our joints, neck, or shoulders, but this pain does not change significantly with the transition to menopause.[35]

Severity of problems such as hot flashes, night sweats, vaginal dryness, and sleep problems increases during the late menopausal transition stage and postmenopause. There are not enough follow-up data to know how long problems persist during the postmenopause.

What we do know is that hot flashes may persist in a moderate proportion of women for at least three years beyond the final menstrual period.[36]

Most problems associated with menopause can be attributed to a variety of factors, including hormone changes, aging, role overload (high demands from multiple roles, such as worker, partner, mother, and caregiver), stress, health history, genetics, and emotional changes.[37] It is crucial that you and your health care provider consider factors other than hormonal changes when trying to understand and treat problems. Not everything that women experience during the menopause transition can be attributed to menopause or hormone changes.

PHYSIOLOGIC CHANGES OF THE MENOPAUSE TRANSITION

Estradiol levels are associated with many physiologic functions in women, including fat deposition, glucose metabolism, bone metabolism, blood clotting, and lipid metabolism. These factors, in turn, have been associated with potential risk for some diseases of advanced age, such as heart disease, diabetes, and osteoporosis.

WEIGHT AND FAT DISTRIBUTION

Adipose (fat) tissue deposits are influenced by estradiol. During adolescence, young women begin depositing fat on their thighs and buttocks and in breast tissue because of estradiol's effect.

Although obesity is becoming much more common among women in the United States, evidence that women gain weight because of the menopausal transition is mixed. Women in the Healthy Women Study experienced an average weight gain of five pounds as they made the transition from menstruating to post-menopause. Nearly 20 percent gained ten or more pounds.[38] In the larger Massachusetts Women's Health Study of Caucasian women, neither menopause transition nor the use of hormone treatment was consistently associated with increased weight beyond the effect of aging. Behavioral factors, especially exercise and alcohol consumption, were more strongly related to weight than was menopausal transition.[39] Women in the ongoing SWAN study do not seem to gain weight as they make the transition to menopause, when aging is taken into account. Factors such as activity and ethnicity are more important than the stage of the menopausal transition.[40]

INSULIN

Insulin is a hormone that is important in transforming our food to energy and in storing energy from food as fat. Rising levels of insulin in the blood during the transition to menopause appear to be associated with weight gain and changes in the distribution of body fat. High insulin levels are associated with diabetes.

Women in the Healthy Women Study experienced an increase in waist circumference and upper body fat during the menopausal transition. Blood insulin levels were highest in women with both a higher body mass index (BMI is higher among women who are heavier for our height) and an increase in abdominal fat.[41] These factors are being tracked in the ongoing SWAN study. Early results suggest that estradiol levels are not associated with resistance to insulin (a body's failure to respond as usual to insulin). The forthcoming results of the SWAN study will be important in our understanding of how metabolism changes across the menopausal transition and as a basis for understanding the development of diabetes. (For more information about diabetes, see page 284.)

BONE MASS

Bone is constantly being built up and broken down. Because estradiol inhibits the breakdown of bone, there is concern that after menopause women are at greater risk of losing bone mass. Indeed, within the first three years following the final menstrual period, we lose bone at a faster rate than we do during the reproductive years. One study indicated that women with higher estradiol and estrone levels have greater bone density, as do women who are overweight.[42] Women in the SWAN study experienced a drop in bone density as the level of follicle-stimulating hormone increased, but there was no relationship of bone density loss to estradiol or testosterone levels.[43] (For more information, see Chapter 16, "Bone Health.")

OTHER CONCERNS

Estradiol promotes blood clotting, which can be good if we need to stop bleeding and heal but can be dangerous if we form blood clots in our leg veins or our lungs (pulmonary emboli) that can interfere with circulation and even cause death. Effects of the menopausal transition on clotting are not yet clear.[44]

Estradiol is associated with increased secretion of lipoproteins, substances in the blood that are related to cholesterol and fat metabolism. It is also associated with lowered serum cholesterol and increased phospholipids levels. There is evidence of a small drop in high-density lipoprotein cholesterol (HDL or "good" cholesterol) levels during the transition to menopause.[45] HDL cholesterol has been linked to a lower incidence of heart disease in women.

Recent data point to changes in cholesterol levels as women progress through the stages of the menopausal transition. Women in the late stage of the menopausal transition compared to those in the early stage have higher total cholesterol levels, higher LDL cholesterol (low-density lipoprotein or "bad" cholesterol), and greater levels of other substances associated with heart disease (ApoB, triglycerides, and VLDL, very-low-density lipoprotein cholesterol).[46] These changes parallel increase in body mass index as women make the transition to menopause. Obesity and fat distribution, low physical activity, cigarette smoking, and alcohol intake also influence HDL cholesterol levels during the menopausal transition.[47] There are substantial increases in LDL cholesterol levels after the menopausal transition,[48] and women in the Healthy Women Study experienced a rise in lipoprotein levels after the last menstrual period.[49] The ongoing SWAN study will help to clarify what cardiovascular changes in lipids, blood pressure, insulin resistance, and clotting occur as women experience the menopausal transition.[50]

These changes may reflect an increasing risk for heart disease as women make the transition to menopause. It will be crucial for the SWAN study to sort out the effects of our eating and activity patterns as well as the influence of aging and changes in hormones on the chemistry in our body that can affect our risk of both diabetes and heart disease.

LEARNING MORE

Women's experiences of menopause and the years that follow it vary widely, and we are only beginning to understand them. It is difficult to separate out the effects of lifestyle, heredity, and aging from those of hormones, since they are all in play.

As more women share our experiences, and more researchers study them, our understanding of the menopause transition will continue to increase. Several large longitudinal studies have focused on women during the menopause transition. These include the Massachusetts Women's Health Study, the Melbourne Midlife Women's Health Project, the Seattle Midlife Women's Health Study, and the Tremin Trust Study. The large, ongoing Study of Women Across the Nation, a multisite study of African-American, Japanese-American, Chinese-American, Hispanic, and Caucasian women, is expected to provide significant findings about menopause in a few more years, as the majority of the participants will have completed the menopause transition. Since many of the earlier studies of the menopause transition followed women for a shorter period of time than SWAN and included mostly white women, this study may deepen our understanding.

NOTES

1. Nancy Fugate Woods and Ellen Sullivan Mitchell, "Anticipating Menopause: Observations from the Seattle Midlife Women's Health Study," *Menopause* 6 (1999): 167–73.

2. L. Hefler, C. Grimm, G. Heinze, C. Schneeberger, M. Mueller, A. Muendlein, J. Huber, S. Leodolter, and C. Tempfer, "Estrogen-Metabolizing Gene Polymorphisms and Age at Natural Menopause in Caucasian Women," *Human Reproduction* 20, no. 5 (2005): 1422–27; J. Murabito, Q. Yang, C. Fox, P. Wilson, and L. Cupples, "Heritability of Age at Natural Menopause in the Framingham Heart Study," *Journal of Clinical Endocrinology and Metabolism* 90, no. 6 (2005): 3427–30; S. Treloar, K. Do, and N. Martin, "Genetic Influences on the Age at Menopause," *Lancet* 352, no. 9134 (1998): 1084–85.

3. Ibid.

4. Kim-Anh Do, S. A. Treloar, N. Pandeya, D. Purdie, A. C. Green, A. C. Heath, and N. G. Martin, "Predictive Factors of Age at Menopause in a Large Aus-

5. M. Soules, S. Sherman, E. Parrott, R. Rebar, N. Santoro, W. Utian, and N. Woods, "Stages of Reproductive Aging Workshop (STRAW)," *Menopause* 1, no. 8 (2001): 402–7.

6. Ibid.

7. E. S. Mitchell, N. F. Woods, and A. Mariella, "Three Stages of the Menopausal Transition from the Seattle Midlife Women's Health Study: Toward a More Precise Definition," *Menopause* 7 (2000): 334–49.

8. A. E. Treloar, "Menstrual Cyclicity and the Pre-Menopause," *Maturitas* 3, nos. 3–4 (1981): 249–64; S. McKinlay, D. Brambilla, and J. Posner, "The Normal Menopause Transition," *Maturitas* 14 (1992): 103–15.

9. E. Mitchell and N. Woods, "Seattle Midlife Women's Health Study" (in progress).

10. Murabito et al.; Treloar et al., "Genetic Influences."

11. S. J. Richardson, "The Biological Basis of the Menopause," *Balliere's Clinical Endocrinology and Metabolism* 7 (1993): 1–16.

12. N. Klein, D. Battaglia, V. Fujimoto, G. Davis, W. Bremner, and M. Soules, "Reproductive Aging: Accelerated Follicular Development Associated with a Monotropic Follicle-Simulating Hormone Rise in Normal Older Women," *Journal of Clinical Endocrinology and Metabolism* 81 (1996): 1038–45.

13. N. Santoro, J. Rosenberg Brown, T. Adel, and J. H. Skurnick, "Characterization of Reproductive Hormonal Dynamics in the Perimenopause," *Journal of Clinical Endocrinology and Metabolism* 81 (1996): 1495–1501.

14. H. Burger, E. Dudley, J. Hopper, N. Groome, J. Guthrie, A. Green, and L. Dennerstein, "Prospectively Measured Levels of Serum Follicle-Stimulating Hormone, Estradiol, and the Dimeric Inhibins during the Menopausal Transition in a Population-Based Cohort of Women," *Journal of Clinical Endocrinology and Metabolism* 84, no. 11 (1999): 4025–30.

15. H. Burger, E. Dudley, J. Cui, L. Dennerstein, J. Hopper, "A Prospective Longitudinal Study of Serum

tralian Twin Study," *Human Biology* 70, no. 6 (1998): 1073–91.

Testosterone Dehydroepiandrosterone Sulphate and Sex Hormone Binding Globulin Levels through the Menopause Transition," *Journal of Clinical Endocrinology and Metabolism* 85 (2000): 2832–2938; B. L. Lasley, N. Santoro, J. F. Randolf, et al., "The Relationship of Circulating Dehydroepiandrosterone, Testosterone, and Estradiol to Stages of the Menopausal Transition and Ethnicity," *Journal of Clinical Endocrinology and Metabolism* 87 (2002): 3760–67.

16. Lasley et al.

17. Burger et al., "A Prospective Longitudinal Study."

18. R. K. Stellato, S. L. Crawford, S. M. McKinlay, and C. Longcope, "Can Follicle-Stimulating Hormone Be Used to Define Menopausal Status?" *Endocrinology Practice* 4, no. 3, (1998): 137–41.

19. J. Randolph, M. Sowers, E. Gold, et al., "Reproductive Hormones in the Early Menopausal Transition: Relationship to Ethnicity, Body Size, and Menopausal Status," *Journal of Clinical Endocrinology and Metabolism* 88, no. 4 (2003): 1516–22.

20. Randolph et al.

21. N. Woods and E. Mitchell, "Symptoms during the Perimenopause: Prevalence, Severity, Trajectory, and Significance in Women's Lives" (submitted).

22. L. Dennerstein, E. Dudley, J. Hopper, J. Guthrie, and H. Burger, "A Prospective Population-Based Study of Menopausal Symptoms," *Obstetrics and Gynecology* 96 (2000): 351–58.

23. E. B. Gold, B. Sternfeld, et al., "Relation of Demographic and Lifestyle Factors to Symptoms in a Multi-Racial/Ethnic Population of Women 40–55 Years of Age," *American Journal of Epidemiology* 152, no. 5 (2000): 463–73.

24. E. W. Freeman, J. A. Grisso, J. Berlin, et al., "Symptom Reports from a Cohort of African American and White Women in the Late Reproductive Years," *Menopause* 8, no. 1 (2001): 33–42.

25. Dennerstein et al., "A Prospective Population-Based Study."

26. Gold et al.

27. Dennerstein et al., "A Prospective Population-Based Study."

28. Dennerstein et al., "Hormones, Mood"; N. Santoro, J. Torren, S. Crawford, J. Allsworth, J. Finkelstein, E. Gold, S. Korenman, W. Lasley, J. Luborsky, D. Mcconnell, M. J. Sowers, and G. Weiss, "Correlates of Circulating Androgens in Mid-Life Women: the Study of Women's Health Across the Nation (SWAN)," *Journal of Clinical Endocrinology and Metabolism* 90, no. 8 (2005): 4836–45; Davis et al.

29. L. Dennerstein, J. R. Guthrie, M. Clark, et al., "A Population-Based Study of Depressed Mood in Middle-Aged, Australian-Born Women," *Menopause* 11, no. 5 (2004): 563–8.

30. N. Avis, S. Crawford, R. Stellato, and C. Longcope, "Longitudinal Study of Hormone Levels and Depression among Women Transitioning through Menopause," *Climacteric* 4 (2001): 243–49.

31. N. Woods, A. Mariella, and E. Mitchell, "Patterns of Depressed Mood across the Menopausal Transition: Approaches to Studying Patterns in Longitudinal Data," *Acta Obstetrica Gynecologica Scandnavica* 81 (2002): 623–32.

32. E. S. Mitchell, N. F. Woods, "Midlife Women's Attributions about Perceived Memory Changes: Observations from the Seattle Midlife Women's Health Study," *Journal of Women's Health and Gender-Based Medicine* 10, no. 4 (2001): 351–62; N. F. Woods, E. S. Mitchell, et al., "Memory Functioning among Midlife Women: Observations from the Seattle Midlife Women's Health Study," *Menopause* 7, no. 4 (2000): 257–65.

33. P. M. Meyer, L. H. Powell, R. S. Wilson, et al., "A Population-Based Longitudinal Study of Cognitive Functioning in the Menopausal Transition," *Neurology* 61 (2003): 801–6.

34. C. M. Sampselle, D. S. Harlow, J. Skurnick, et al., "Urinary Incontinence Predictors and Life Impact in Ethnically Diverse Perimenopausal Women," *Obstetrics and Gynecology* 100, no. 6 (2002): 1230–38.

35. Gold et al.

36. L. Dennerstein et al., "A Prospective Population-Based Study."

37. Gold et al.

38. R. R. Wing, K. A. Matthews, L. H. Kuller, E. N. Meilahn, and P. L. Plantinga, "Weight Gain at the Time of Menopause," *Archives of Internal Medicine* 151, no. 1 (1991): 97–102.

39. L. H. Kuller, E. N. Meilahn, J. A. Cauley, J. P. Gutai, K. A. Matthews, "Epidemiologic Studies of Menopause Changes in Risk Factors and Disease," *Experimental Gerontology* 29 (1994): 495–509.

40. K. Matthews, B. Abams, S. Crawford, T. Miles, R. Neer, L. Powell, and D. Welsey, "Body Mass Index in Mid-Life Women: Relative Influence of Menopause, Hormone Use, and Ethnicity," *International Journal of Obesity* 25 (2001): 863–73.

41. R. R. Wing, R. W. Jeffery, L. R. Burton, C. Thorson, L. H. Kuller, and A. R. Folsom, "Change in Waist-Hip Ratio with Weight Loss and Its Association with Change in Cardiovascular Risk Factors," *American Journal of Clinical Nutrition* 55 (1992): 1086–92.

42. Kuller et al.

43. M. Sowers, J. Finkelstein, B. Ettinger, I. Bondarenko, R. Neer, J. Cauley, S. Sherman, and G. Greendale, "The Association of Endogenous Hormone Concentrations and Bone Mineral Density Measures in Pre- and Perimenopausal Women of Four Ethnic Groups: SWAN," *Osteoporosis International* 14, no. 1 (2003): 44–52.

44. E. N. Meilahn, L. H. Kuller, K. A. Matthews, and J. E. Kiss, "Hemostatic Factors according to Menopausal Status and Use of Hormone Replacement Therapy," *Annals of Epidemiology* 2 (1992): 445–55; see also M. Sowers, C. Derby, M. Jannausch, J. Torrens, and R. Pasternak, "Insulin Resistance, Hemostatic Factors, and Hormone Interactions in Pre- and Perimenopausal Women: SWAN," *Journal of Clinical Endocrinology and Metabolism* 88, no. 10 (2003): 4904–10.

45. J. A. Cauley, J. P. Gutai, L. H. Kuller, J. G. Powell, "The Relation of Endogenous Sex Steroid Hormone Concentrations to Serum Lipid and Lipoprotein Levels in Postmenopausal Women," *American Journal of Epidemiology* 132 (1990): 884–94.

46. M. Carr, K. Kim, A. Zambon, N. Woods, et al., "Changes in LDL Density across the Menopausal Transition," *Journal of Investigative Medicine* 48 (2000): 245–50.

47. E. N. Meilahn, L. H. Kuller, K. A. Matthews, R. R. Wing, A. W. Caggiula, and E. A. Stein, "Potential for Increasing High-Density Lipoprotein Cholesterol, Subfraction HDL_2-C and HDL_3-C, and Apoprotein A1 among Middle-Age Women," *Preventive Medicine* 20 (1991): 462–73.

48. Cauley et al.

49. Meilahn et al., "Hemostatic Factors."

50. M. Sowers, S. Crawford, B. Sternfeld, D. Morganstein, E. Gold, G. Greendale, D. Evans, R. Neer, K. Matthews, S. Sherman, A. Lo, G. Weiss, and J. Kelsye, "SWAN: A Multicenter, Multiethnic Community-Based Cohort Study of Women and the Menopausal Transition," in R. Lobo, J. Kelsey, and R. Marcus, *Menopause: Biology and Pathobiology* (San Diego: Academic Press, 2000), 175–88.

CHAPTER 4

Sudden and Early Menopause

For many women, menopause is not a midlife transition. Our periods may end suddenly due to medical treatments or stop gradually but earlier than usual for no known reason. In either case, menopause can come as a surprise. A thirty-year-old woman who recently learned that she has gone through a natural early menopause says,

I had all of the symptoms since I was probably twenty-five or twenty-six. It never once occurred to me that I could be going through menopause. Menopause happened to women twice my age! I kept thinking it was stress or something like that. So did my doctors, actually.

A woman whose uterus and ovaries were removed, causing what is called surgically induced menopause, explains,

When I was thirty-five, I had a hysterectomy because I just couldn't live with the pain and bleeding from endometriosis, and nothing else worked. Before the hysterectomy, the surgeon told me that it would be better to remove my ovaries at the same time, in order to prevent any problems in the future. But wow! Was I surprised when I woke up after surgery feeling like a french fry from the hot flashes!

WHAT IS "EARLY MENOPAUSE"?

Most women experience menopause between the ages of 45 and 55. The average age in the United States is 51 years old. Yet many of us face menopause at a much earlier age. Menopause is considered "premature" when it takes place before the age of 40. Although this is not typical, it is also not rare.

It is hard to know how many American women reach menopause suddenly through gynecological surgery or medical treatments. One in three American women undergoes hysterectomy by age 60;[1] a little more than half of all hysterectomies are performed on women under age 45;[2] and 40 percent of women who have a hysterectomy between the ages of 15 and 44 have both ovaries removed at the time of the surgery.[3]

In addition, women's ovaries can stop functioning at an early age because of genetic factors or autoimmune disorders. In the United States, this includes 1 in 10,000 women by age 20, 1 in 1,000 women by age 30, 1 in 250 women by age 35, and 1 in 100 women by age 40.[4]

WHAT CAUSES EARLY MENOPAUSE?

There are several possible causes of early menopause, including surgery, medical treatment, and early changes in ovary function.

SURGICAL MENOPAUSE

The removal of your ovaries (oophorectomy) or injury to your ovaries from other surgeries can cause what is known as surgical menopause. Some women's ovaries are removed because they are damaged or cancerous. In addition, many women's healthy ovaries are removed in conjunction with removal of the uterus (hysterectomy) or to prevent recurrence of estrogen receptor–positive breast cancer. Ovaries also may be removed during surgeries to treat colon, rectal, and cervical cancer.

Removal of Both Ovaries (Bilateral Oophorectomy)

If your uterus and both of your ovaries are removed, you will never again menstruate, and, because of the abrupt loss of ovarian hormones, you will undergo menopause-related changes almost immediately. This result is referred to as sudden menopause or surgically induced menopause. It is in strong contrast to natural menopause, which is often a very gradual process, spread over a long period of time in women who have the continued function of their uteruses and ovaries. The surgery will probably cause you to experience more sudden and severe vasomotor signs (like hot flashes and night sweats) than are typically experienced in natural menopause. While postmenopausal ovaries still continue to produce some estrogens and androgens, removal of the ovaries immediately and permanently eliminates this major source of hormone production.

A thirty-two-year-old woman who underwent bilateral oophorectomy says,

My doctor said surgical menopause is like a car driving seventy miles per hour and then slamming into a brick wall. I don't think you can ever be prepared for it—the immediateness of sudden menopause via surgery, especially when you're young like I was. It's a life-changing event. I'm learning to cope, but it's been pretty devastating.

Because of the abrupt and untimely loss of ovarian hormones, removal of the ovaries may also cause a variety of serious long-term effects, including an increased incidence of heart disease, osteoporosis,[5] and Parkinson's disease.[6] If your ovaries were removed prior to natural menopause, you probably should be closely monitored for symptoms of these conditions.

In some gynecological surgeries, blood flow to the ovaries is compromised or lost, or the ovaries themselves are damaged. Procedures such as cyst removal or tubal ligation (getting your "tubes tied") have been linked to effects on ovarian hormone production.

Removal of the Uterus (Hysterectomy)

Hysterectomy is the second most common surgery in the United States, affecting more than 600,000 American women per year.[7] By the age of sixty, about one out of every three American women undergoes hysterectomy.[8] The most recent government health data indicates that 52 percent of all hysterectomies are performed on women younger than forty-four, most of whom are premenopausal.[9] Women have hysterectomies for various reasons, including extremely heavy periods not controlled by less invasive means, fibroids, endometriosis, uterine prolapse, and malignant or premalignant changes of the uterus, cervix, or ovaries. Only 10 percent of hysterectomies are performed because of cancer or suspected cancer.[10]

Not all of us who undergo hysterectomy have our ovaries removed at the same time. However, 40 percent of American women under age forty-five who have hysterectomies have our ovaries removed at the time of the surgery.[11]

If your ovaries are left in place and continue to produce hormones, menopause usually will not occur immediately, but menstrual bleeding stops and your fertility ends. Nevertheless, even if your ovaries are not removed and do con-

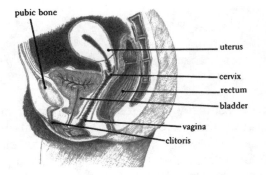

© Peggy Clark

A partial hysterectomy: After surgery, the cervix and the stump of the uterus remain, requiring regular Pap tests. (Ovaries and fallopian tubes are also sometimes removed.)

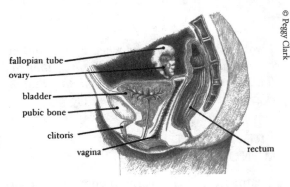

© Peggy Clark

A complete hysterectomy: The uterus is removed, including the cervix. Regular Pap tests are required only if the woman had previous treatment for precancerous changes of the cervix. (Ovaries and fallopian tubes are attached to the top of the vagina in this image, but some women elect to have them removed as well.)

tinue to function appropriately, hysterectomy generally causes menopause to occur more than three and a half years earlier than it would be expected to otherwise.[12] This is most likely because the blood supply to the ovaries has been disturbed and/or because the ovaries may require stimulation from prostaglandins (hormonelike substances produced by the uterus) in order to work properly.

Three years after her hysterectomy, one young woman says,

I was shocked and grieved when I found out my ovaries no longer produced eggs. Even though I had a hysterectomy, I still had a fantasy that my eggs could be harvested or something.

TREATMENT-INDUCED MENOPAUSE

Treatment-induced early menopause occurs most commonly as the result of chemotherapy, radiation therapy, or drug therapy related to cancer treatment. Early menopause may occur because the same treatments that are used to kill cancer can also damage your ovaries. The severity of the consequences depends on many factors, including the drugs used, the dosage, your age, and your general health.

Chemotherapy

The effects of chemotherapy on ovaries (often referred to as *chemopause*) usually occur over several months, rather than immediately. However, these effects are often considered sudden menopause because the changes don't happen over a period of three to five years as with natural menopause. It is more likely that

chemotherapy will induce menopause in women closer to the age of natural menopause. But younger women, who have higher hormone levels before chemotherapy, are more likely to experience harsher menopause-related effects.

A woman who was diagnosed with breast cancer premenopausally and was treated with the drug Lupron, requiring an injection once a month to cause her ovaries to stop producing estrogen, describes her experience:

The first month I didn't really notice anything much, but shortly after my second month's shot, the proverbial shit hit the fan. I began having major hot flashes, yes, but worse than that, it felt like my whole body was buzzing, as if I were running on overdrive. One of my doctors said to me, "Some women's brains are just very sensitive to estrogen levels." I guess mine is one of those.

The interruption of your working ovaries may be only a temporary condition, particularly if the treatment is low-dose or short-term. Your menstrual periods may return to normal, generally within four months of treatment.

Radiation Therapy

The effects of radiation depend largely on the location of your treatment. Pelvic or ovarian radiation can cause a rapid and dramatic decline in estrogen levels. You may experience relatively sudden signs of menopause such as hot flashes and vaginal dryness, which may be more severe than those experienced after chemotherapy. You may also stop menstruating. These changes usually occur during the course of treatment or within three to six months following radiation. In the case of pelvic or ovarian radiation, your reproductive system is nearly always permanently affected, leading to early menopause.

"PREMATURE OVARIAN FAILURE" (POF)

If you are under forty years old, your ovaries have stopped working as they usually do, and you have not had gynecological surgery, chemotherapy, or radiation treatment, you may be diagnosed with *premature ovarian failure (POF)*. Some health care providers also use the term *ovarian insufficiency* to describe this condition. POF may occur years or decades before the typical age for menopause. Sometimes your menstrual periods may completely stop, but often with POF you may still menstruate sporadically. In fact, sometimes POF is not classified as strictly early menopause, because the biological causes can be different.

Researchers have not been able to determine exactly why some women's ovaries stop working as usual at an early age. While autoimmune disorders, chromosomal disorders, smoking, and certain viruses have been implicated, some of us may just be genetically programmed to go through menopause at a younger age than others. In this case, despite the medical terminology, your ovaries have not really "failed," they have simply completed their mission earlier than usual. Just as women begin menstruation at different ages, women also reach menopause at different ages. Also, sometimes ovarian function may be temporarily disrupted and may resume again.

Early natural menopause appears to be least common among Japanese-American women (0.1 percent of whom experience early natural menopause, according to a recent study) and most common among African-American women and Latinas (with 1.4 percent of women in these groups experiencing early natural menopause).[16] About 1 percent of white American women and 0.5 percent of Chinese-American women experience early natural menopause. Early natural menopause is also more common among women who are poor.[17]

It is not usually possible to know whether your POF is temporary. In addition, the specific cause of your POF may never be found. A thirty-six-year-old woman with premature ovarian failure describes her frustration with this uncertainty:

When I finally got the POF diagnosis, after years of these weird and awful symptoms, I was in shock. I could not believe I was sitting there and my doctor was telling me, "Yes, it's POF but we really can't tell you how you got it." I was like, "What? You're the doctor. Tell me how I got this awful thing!" I truly think that's one of the worst parts of the diagnosis—not knowing.

Some women may blame ourselves for behaviors or risks that we think may have brought on our POF. We often try to find a "reason" when there doesn't appear to be a definite cause. Most causes of early menopause are beyond our control. Some factors that may affect POF are discussed in the following pages.

Autoimmune Disorders

Autoimmune disorders probably account for a large proportion of premature ovarian failure (POF) cases. An autoimmune disorder causes your body to produce abnormal antibodies, which can attack your tissues, including your ovaries. The most common autoimmune disorders linked with premature ovarian failure are thyroid dysfunction (including Graves' disease); Addison's disease (adrenal insufficiency); polyglandular failure I and II; hypoparathyroidism; diabetes (particularly insulin-dependent diabetes mellitus or Type I diabetes); lupus; rheumatoid arthritis; inflammatory bowel syndrome; and myasthenia gravis. In addition, research indicates that if you develop premature ovarian failure due to an autoimmune disorder, it is more likely that you could develop *other* autoimmune disorders.[18] You and your health care provider should be aware of this possibility, so that you can be checked.

One thirty-year-old woman says,

I had POF symptoms since my early twenties and was finally diagnosed last year, from possible autoimmune factors. Since then I've developed other autoimmune disorders here and there, like fibromyalgia and asthma. My doctor tells me it's pretty typical to have autoimmune disorders, and then get even more after the diagnosis!

Family History/Genetics

Following autoimmune disorders, the next most common cause of premature ovarian failure (POF) is genetics. Approximately 30 percent of women with POF have an affected female relative, and new information has identified a gene mutation that may bring about early menopause.[19] Although there is some variation, most women go through menopause at about the same age as our mothers, so if there's a family history of POF, you may experience it as well.[20]

Chromosomal Irregularities

Some cases of inherited premature ovarian failure are caused by chromosomal irregularities. Two major conditions linked to POF are fragile X syndrome and Turner's syndrome, each of which is related to defects on an X chromosome. Specific testing can determine if you have either of these conditions.

Smoking

Research shows that smoking cigarettes is associated with an earlier age of menopause, by a few years, and the problems associated with menopause may be more severe for smokers.[21]

Viral Infections

Some viral infections (such as mumps or cytomegalovirus) may affect your ovaries and trigger premature ovarian failure. Also, certain viral infections in pregnant women can affect ovarian development in their female fetuses. Therefore, their daughters may be born with fewer viable eggs than usual, which can bring about POF.

Stress

A great deal of research has shown the connection between emotional and physical health. Although stress doesn't actually cause early menopause, it can make some problems associated with it worse. For example, stress may increase the severity of hot flashes and sleep disturbances and negatively affect sexual desire. A twenty-eight-year-old woman diagnosed with early menopause says,

You always hear that stress affects your health. I just never realized, until I was diagnosed, how much of a difference it makes in my day-to-day living. I've started some stress management tech-

niques that have made a huge difference in coping with my premature menopause.

Environmental Toxins

A variety of potentially harmful chemicals are used to manufacture all types of products, including pesticides, plastics, computer chips, soaps, and many others. Environmental toxins can interfere with the normal functioning of your body. A particular group of chemicals, *xenoestrogens* (which mimic estrogen in the human body), are suspected of contributing to the incidence of POF, although this link has not been completely confirmed by research.[22]

Reproductive Factors

Some research indicates that other factors may contribute to early menopause, including having a history of irregular menstrual cycles, having no children or only one, and having a long gap between a first and second birth.[23]

WHAT IS UNIQUE ABOUT EARLY MENOPAUSE?

Early menopause carries a distinctive set of physical and emotional concerns. There can be confusion caused by the sometimes vague and unexpected physical changes that accompany early menopause that is not prompted by surgery or medical treatment. Health care providers don't usually consider the diagnosis of menopause for women under forty. A thirty-two-year-old woman remembers,

For about two years, maybe three, even though I didn't know it, I was going through premature menopause. I had all kinds of different symptoms—aching joints, sleepless nights, terrible night sweats, gaining weight even though I was eating normally, and really bad mood swings that affected my family and me badly. Since I was so

young, I never thought of menopause. Neither did my doctors.

SIGNS OF EARLY MENOPAUSE

Women who enter menopause naturally, whether at the average age or earlier, tend to experience certain physical changes gradually. These changes can include irregular menstrual periods, heavier or lighter menstrual flow than is normal for you, hot flashes, night sweats, and vaginal dryness.

Women going through the menopause transition also sometimes report urinary problems (including frequency of urination, urinary stress incontinence, and pain on urination), abrupt mood swings, problems concentrating or remembering things, and loss of sexual desire or response, but the connection between such changes and menopause is not as clear; aging or other life stresses may be the cause. (For more information, see longer discussions of these issues in other chapters.) Additional changes that some women note at the time of menopause include migraine headaches or head pressure, dryer and thinner skin, thinner and more brittle hair, weight gain, and/or breast swelling and tenderness. Any of these changes can be indications of other conditions, and not all women going through the menopause transition experience all of these.

Many young women mistake the early signs of menopause for PMS. If you have a combination of several signs of menopause that occur throughout the month (rather than beginning prior to menstruation and ending shortly after menstruation begins), they may indicate menopause rather than PMS. A thirty-one-year-old woman who went through a natural early menopause describes her experience:

My periods were always so irregular, and I had so few other symptoms, that I never really noticed anything that screamed "Symptom!" before I was diagnosed with premature menopause. I always felt pretty healthy overall.

Some women never experience a single hot flash; they just stop menstruating. Others experience minimal hot flashes or other minor symptoms for a short time, stop menstruating, and never again have any symptoms. However, if you are younger than the typical age for menopause, it is likely that you will experience more severe problems than other women.[24]

IS IT REALLY EARLY MENOPAUSE?

If you experience early menopause that is not related to surgery or medical treatment, you may have some difficulty getting your condition recognized because the signs are so varied and you are not the typical age for menopause. Many women describe knowing something was going on, physically and emotionally, but never considering menopause as a possible cause.

Most health care providers do not see a large number of women with early menopause, so they may not have enough experience to diagnose, answer questions about, or provide an accurate evaluation of your condition. This means that it's very important for you to know the signs of your condition (see "Signs of Early Menopause," page 63), as well as to seek out current resources to find the most informed medical providers (see "Resources," page 317, and "Treatment and Support," page 69).

When you visit your health care provider, be prepared to describe your menstrual cycle changes, signs of menopause such as hot flashes, and any history of ovarian surgery, radiation, or chemotherapy. Tell your provider if you've had an endocrine disorder, any recent infections, or a family history of gynecological

problems, including premature ovarian failure. You can ask your health care provider to administer specific diagnostic tests or to refer you to a gynecologist or endocrinologist who can perform them. A thirty-one-year-old woman with signs of early menopause says,

My advice? Educate yourself. Read, read, read! Keep a medical journal and get to know your body. And get second and third opinions if you have to. Remember that you probably know your body better than anyone.

Early menopause or premature ovarian failure can be diagnosed using a number of tests. Your health care provider should initially perform a thorough physical exam, in which she or he will draw blood and take your medical and family histories in order to rule out other possible conditions such as pregnancy, extreme weight loss, thyroid disease, or other hormone disturbances. Your provider may also order a test to measure your levels of *estradiol,* a form of estrogen. Low levels of estradiol can indicate that your ovaries are starting to fail and may signal that you are perimenopausal or menopausal. Other assessments may include thyroid tests, vaginal acidity analysis, ultrasound, and tests of blood levels of prolactin and luteinizing hormone.

The most important test used to diagnose early menopause is a blood test that measures your level of follicle-stimulating hormone (FSH). FSH causes your ovaries to produce estrogen. When your ovaries slow down or begin to fail, your levels of FSH increase. If your FSH levels rise above 30 or 40, it is generally a sign that you are entering menopause. However, because your hormone levels may fluctuate from one week to the next, the results of the first test can be misleading. Therefore, you should have this testing done for at least two consecutive months. It is considered more reliable three or four days after the start of a period.

TEMPORARY CONDITIONS THAT ARE NOT EARLY MENOPAUSE

As with some cases of premature ovarian failure, the normal functioning of your ovaries can be interrupted for various reasons, causing your menstrual periods to stop temporarily. This is typically referred to as *temporary menopause*, although it is not really menopause because your menstrual periods eventually resume.

The "Treatment-Induced Menopause" section (page 60) discusses the sometimes temporary effects of chemotherapy and radiation. In addition, tamoxifen is often used either to prevent breast or endometrial cancer or to increase the survival rates of women with these cancers. Tamoxifen can cause some problems that are associated with menopause.[25] As a woman in her thirties found:

Taking tamoxifen has made for a rocky time. Immediately, I started having hot flashes, night sweats, vaginal discharge, and vaginal dryness.

The menopause-like effects from using tamoxifen are generally temporary. Your ovaries will usually begin working again after treatment ends, particularly if you are young. The closer you are to the age of a natural menopause, the more likely it is that the ovaries will not resume their previous function.

Many premenopausal women who have endometriosis (a benign condition that can cause great pain and bleeding) or benign uterine fibroids take hormonal treatment that tem-

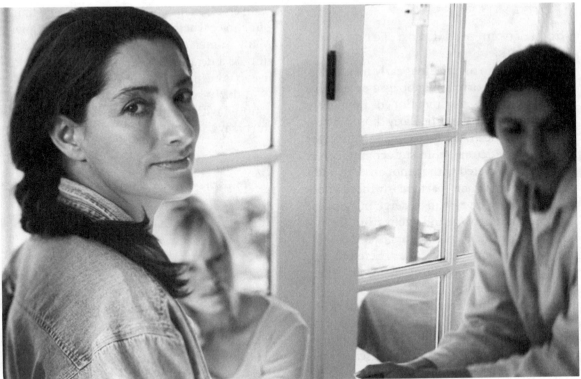

porarily stops menstrual periods. If you are treated with progestin, danazol (Danocrine), or GnRH (gonadotropin-releasing hormones) agonists (including Synarel or Lupron), your periods usually will resume once you end this therapy. Similarly, if you go on continuous birth control medication (such as Seasonale), your menstrual periods should return after you finish taking it.

Illness, high levels of emotional stress, over-exercise, and excessive dieting (particularly eating disorders such as anorexia and bulimia) can all cause your menstrual periods to stop. Usually, once your health improves or you have resumed healthy lifestyle habits, your periods will begin again.

MENOPAUSE CONCERNS FOR YOUNG WOMEN

MEDICAL ISSUES

Short-Term and Long-Term Problems

It is a mistake to assume that early menopause is the same as normal menopause except that it occurs earlier. As mentioned previously, women under forty (particularly those who experience surgically induced menopause) are likely to suffer from more sudden and severe problems associated with menopause. In addition, younger women (particularly those under the age of thirty-five) who undergo menopause have not had the time to benefit from the full number of years of premenopausal estrogen, progesterone, and testosterone. Therefore, you may be at greater long-term risk for heart disease and osteoporosis.[26]

In fact, women who experience surgically induced menopause or early menopause prior to the age of thirty-five may have a seven times greater risk of coronary heart disease than women who undergo natural menopause after that age.[27] Some recent research indicates that, although those of us who undergo menopause earlier have a reduced risk of death due to uterine or ovarian cancer, we have a somewhat shorter lifespan than those who undergo menopause later, due in large part to heart disease and stroke.[28] Make sure that your health care provider monitors these possible health problems so that you can get treatment if necessary.

Pregnancy

Many of us discover that we are in early menopause because we have been unable to become pregnant. While some women are relieved to no longer have to worry about pregnancy, for most of us, the single most devastating part of early menopause is losing the ability to give birth. This can affect us even if we already have children. Some of us who previously did not want children may feel regret that it is no longer our choice whether or not to become pregnant. Many women describe the untimely loss of fertility as a death and a feeling that part of their lives has been taken away.

A thirty-seven-year-old married woman diagnosed with premature ovarian failure at age thirty says,

My husband and I had talked about kids, sure, but it was always way down the road. And then it was like, one minute I could have children and then—boom—that's over. The best way I can describe it is it felt like something was just physically ripped away from me.

Approximately 5 to 10 percent of women diagnosed with some forms of premature ovarian failure do become pregnant every year.[29] It appears that some women's ovaries can spontaneously begin to work again, particularly while they are taking estrogen. It is important to remember, though, that even if your periods have resumed, you may not actually be ovulating or capable of becoming pregnant.

There are options for women who want to become mothers despite early menopause. If you still have your uterus, you might consider trying induced ovulation, egg donation, autoimmune suppression, or ovarian tissue transplant. You should consult with a reproductive endocrinologist to explore these or other assisted reproductive technologies, which can be somewhat complicated. If you have undergone hysterectomy, you may want to attempt to have another woman bear your child. Finally, many women have found that adoption is a wonderful way to become a mother and simultaneously provide a family for a child who needs one. You can learn more about this option through public and private adoption agencies. However, it is important to fully mourn your inability to have a child in the way you had hoped for, before pursuing other options.

Sexuality

If you reach menopause early, you may be particularly upset if your sexual urges and responses change for the worse. You may experience changes that interfere with your ability to enjoy sex as you once did, such as hot flashes, vaginal dryness, or decreased libido. You could also feel that you have aged prematurely and that you have therefore lost your sex appeal.

On the other hand, some women feel more comfortable and enjoy sex more after early menopause. This is especially true for those of us who did not want to become pregnant or who suffered from painful gynecological conditions or breakthrough bleeding prior to menopause. A woman who had a hysterectomy and surgical removal of her ovaries because of benign fibroid tumors says,

When I got into my thirties, I started having pain when I had penetrative sex. It would hurt afterwards, in a weird echo-y, almost crampy way, often the next day. . . . Sex is so much better now. It's completely amazing how useful it is to be pain-free.

Many women notice no difference in sexual desire or response following early menopause. Sexuality is very complicated, and it can be affected by a number of factors besides a change in hormonal balance. Hormone treatment may help some young women who are experiencing problems with sexuality. (For more information, see Chapter 9, "Sexuality," and Chapter 7, "Hormone Treatment.")

PSYCHOLOGICAL CONCERNS

Feelings of Loss

Those of us who experience early menopause often describe it as a shock because we didn't think we would have to face this change for many years. Despite some relief that we no longer have to put up with menstrual problems, many young women miss our periods as a source of regularity in our lives and as a sign that we are still youthful. Fertility is often linked to youth and womanhood, so it is not surprising that we often feel diminished or deficient because we have gone through early menopause.

It is very important to allow yourself to grieve the losses you have suffered, and to have your emotions acknowledged and validated. You may feel sadness, exhaustion, and even periods of hopelessness. A twenty-eight-year-old woman, recently diagnosed, says,

I don't even remember the months after I was diagnosed. I basically didn't leave the house. I was heartbroken, depressed, ashamed, in pain— physical as well as emotional. You have to mourn

what you have to mourn and that's it. You can't just hide your feelings with "make your life happy" pills.

From day to day, you may go back and forth between feeling better and then worse again. These emotions are understandable reactions and nothing to feel ashamed or guilty about. You may need to go through an adjustment process, and you will probably rebound over time. However, you should give yourself this time. The psychological effects of early menopause can be just as difficult to deal with as the physical impact.

Depression

Women who undergo surgical or early menopause are far more likely to become clinically depressed than women who are the typical age for menopause; this is probably because depression can be associated with both a sudden drop in hormones and emotional trauma.[30] Women who previously experienced depression premenstrually or postpartum or both are most likely to experience depression associated with early menopause.[31] Also, women who have undergone multiple surgeries or lack social supports are more likely to become clinically depressed.[32]

Since recent popular and medical articles have stressed that menopause does not automatically cause depression, some people, including some health care providers, may not understand depression associated with sudden and early menopause. It is important to recognize that, in the case of early menopause, depression can be a predictable reaction to an untimely and atypical physical occurrence. Although some women may feel embarrassed or even ashamed to talk about mental health problems, you should never suffer in silence. Make sure that you get the help you need. (For more information on depression, see Chapter 15, "Memory and Mood.")

SOCIAL DIFFERENCES

Early menopause often makes young women feel "out of step" with those in our peer group. We are experiencing a life change that ordinarily happens to much older women. This may hit you if a friend asks to borrow a tampon or a sister-in-law announces that she is pregnant. They are still menstruating and still fertile. In addition, they are not suffering from hot flashes and don't look older as the result of hormonal changes. You may feel that, in certain ways, you no longer fit in. You may find it difficult to talk with others who can't fully understand what you are going through.

A twenty-two-year-old woman diagnosed with premature ovarian failure describes her frustration:

After a few months a lot of my friends were basically just telling me to "get over it." They just didn't get it. How am I supposed to get over things like hot flashes, infertility, and losing my hair—at twenty-two years old?

It may, for example, upset you to attend a baby shower right after you have been diagnosed with early menopause or experienced sudden menopause following a hysterectomy or other treatment. You may have to give yourself time to heal before you ease into these types of situations. You have suffered a real setback, and it can be helpful to lower your stress level.

As with other unexpected life events, talking things through can be especially valuable. Joining a support group of women experiencing the same things may help you cope with your diagnosis. Support groups are a unique way to feel connected. They allow you to ask questions, share your experiences, and get advice from other women who understand (see "Support Groups," page 70).

TREATMENT AND SUPPORT

HORMONAL TREATMENT

The most commonly prescribed treatment for women undergoing early menopause is hormone therapy. You can read about the pros and cons of hormone therapy in Chapter 7, which discusses the Women's Health Initiative (WHI) finding that the risks of hormone therapy exceed the benefits. However, it is important to bear in mind that the WHI studied the effects of hormone therapy on women fifty to seventy-nine years old. We don't know the consequences of this therapy for younger women who have undergone surgical or treatment-induced menopause or premature ovarian failure. The WHI recommendations focus on "routine" use of these therapies; early menopause, particularly through surgery, is arguably not routine. In fact, the benefits of hormone therapy for women under forty may well exceed the risks.[33]

Women who go through menopause at middle age cope with a gradual, natural lowering of hormone levels. In fact, the medical community now generally refers to "hormone therapy" rather than "hormone replacement therapy" for these older women because it is no longer believed that midlife women need to "replace" naturally decreasing hormones. However, for younger women, hormone therapy can actually be a replacement for what we have lost prematurely. This is particularly true for women who have had our ovaries removed. Following natural menopause, the ovaries continue to produce low levels of hormones (including estrogen, progesterone, and testosterone). While your body has other minor sources of hormone production, if your ovaries were removed, this major source is gone.

Even before the announcement of the Women's Health Initiative results, younger women who experienced early natural menopause or had their ovaries removed were much more likely to fill prescriptions for hormone therapy than were those women who underwent natural menopause at the average age.[34] The problems associated with surgically induced menopause, treatment-induced menopause, and early natural menopause are often more abrupt, severe, and frequent than those of natural menopause. In addition, you are at greater risk for many long-term health problems. (See "Medical Issues," page 66).

Many medical researchers argue that if you take hormone treatment to minimize the consequences of early menopause, you are not prolonging your exposure to these hormones. In fact, the amount of estrogen in hormone treatment is only about one quarter of the amount made, on average, by the ovaries of a menstruating woman. So you are not even maintaining what would have occurred naturally if you had reached the typical age of menopause. Because you face many more years without your ovarian hormones, it is often recommended that you take hormone therapy until about age fifty, and then consult the most current research and make a decision with your health care provider about whether to continue.[35] You may decide to decrease the level of hormone therapy gradually, to mimic the gradual decrease of hormones in natural menopause. Your assessment of whether to start or continue hormone treatment should center on whether the benefits exceed the risks for you as an individual. This assessment should be reviewed regularly in light of new information. Alternative medical therapies for osteoporosis, like bisphosphonates, may be more appropriate for you than hormone treatment. It is particularly important to discuss your situation with a health care provider who has extensive experience with early menopause as well as to familiarize yourself with the most current studies.

You may decide that you prefer nonhormonal or "natural" remedies to cope with problems associated with early menopause. Such complementary and alternative practices might include herbal medicine, phytoestrogens, special healthy diets, acupuncture, chiropractic, homeopathy, and stress reduction techniques such as meditation, hypnosis, yoga, and massage therapy. These natural remedies can be used instead of or in addition to medical therapies. It is valuable to inform yourself about their possible benefits and risks, just as you would with conventional medical treatments. (For more information on making health care decisions, see Chapter 2, "Making Health Care Decisions"; for more information on stress reduction techniques, see Chapter 11, "Emotional Well-Being and Managing Stress.")

A thirty-three-year-old, diagnosed with early menopause at nineteen, explains,

After talking with a lot of women with POF, I've found that each woman has to go through her own discovery process of what does and does not work for her. I work with a naturopath and my endocrinologist and that works for me. I learned long ago that ultimately I'm in charge of my health.

Women who have undergone sudden menopause may be less interested in "natural" remedies than other women who go through menopause, since our menopause was so unnatural.[36] Yet we may find that integrating various techniques allows us to manage menopausal changes more easily and use lower doses of medications to achieve relief. Many of us who experience early menopause find that exercise and diet can help us feel and look our age, as well as promote our long-term health.

COUNSELING, THERAPY

Surgical or treatment-induced menopause or a diagnosis of premature ovarian failure often instigates a period of grieving, and this can sometimes develop into depression. Depression should not be ignored. Many women (and our partners) find that professional counseling can help us deal with our feelings. Therapy is an opportunity to discuss your problems and fears, in an atmosphere that is nonjudgmental and supportive. It is important to find the right person. Your health care provider, friends, or relatives can help you locate a trained therapist or counselor.

SUPPORT GROUPS

Many women going through sudden or early menopause find it helpful to connect with others in the same situation. In a support group, we can talk honestly about what is happening and how we feel. Sharing our experiences with other women we trust helps us feel that we are not alone.

A thirty-four-year-old woman recently diagnosed with early menopause says,

I must have spent four hours online the first time I found the Web discussion board! Honestly, I've never known support like this. I've made friends not only across the country but around the world—people who get me, and get my condition.

Support groups, both online and in person, are constantly developing and evolving. They are often started at a small, grassroots level by women wanting to make contact with others. Make sure that you look for a group composed of women who are facing menopause at an early age. Attending a group with midlife women may increase your feeling of isolation.

RESOLUTION

It is important to remember that, even though you may be experiencing physical symptoms and biological changes that most women don't face until later in life, you are still young in many other respects. Some of us find that there are some positive sides to early menopause, even though it was not what we expected or would have wanted. Menopause at an early age may encourage us to consider what we want to do with the rest of our lives. We may improve our eating and exercise habits, we may start new careers, or we may face our infertility and adopt children while we are still young enough to have many years left to enjoy with them.

One woman diagnosed with premature ovarian failure says,

For about a week I cried and cried. I felt like my youth was gone, all those dreams and hopes and excitement of what lies ahead. . . . [Six months later,] now that I've gotten over a lot of the sorrow and feeling of loss, the mourning over my lost youth, I feel so much stronger and better and I love myself even more.

Another woman, who had her uterus and ovaries removed in her thirties, realized almost twenty years later,

You never know what can happen in life. Surgical menopause was a "wakeup call" for me that made me reevaluate my situation. Yes, it was a change—a traumatic one at the time—but ultimately one that was not completely negative. What I thought was the worst thing that had ever happened to me led me to make some very positive changes. I left a bad marriage, went back to school, and started on the path to a new life that was better in many ways than the old one.

NOTES

1. National Women's Health Information Center, "Hysterectomy," 2002, accessed at womenshealth.gov/faq/hysterectomy.htm on September 10, 2005.
2. Homa Keshavarz, Susan D. Hillis, Burney A, Kieke, Polly A. Marchbanks, *Hysterectomy Surveillance—United States, 1994–1999* (Maryland: Centers for Disease Prevention, 2002), 1.
3. Ibid., 4.
4. National Institutes of Health National Institute of Child Health and Human Development, "Fast Facts about Premature Ovarian Failure," accessed at www.nichd.nih.gov/publications/pubs/pof/sub1.htm on June 1, 2005.
5. Jonathan S. Berek, ed., *Novak's Gynecology*, 13th ed. (Philadelphia: Lippincott Williams, 2002), 1111; David McKay Hart and Jane Norman, *Gynaecology Illustrated*, 5th ed. (London: Churchill Livingston, 2000), 424–25.
6. Mayo Clinic, "Ovary Removal Elevates Risk for Parkinson's Disease and Parkinsonism," April 15, 2005, accessed at www.mayoclinic.org/news2005-rst/2751.html on August 1, 2005.
7. Keshavarz et al., 2.
8. National Women's Health Information Center, "Hysterectomy."
9. Keshavarz et al., 4.
10. Natalie Angier, "In Culture of Hysterectomies, Many Question Their Necessity," *New York Times*, February 17, 1997, Section A: 1, 1; see also National Women's Health Information Center, "Hysterectomy," accessed at www.4women.gov/faq/hysterectomy.htm on July 15, 2005.
11. Keshavarz et al., 4.
12. Cynthia M. Farquhar, Lynn Sadler, Sally A. Harvey, Allistair W. Stewart, "The Association of Hysterectomy and Menopause: A Prospective Cohort Study," *BJOG: An International Journal of Obstetrics and Gynecology* 112, no. 7 (July 2005): 956.
13. William H. Parker, Michael S. Broder, Zhimei Liu, Donna Shoupe, Cindy Farquhar, and Jonathan S. Berek, "Ovarian Conservation at the Time of Hys-

terectomy for Benign Disease," *Obstetrics and Gynecology* 106, no. 2 (August 2005): 219–26.

14. Parker et al.

15. Eliana Aguair Petri Nahás, Anaglória Pontes, Jorge Nahás-Neto, Vera Therezinha Medeiros Borges, Rogerio Dias, and Paulo Traiman, "Effect of Total Abdominal Hysterectomy on Ovarian Blood Supply in Women of Reproductive Age," *American Institute of Ultrasound Medicine* 24 (2005): 169–74; see also E. Nahás, A. Pontes, P. Traiman, J. Nahasneto, I. Dalben, and L. DeLuca, "Inhibin B and Ovarian Function after Total Abdominal Hysterectomy in Women of Reproductive Age," *Gynecological Endocrinology* 17, no. 2 (April 1, 2003): 125–31; Furrat Amen, "Hysterectomy and Ovarian Preservation," accessed at www.medworks.co.uk/hyster.htm on July 13, 2005; "Ovarian Failure Following Hysterectomy," accessed at www.menopause/hysterectomy.com/ovarian 2 on July 13, 2005; M. Parker, J. Bussher, D. Barnhill, et al., "Ovarian Management during Radical Hysterectomy in the Premenopausal Patient," *Obstetrics and Gynecology* 82, no. 2 (1993): 187–90; "Annual Meeting of the Northern Obstetrical and Gynaecological Society, Perth Royal Infirmary, 18 May 2001," *Journal of Obstetrics and Gynaecology* 22, no. 1 (January 1, 2002): 107–11; P. Loizzi, C. Carriero, A. DiGesu, et al., "Removal or Preservation of Ovaries during Hysterectomy: A 6 Year Review," *International Journal of Gynecology and Obstetrics* 31 (1990): 257–61; Vicki Hufnagel, *No More Hysterectomies* (New York: New American Library, 1998).

16. J. L. Luborsky, P. Meyer, M. F. Sowers, E. B. Gold, and N. Santoro, "Premature Menopause in a Multi-Ethnic Population Study of the Menopause Transition," *Human Reproduction* 18, no. 1 (2002): 201.

17. Ibid., 204.

18. Lawrence M. Nelson, "Spontaneous Premature Ovarian Failure: Young Women, Special Needs," accessed at www.nichd.gov/publications/pubs/pof on June 1, 2005.

19. *Scientific American*, "Premature Menopause Gene," January 31, 2001, accessed at www.sciam.com/ article,cfm?articleID=00073EC2-9CBD-1C5A-B882 809EC588ED9F on June 2, 2005.

20. J. P. Bruin, H. Bovenhuis, P. A. H. van Noord, P. L. Pearson, J. A. M. van Arendonk, E. R. te Velde, W. W. Kuurman, and M. Dorland, "The Role of Genetic Factors in Age at Natural Menopause," *Human Reproduction* 16 (September 2001): 2014–18; Joanne M. Murabito, Qiong Yang, Caroline Fox, Peter W. F. Wilson, and L. Adrienne Cupples, "Heritability of Age at Natural Menopause in the Framingham Heart Study," *Journal of Clinical Endocrinology & Metabolism* 90, no. 6 (2005): 3427–30.

21. Centers for Disease Control, "Women and Smoking: A Report of the Surgeon General," 2001, accessed at www.cdc.gov/tobacco/sgr/sgr_forwomen/factsheet_ consequences.htm on June 2, 2005.

22. Kathryn Petras, *The Premature Menopause Book: When the Change of Life Comes Too Early* (New York: Avon Books, 1999).

23. Marlies E. Ossewarrd, Michele L. Bots, Andre L. M. Verbeek, Petra H. M. Peeters, Yolanda van der Graaf, Diederick E. Grobbee, Yvonne T. van der Schouw, "Age at Menopause, Cause-Specific Mortality and Total Life Expectancy," *Epidemiology* 16, no. 4 (July 2005): 556–62.

24. National Institutes of Health, "Fast Facts about Premature Ovarian Failure"; Sara Rosenthal, *The Gynecological Sourcebook,* 3rd ed. (New York: McGraw Hill/Contemporary Books, 1999); Susan Love with Karen Lindsey, *Dr. Susan Love's Menopause and Hormone Book: Making Informed Choices* (New York: Three Rivers Press, 2003); "Managing Treatment Induced Menopause," accessed at www.umanitoba.ca/ women'shealth/meno1.htm on July 13, 2005; "Premature Menopause," accessed at www.project-aware. org/Experience/premature.shtml on August 2, 2005.

25. Breast Cancer.org., "Side Effects of Tamoxifen," accessed at www.breastcancer.org/tre_sys_tamox crzySide.html on June 2, 2005.

26. Nada L. Stotland and Donna E. Steward, *Psychological Aspects of Women's Health Care: The Interface between Psychiatry and Obstetrics and Gynecology,* 2nd ed.

(Washington, DC: American Psychiatric Press, 2001), 242; Hart and Norman, 425.

27. Hart and Norman, 425.

28. Ossewarrd et al.

29. Nelson.

30. Association for the Study of Reproductive Medicine, "Premature Ovarian Failure Is Not Early Menopause," accessed at www.asrm.org/Professionals/Meetings/philadelphia2004/POFworkshop.pdf on April 15, 2005; see also Carol Lyndaker and Linda Hulton, "The Influence of Age on Symptoms of Perimenopause," *Journal of Obstetric, Gynecologic, and Neonatal Nursing* 33 (2004): 340–47; J. B. McKinlay, S. M. McKinlay, and D. J. Brambilla, "Health Status and Utilization Behavior Associated with Menopause," *American Journal of Epidemiology* 125, no. 1 (1987): 110–21; Stotland and Steward, 295.

31. McKinlay et al.; see also Stotland and Steward, 293.

32. Stotland and Steward, 295.

33. Philip M. Sarrel, Lila E. Nachtigall, Martin Irvine (moderator), "Individualizing Hormone Therapy for Surgically Menopausal Women," Transcript of Archived Web Conference, October 20, 2004, accessed at www.medscape.com/viewprogram/3504 on June 1, 2005; Hysterectomy Association, "Learn about HRT," accessed at www.hysterectomy-association.org.uk/learn/hrt/; National Institute of Health National Institute of Child Health and Human Development, "Fast Facts about Premature Ovarian Failure: Are There Treatments for the Symptoms of POF?" accessed at www.nichd.nih.gov/publications/pubs/pof/sub2.htm on June 1, 2005.

34. Christine Finley, Edward W. Gregg, Laura J. Solomon, and Elaine Gay, "Disparities in Hormone Replacement Therapy Use by Socioeconomic Status in a Primary Care Population," *Journal of Community Health* 26, no. 1 (February 2001): 39–50.

35. National Institutes of Health, "Fast Facts."

36. Jean Elson, *"Am I Still a Woman?" Hysterectomy and Gender Identity* (Philadelphia: Temple University Press, 2004).

CHAPTER 5

Hot Flashes, Night Sweats, and Sleep Disturbances

The hallmarks of menopause in popular thinking are hot flashes, night sweats, and sleep disturbances, even though many women do not experience them.

THE HEAT SPECTRUM

Variously called hot flashes, hot flushes, night sweats, and vasomotor symptoms, sensations of heat during the menopause transition can occur occasionally or frequently and range from mild to intense. For a small number of women, flashing can become a regular occurrence, day and night. For some, these episodes are associated with heart palpitations or a sense of panic or dread.

If you have been experiencing hot flashes for a while now or you're suddenly finding yourself shedding layers of clothing during an episode, you are not alone. Studies have shown a wide variation in the incidence of hot flashes, from a low of about 35 percent to a high of 80 percent.[1] Women who have hot flashes experience them on average for slightly less than four years, but they can persist even longer; a small number of women may still have hot flashes in their seventies and eighties.[2]

Some women are relieved to feel some heat after years of enduring cold hands and feet.

I have experienced a few hot flashes and night sweats, but nothing too concerning. I've been cold all my life, so I welcome a little warmth.

Others view the surges as powerfully sensual experiences. Still other women find the unpredictability and intensity upsetting.

I was experiencing hot flashes to the extent that they were interfering with my business. While doing real-estate presentations for my clients, for example, I'd break out in a drenching sweat and my glasses would fog over. I felt embarrassed.

WHAT IS A HOT FLASH?

A *hot flash* is a sudden sensation of heat, usually in the upper body, that may rise up from the abdomen—or in some cases emanate from the toes—into the chest, back, and head, and may be accompanied by perspiration. Other sensations may include heart palpitations and anxiety. A hot flash may last from about one to five minutes.[3] Once the flash is over, some women may also feel chilled. Women with physical disabilities such as spinal cord injuries may experience hot flashes in different parts of the body or only on one side.[4]

The reasons women have hot flashes have not been fully explained. In the past, doctors postulated that the onset of hot flashes had everything to do with the decrease in estrogen as a woman approached menopause. However, not all women get hot flashes. What's more, researchers have found that the levels of estrogen do not differ substantially between women who have hot flashes and those who don't.[5]

Other factors that may be involved in hot flashes include the body's core temperature regulation and brain chemicals. The body's thermostat has an upper set point, at which the body's blood vessels open up and perspiration occurs, in an effort to release heat. There is also a lower threshold, at which shivering begins to generate heat. Between these two extremes is a temperature zone at which the body normally functions. Doctors now theorize that the zone between the high and low set points in peri- and postmenopausal women who experience hot flashes is narrower than in women who don't experience any hot flashes. A slight increase in core body temperature, therefore, could be causing a sensitized woman to experience a hot flash as her body tries to reduce its temperature.[6] Another factor that could be affecting the body's core temperature regulation is the brain neurotransmitter norepinephrine. Levels seem to be higher in some peri- and postmenopausal women who experience hot flashes.[7]

WHAT IS A HOT FLUSH?

While the terms *hot flash* and *hot flush* are often used interchangeably, some experts define hot flushes as the heat that dilates blood vessels, causing some women to turn red in the chest and face. Not all hot flashes are accompanied by flushing.

WHAT IS A NIGHT SWEAT?

A night sweat is a hot flash experienced at night that usually causes perspiration in the back of the head and chest and dampens sleepwear, pillows, and sheets. A woman may wake up and have to change her clothing and bedding. Some women may have difficulty falling back to sleep after a night sweat.

I've been tracking my night sweats for a few months and sure enough, I get them a lot right before my flow starts. Sometimes, I just roll over to another part of my king-size bed. If that's not good enough, I flip my duvet from top to bottom to snuggle under a dry patch. If it really gets bad, then I wear my new pajamas, which I made out of that soft cottony fabric that wicks away the sweat and dries quickly.

For night sweats, I found that sleeping in cotton pj bottoms but only a bra on top helped me because there was no wet top to wake me up, which I would then have to take off.

WHO EXPERIENCES HOT FLASHES?

Studies over the years have shown that women from various ethnocultural backgrounds are affected differently. In the U.S. Study of Women's Health Across the Nation (SWAN), a survey of 16,065 women aged forty to fifty-five, African-American women reported hot flashes most frequently (45.6 percent), whereas Japanese-American women reported the lowest incidence (17.5 percent). After African-Americans, the next highest groups were Latinas at 35.4 percent, white women at 31.2 percent, and Chinese-Americans at 20.5 percent.[8] In a separate study of 841 white women with physical disabilities in peri- and postmenopause across the United States, 64.9 percent reported having hot flashes.[9]

Women with medical conditions may have high rates of hot flashes. As many as 90 percent of women who have our ovaries removed experience hot flashes, according to one study; hot flashes occur more often and are of greater severity in younger women who have experienced a sudden onset of menopause due to surgery, medical conditions, or treatments than in women who have experienced natural menopause.[10] Thyroid disease, epilepsy, leukemia, and autoimmune disorders, among others, can also bring on hot flashes; women with breast cancer who have undergone chemotherapy or use medications such as raloxifene or tamoxifen may have a higher number of hot flashes.[11]

Women who smoke and women who are obese also report higher than usual rates of hot flashes.[12]

WHAT CAN I DO ABOUT HOT FLASHES?

There are several effective, natural ways to cope with hot flashes. Wearing layers of clothing that can easily be removed when the heat becomes intense is an option. Many women opt to wear lighter fabrics like cotton—even in winter—because cotton absorbs perspiration.

What I do to cope with public experiences of hot flashes is to use a beautiful fan I bought in Oaxaca, Mexico. No matter where, at the theater, in movies, lectures, or restaurants, I just pull it out as required and treat myself to an instant breeze. I think of my fan as both a practical and a fashion statement.

I find that putting my palms on a table surface and my bare feet on a cool floor helps to release the heat. I move them to a cool spot every minute or so until the hot flash eases.

While some women find such coping strategies effective, others may want to adopt a more preventive approach. Several options exist, including lifestyle changes, paced respiration, complementary health practices, and prescription medications, including hormone treatment.

LIFESTYLE CHANGES

The Smoking Link
The Study of Women's Health Across the Nation (SWAN) found that women smokers tend to have more hot flashes than nonsmokers. The more women smoked, the more intense the flashes.[13] *Options:* Cutting down or quitting smoking can go a long way toward calming flash severity and frequency. Ask your health

care professional for guidance. (To learn more about quitting smoking, see page 279.)

Diet

Some women find that limiting or totally avoiding spicy foods, hot drinks, soups, alcohol, sugary snacks, chocolate, and caffeine (in coffee, tea, cola, and headache preparations) may help. However, no research has shown that these foods aggravate hot flashes.[14] *Options:* Experiment with eliminating such foods from your diet. (To learn more about how diet may influence hot flashes and other signs of menopause, see Chapter 12, "Eating Well.")

The Weight Connection

Women who are under or over a healthy weight may experience more frequent and intense hot flashes. The SWAN study showed that perimenopausal women with a body mass index (BMI) of more than 30 experienced more hot flashes than women with a lower BMI.[15] (BMI is a measure of weight in relation to height. For more information, see page 249). *Options:* Achieving a healthier weight through improved nutrition and regular exercise has many health benefits, including the potential to ease hot flashes.

The Exercise Effect

Although there is mixed data on the subject of exercise and hot flashes, the SWAN study showed that daily exercise is associated with an overall decreased incidence of hot flashes.[16] *Options:* If you've been meaning to start exercising, you may want to choose an activity that you will enjoy on a regular basis—gardening, biking, walking, or swimming—and find a friend or family member to help you stick to it. (See Chapter 13, "Staying Active.")

The Stress Factor

If you're overwhelmed by life's ups and downs—whether you are trying to provide for your family or coping with a recent divorce or a diagnosis of a serious illness—you may find it difficult to handle menopausal changes such as hot flashes. A study published in 2005 of 535 African-American and white women followed for six years found that women with the highest anxiety levels reported nearly five times more hot flashes than women with lower levels of anxiety.[17] The study showed that anxiety and hot flashes were correlated and that the anxiety preceded the hot flashes, but it did not prove a cause-effect relationship; it is possible that other social or physical factors caused both. Feeling discomfort with uncertainty and finding oneself in uncomfortable social situations may make flashes more distressing.

Options: Practicing relaxation techniques such as paced respiration, yoga, tai chi, and meditation may help. Counseling with a health care provider such as a psychologist or social worker may be beneficial. You may also want to look into cognitive therapy, a treatment method that helps to change a person's inaccurate beliefs and thoughts. It includes learning positive self-talk and problem-solving skills to handle troublesome social situations. (For more information, see Chapter 11, "Emotional Well-Being and Managing Stress.")

PACED RESPIRATION

Several studies have shown that the simple act of breathing from the diaphragm in a regulated way may reduce the incidence of hot flashes by up to 60 percent.[18] (See "Cool Off!" page 78.)

COMPLEMENTARY HEALTH PRACTICES

Since the 2002 release of the Women's Health Initiative Study, which linked hormone treatment with increased risks for breast cancer, cardiovascular disease, and other health problems

COOL OFF!

In two clinical trials, paced respiration has been shown to be effective in controlling the frequency and intensity of hot flashes, with decreases averaging between 50 and 60 percent.[19] Here's how to do it:

Practice: Before trying to use paced respiration to help moderate your hot flashes and night sweats, you may want to practice first. Find a quiet, private place where you won't be interrupted by anyone or anything, including the phone.

Find your diaphragm: Place your hands on your diaphragm, which is located just below your rib cage. Breathe slowly in and out. Try to keep your rib cage still. Feel the slow rise and fall of your diaphragm. (If you're having trouble locating your diaphragm, lie down on your back and place your hands on your belly under your rib cage.)

Count: In a seated or lying position, inhale slowly through your nose, counting to five, then exhale slowly through your mouth, counting back down to one. Repeat for 15 minutes.

Keep it up: Practice twice a day, sitting or standing, for 15 minutes, for about a week. You can do this while you're having a hot flash or night sweat, but it is not necessary.

Use it: Once you have mastered the technique, you can use it whenever you feel heat rising—on the subway, standing in line at the grocery store, at work, or in bed. Place your hand on your diaphragm, start the paced breathing, and continue until you feel the hot flash has faded.

(see Chapter 7, "Hormone Treatment"), women with hot flashes have increasingly turned to nonmedical methods for relief. Complementary health practices range from remedies such as black cohosh and red clover to hypnosis and acupuncture. Although some of these alternatives may be beneficial, many have not been scientifically studied. Several that have been tested have been shown to be no more effective in reducing hot flashes than taking a placebo (or inactive pill). On average, women taking a placebo in a research study experience a 20 to 30 percent reduction in hot flashes. One woman in four taking a placebo reports a 50 percent reduction.[20] Complementary health products and practices that have been found to be no better or worse than a placebo include dong quai (a Chinese herb), ginseng, evening primrose oil, magnets, and reflexology.[21] Many complementary health practices are not regulated. Botanical and herbal remedies are sold as dietary supplements and, as a result, are not standardized or monitored for quality, safety, or effectiveness in North America. New regulations are being developed in the U.S. and Canada.

Black Cohosh

A relative of the buttercup family, black cohosh is a native North American plant. Native peoples and modern-day alternative health practitioners have used the roots and underground stems in various preparations such as pills and liquids to treat a variety of conditions, from infertility and labor pains to menopause-related problems.[22]

In Europe, especially Germany, many women over the years have used black cohosh during the menopause transition. In North America, women have only recently been using the plant for menopause-related problems. It has not been extensively studied. In three randomized, double-blind, placebo-controlled clinical trials in the United States that compared estrogen with black cohosh, very little effect was seen on hot flashes with use of black cohosh, although in one trial there was some reduction in perspiration.[23] A more recent study found that women taking a combination of St. John's wort and black cohosh reported fewer hot flashes and less depression. But few studies exist that confirm black cohosh's consistent ability to reduce hot flashes or its safety over the long term. (Most studies have lasted no more than six months.) Results may be inconclusive because the preparations (pill or liquid form), dosages, and study durations have not been consistent. Several clinical trials across the United States and Canada are currently investigating black cohosh for menopause-related problems.

Some women have found some relief from hot flashes using black cohosh.

I took black cohosh for about six months and it worked beautifully. After six months, it stopped working.

Options: Consider making an appointment with a naturopath or other licensed health practitioner specializing in herbal preparations to discuss whether black cohosh is right for you. Let your health care provider know about any alternative remedies you are taking. Negative effects may include stomach upset, headaches, and dizziness.[24] Although black cohosh does not seem to contain estrogenlike substances[25] (studies have been contradictory), women with breast cancer may want to check for the latest studies and speak to a health care provider before using this product.

Phytoestrogens: Red Clover and Soy

At the age of fifty-two, and a year into menopause, I had such severe hot flashes that I took a facecloth to work so I could go into the women's room, take off my top, and have a mini sponge bath. I put facial tissue between my breasts to keep the perspiration from running down. At night I dreamed of dampness, of being in a wet sleeping bag and of lying in the bottom of a leaky canoe.

I was so miserable that I made an appointment with my physician to ask for hormone replacement therapy. Wise woman that she is, she suggested I go on a phytoestrogen-heavy diet. This sounded more like a folk remedy than anything scientific, but as I had nothing to lose, I proceeded to stock up on black cohosh supplements, soy products, and flaxseed.

I cannot believe how well it worked. I went from having a severe hot flash about every two hours to having a barely noticeable one occasionally. I always knew diet was important, but I never thought I'd see simply diet make a change like this.

Phytoestrogens are plant-based compounds that have weak estrogen effects in the body. They can be found in a variety of foods, from soy beans and other legumes to flaxseed and red clover. To treat hot flashes and other menopause-related problems, many women include soy products in our regular diet or take red clover. However, an analysis of twenty-five randomized, placebo-controlled trials of soy foods, beverages, or powders, and red clover ex-

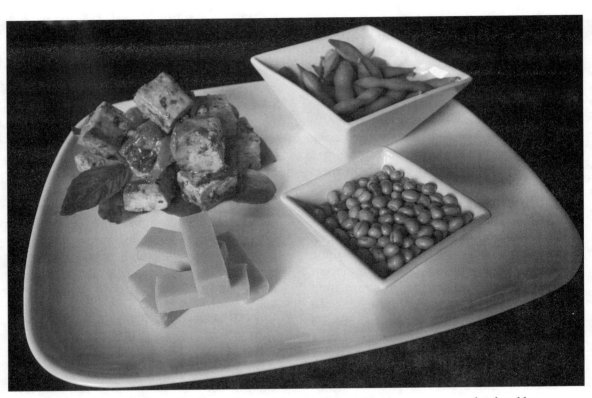

Many of us include soy products in our diets to reduce hot flashes and other menopause-related problems, though studies have not proved their effectiveness.

tracts found no significant differences in hot flash frequency between groups who took them and groups who took a placebo.[26]

Other Supplements

Dong quai, evening primrose oil, ginseng, licorice root, and many other herbal and homeopathic remedies have rarely been properly or extensively studied to determine their effectiveness in treating hot flashes. The few studies that have been published on these supplements have shown very little benefit over placebo.[27]

Acupuncture

Acupuncture is an ancient Eastern healing technique that aims to balance energy meridi-

ans in the body to promote healing. Sterile, fine needless are painlessly inserted at key points corresponding to body organs to relieve pain and treat disease. Related techniques include electroacupuncture (using low voltage electric current) and acupressure (using a form of massage). Few studies exist on acupuncture for hot flash treatment. One randomized study of twenty-four postmenopausal women using electroacupuncture found no statistical difference in hot flash relief between those getting the treatment and a control group.[28] However, more studies on acupuncture and hot flash relief in women with breast cancer are under way at Detroit's Henry Ford Health System and at the Memorial Sloan-Kettering Cancer Center in New York.

Hypnosis

According to the American Psychological Association Division of Psychological Hypnosis, hypnosis "is a procedure during which a health professional or researcher suggests while treating someone that she experience changes in sensations, perceptions, thoughts, or behavior. Although some hypnosis is used to make people more alert, most hypnosis includes suggestions for relaxation, calmness, and well-being." [29] Although no randomized, placebo-controlled trials have been conducted on hypnosis for hot flashes, some small-scale studies and anecdotal reports hold out promise to women experiencing mild to severe hot flashes, especially women with breast cancer.

PRESCRIPTION MEDICATIONS

Several prescription medications can be used to help women control hot flashes. Their safety and effectiveness vary. Hormone treatments can reduce the frequency and severity of hot flashes. Nonhormonal medications such as antidepressants, antileptics, and blood pressure medications are also helpful for some women, although they are not as effective.

Hormone Treatment

For almost six decades, doctors have been prescribing estrogen therapy or estrogen plus progestogen therapy ("combined" hormone treatment) to treat hot flashes. The Cochrane Database of Systematic Reviews analyzed twenty-one randomized, double-blind, placebo-controlled studies of both forms of hormone treatment, representing a total of 2,511 women, and found that both estrogen alone and estrogen plus progestogen are effective in reducing the frequency (77 percent) and severity (87 percent) of hot flashes.[30] Since the Women's Health Initiative Study in 2002 showed that both forms of hormone treatment increased the risk of cardiovas-cular disease and that estrogen plus progestogen increased the risk of breast cancer, among other problems, women have become more cautious about hormone treatment. Progestogens alone are also effective for hot flashes, although the results of the WHI suggest they have adverse effects.

Both the American and Canadian associations of obstetricians and gynecologists recommend that their members carefully weigh the benefits and risks of hormone treatment for each individual woman before prescribing hormones. The associations also recommend the lowest dose for the shortest possible time. (For more information, see Chapter 7, "Hormone Treatment.")

Antidepressants

Recent evidence points to brain chemicals as a possible factor in hot flash frequency and severity (see "What Is a Hot Flash?" page 75), and several antidepressants have proven to be effective in treating hot flashes. Venlafaxine (Effexor), a combined serotonin and norepinephrine reuptake inhibitor (SNRI), was studied in a randomized, double-blind, placebo-controlled trial of 229 women. Those taking venlafaxine experienced a reduction of hot flashes of 37 to 60 percent, depending on dosage.[31] Other antidepressants such as paroxetine (Paxil) and fluoxetine (Prozac) have had similar, though less effective, results.[32] Women who are taking tamoxifen should inquire about possible drug interactions before taking Paxil. Antidepressants have downsides and should be used with caution. As with other medications, they should be used only for as long as they are needed and useful. (For more information, see "Antidepressant Medications," page 228.)

Gabapentin

On the market since the mid-1990s, gabapentin (sold under the brand name Neurontin) has been prescribed primarily to control seizures in people with epilepsy and to ease chronic pain. This drug has also been tested for treating hot flashes, although its ability to do so is not well understood. Eight weeks of gabapentin therapy in 420 women with breast cancer in a double-blind, placebo-controlled trial produced up to a 49 percent reduction in hot flash frequency and severity in those who took a 900 mg dose.[33] Several clinical trials in the United States and Canada are studying this drug in the treatment of hot flashes. Unwanted effects may include sleepiness, dizziness, clumsiness, edema (swelling caused by accumulation of fluids), urinary frequency, and incontinence.[34]

Blood Pressure Medications

Hypertension, also known as high blood pressure, is a condition in which the pressure against arterial walls is high, increasing the risk of heart attack and stroke. Blood pressure medications work by decreasing the body's release of adrenaline and other hormones that increase blood pressure, heart rate, and anxiety or by stimulating the brain to send nerve signals to the blood vessels, making them relax and widen. Two blood pressure drugs have been studied for the treatment of hot flashes: clonidine (sold under the brand name Catapres) and methyldopa (sold under the brand name Aldomet). In randomized, double-blind, placebo-controlled trials, both medications helped to reduce the frequency of hot flashes by 46 to 80 percent in healthy women and those with breast cancer.[35] Negative effects for clonidine and methyldopa include dizziness, unusual tiredness, and weakness. Check with your provider if you experience cold hands and feet; swelling of the ankles, feet, and lower legs; heart palpitations; or chest pain.[36]

Other Considerations

Prescription medications may cause adverse effects while they are being taken and during withdrawal. Also, studies of medications for hot flashes show a strong placebo effect, with as many as 30 percent of women who take "dummy" pills reporting hot flash relief. Hot flashes, hot flushes, and night sweats usually abate over time in almost all postmenopausal women without treatment.

INSOMNIA AND OTHER SLEEP DISTURBANCES

As we progress through the menopause transition, many of us experience sleep problems for the first time, or have trouble getting a good night's sleep more often than we used to.[37] A variety of factors, from having to get up in the night to go to the bathroom (see "Bladder Health," page 213) to night sweats, may cause a woman to experience lighter sleep, early morning waking, or insomnia. In one study of women in midlife, 38 percent reported difficulty sleeping due to night sweats and other reasons. Late perimenopausal women had the highest rate at 45 percent.[38] Other studies, however, have questioned whether there is a direct link between night sweats and sleep disturbances.[39] Extensive serious research in this area is relatively new.

Menopause is not the only cause of sleep disturbances at this time in a woman's life. Sleep disturbances can result from medical conditions such as heart disease, high blood pressure, or hyperthyroidism; physical reactions to medications such as antidepressants and cholesterol-lowering statins, to alcohol, or to stimulants such as nicotine or caffeine; a changing sleep schedule or poor sleep habits; psychological factors such as stress, anxiety, or depression; or sleep disorders such as sleep apnea or restless leg syndrome.

WHAT IS INSOMNIA?

Most of us need between seven and nine hours of sleep a night to function at our best, although some people feel alert and rested after fewer hours. Insomnia is the inability to obtain adequate sleep. People experience insomnia in a variety of ways, including having difficulty falling or staying asleep, waking too early in the morning, and waking up feeling unrefreshed. Almost everyone experiences occasional bouts of insomnia. If your sleep is disrupted for three or more nights a week for more than one month at a time, you have what is considered chronic insomnia. Chronic insomnia often causes problems during the day, such as sleepiness, fatigue, difficulty concentrating, and irritability. It can contribute to poor performance on the job and to car accidents, and profoundly affects our sense of well-being and general health.

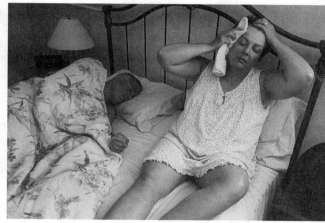

© Donna Alberico

IMPROVING YOUR SLEEP

Certain lifestyle factors are known to interfere with sleep. These factors include:

- *Medications* such as antidepressants and blood pressure, heart, and thyroid drugs. Research any drugs you take—including over-the-counter medications and supplements—to see if potential adverse effects include sleep difficulties, and discuss alternatives with your health care provider.
- *Alcohol.* Women metabolize alcohol less efficiently than men, and this difference becomes more pronounced as we grow older. Although alcohol initially is sedating, as it is broken down by the body it becomes a stimulant and can be responsible for us waking in the middle of the night.
- *Caffeine.* Caffeine is a stimulant that women metabolize less effectively as we age; even coffee, chocolate, soda, or tea at lunchtime can affect sleep at night. Caffeine is also present in some over-the-counter medications including the popular pain relievers Excedrin and Anacin.
- *Smoking.* Nicotine is also a stimulant.

Other lifestyle changes may help improve sleep, including:

- *Physical activity.* Moderate exercise, particularly when it is done early in the day, may help you sleep better at night. Avoid exercising within three hours of going to bed, as this can have the opposite effect.
- *Relaxation,* massage, meditation, or other stress reduction techniques.
- *Sunshine.* Exposure to light during waking hours helps to set your body clock.
- *Sleep hygiene techniques* (see "Squeaky Clean Sleep," page 84).

DIAGNOSABLE SLEEP DISORDERS

Sleep disruption can be caused by a wide variety of factors. If you have made lifestyle changes, incorporated sleep hygiene techniques, and still have difficulties sleeping, you may want to consider consulting a sleep specialist and undergoing a sleep study, an overnight recording of sleep patterns and behaviors associated with sleep. Two sleep disorders that can be diagnosed through a sleep study are sleep apnea and restless leg syndrome.

SQUEAKY CLEAN SLEEP

Some women find that following a prescribed pattern of habits before going to bed—known as *sleep hygiene*—helps us fall and stay asleep. The habits are:

- Going to bed and waking up at about the same time every day, including weekends.
- Creating quiet time—at least an hour before you get into bed—for activities such as reading a nonstimulating book or listening to soft music. Turning off the TV, cell phones, computers, and other electronic equipment may also help.
- Reserving your bedroom for sleep and sex only. It may be helpful to keep television sets, telephones, pets, or anything else that may disturb your sleep in other areas of your home.
- Wearing socks to bed if cold feet tend to wake you.
- Keeping the temperature in your bedroom cool.
- Using light sheets and blankets for bedding.
- Dressing in light cotton or other material that wicks away perspiration.
- Placing a chilled gel pack under your pillow. When a night sweat occurs, you can simply turn your pillow over for a quick, cool hit. Even without a gel pack, sometimes just turning the pillow over is enough, or having a second pillow for switching off during the night helps.
- Installing thick shades on bedroom windows to block out all light.
- Using an eye mask and earplugs.
- Practicing meditation, paced respiration, cognitive therapy self-talk, or self-hypnosis techniques to calm worries and concerns that may cause sleeplessness.
- Turning the alarm clock toward the wall so you will refrain from looking at it, which may make you fret.
- Taking a hot shower or bath right before bedtime. This increases your body temperature. When you dry off, your body temperature begins to drop and thus starts the internal physiological process that is the beginning of sleep. However, getting under a down comforter when you are hot could trigger hot flashes.

Both tend to occur more frequently at about the same age as most women experience the menopause transition.

Sleep Apnea

Snoring, interrupted breathing during sleep, and daytime fatigue are distinct markers of the sleep-breathing disorder known as sleep apnea.

Until about a decade ago, doctors thought that sleep apnea affected only overweight men. But new research has shown that at age fifty, women represent the same number of new sleep apnea cases as men,[40] and a study of midlife women found that the menopausal transition was significantly associated with an increased risk of sleep-disordered breathing.[41] Two causes may be at work. First, the levels of sex hormones that are thought to protect women against sleep apnea decrease; second, during the menopause transition many women gain weight, which increases risk for sleep apnea.

Treatments may include avoiding alcohol, losing weight, or being fitted with a dental appliance resembling a mouth guard, which is worn during sleep to bring the jaw up and forward, opening the breathing passage. If these solutions don't produce results, a continuous positive airway pressure (CPAP) machine may be recommended. The sleeper wears a mask that covers the nose, and sometimes the mouth, forcing oxygen down the breathing passage.[42]

Restless Legs Syndrome

Restless legs syndrome (RLS) is a neurological disorder characterized by uncomfortable sensations in the legs, accompanied by an irresistible urge to move about in an effort to relieve these feelings. Symptoms include crawly, tingling skin, excessive twitching, and involuntary leg twitching or jerking movements during sleep. These abnormal muscle spasms, which can occur as often as every twenty to sixty seconds, can interfere with normal sleep. The incidence of RLS increases with age, and it affects more women than men.

RLS is associated with chronic illnesses such as kidney failure, diabetes, Parkinson's disease, peripheral neuropathy, and gastroesophageal reflux disease (GERD). Caffeine, alcohol, tobacco, and other stimulants may aggravate or trigger symptoms, as can some drugs used to treat high blood pressure, heart conditions, nausea, colds, allergies, and depression.

Treatments include reducing or eliminating any stimulants in your diet. Because RLS may be caused or exacerbated by iron or vitamin deficiencies, iron, folate, and magnesium supplements may help.

Other treatments include a class of drugs known as dopamine agonists (used primarily to treat the uncontrollable movements of Parkinson's). These drugs, which include ropinirole (sold under the brand name Requip), perogolide (Permax), and pramipexole (Mirapex), have been shown to be effective. Negative effects include headache, nausea, and sudden drop in blood pressure. A 2005 study showed that one in five people taking the above-named brands may experience attacks of sudden sleepiness while performing such functions as driving a car. (No other dopamine agonists were implicated.)[43]

SLEEP REMEDIES AND MEDICATIONS

Complementary Treatments

Your grandmother may have suggested that you sip a warm glass of milk or a cup of chamomile or valerian tea to help you sleep. While some women find these helpful, no studies consistently confirm their effectiveness.[44] Melatonin has only limited or no benefit in the treatment of sleep disorders, although it can be helpful for jet lag.[45]

Medications

There are many medications, both prescription and over the counter, that can be taken to improve sleep. Because many sleep medications are addictive or can have other serious adverse effects, it is wise to make lifestyle changes and try self-care treatments such as sleep hygiene techniques before considering medications. Sleep medications generally should not be taken for more than a few weeks.

Over-the-Counter Sleep Aids

Over-the-counter sleep aids are readily available to help alleviate sleep problems in the short term. Many contain antihistamines with sedative effects. Antihistamines are central nervous system suppressants and may have a carryover effect the next morning, potentially causing short-term memory problems, confusion, and headaches. It is important that sleep aids be used according to directions and not taken with alcohol or other drugs with sedating effects such as tranquilizers.

Prescription Drugs

Prescription medications are also available to treat insomnia. While these medications can be helpful in the short term, the risks should be well understood before taking them.

The most common drugs prescribed for short-term treatment of insomnia are benzodiazepines such as temazepam (sold under the brand name Restoril), flurazepam (Dalmane), and triazolam (Halcion). Benzodiazepines (also sometimes called tranquilizers or sedatives) are considered either short-acting or long-acting, depending on how long they are active in your body. In general, short-acting benzodiazepines are used to treat insomnia, while longer-acting ones are used for anxiety and other problems. While these medications can improve sleep, they also carry significant risk, as even short-term use of tranquilizers can cause daytime sleepiness and harm memory and reasoning, balance, and coordination. More serious, longer-term use of tranquilizers can lead to tolerance and dependence, and discontinuing the medication can cause rebound insomnia, anxiety, and a host of other withdrawal effects. Because of the risks, these medications should be used only in the short term. If your insomnia is chronic and other treatments have been ineffective, consider taking these medications intermittently (perhaps every other or every third day) rather than every night.

Another class of drugs prescribed to improve sleep is tricyclic antidepressants such as amitriptyline (brand name Elavil) and doxipin (Sinequan). These drugs are sedating and sometimes are used in low doses to improve sleep, particularly for people with chronic pain conditions. The antidepressant desyrel (Trazodone) may also be helpful. These drugs can cause daytime drowsiness and sedation. In rare cases they can also cause low blood pressure, rapid heart rate, fainting, constipation, urinary retention, and blurred vision.

More recent, new nonbenzodiazepines have come on the market. They include zolpidem (sold under the brand name Ambien), zaleplon (Sonata), and eszopiclone (Lunesta). These drugs have been heavily marketed to consumers, with the claim that they are less likely than benzodiazepines to cause next-day drowsiness. However, a 2005 meta-analysis of sleep medication usage in older people found no significant difference in the adverse effects of the older drugs compared to the newer ones.[46]

Another class of sleep medication, Selective Extrasynaptic GABA$_A$ Agonists, with the generic name gaboxadol, is undergoing clinical trials. Preliminary findings show that gaboxadol does not seem to disrupt the dream stage known as REM, which other sleeping pills do, nor did it cause next-day sedative effects, although other negative effects included abdominal pain, dizziness, and headache.[47]

While sleep medications can at times provide relief, it is important to be aware that some new and highly promoted drugs are no better than older drugs for which we have a longer safety track record. In an era where pharmaceutical companies market new drugs in the absence of adequate safety data and the FDA frequently fails to carry out its mandate of protecting consumers, it is wise to be cautious about new drugs. If you are considering taking sleep medication, become well-informed about the drug's risks and benefits and work with your provider to determine the lowest effective dose.

NOTES

1. National Institutes of Health State-of-the-Science Panel, "National Institutes of Health State-of-the-Science Conference Statement: Management of Menopause-Related Symptoms," *Annals of Internal Medicine* 142, no. 12 (June 21, 2005): 1003–13.

2. Nancy E. Avis, Sybil L. Crawford, and S. M. McKinlay, "Psychosocial, Behavioral, and Health Factors Related to Menopause Symptomatology," *Women's Health* 3, no. 2 (Summer 1997): 103–20; see also Denise Goldani von Muhlen, Donna Kritz-Silverstein, and Elizabeth Barrett-Connor, "A Community-Based Study of Menopause Symptoms and Estrogen Replacement in Older Women," *Maturitas* 22, no. 2 (September 1995): 71–78.

3. Fredi Kronenberg, "Hot Flashes: Epidemiology and Physiology," *Annals of the New York Academy of Sciences* 592 (June 13, 1990): 52–86.

4. Claire Z. Kalpakjian, Elisabeth H. Quint, Denise G. Tate, Sunny Roller, and Loren L. Toussaint, "The Experience of Menopause in Women with Physical Disabilities," Final Report, Department of Physical Medicine, University of Michigan, Ann Arbor, May 2004.

5. Alexandra Block, "Self-Awareness during the Menopause," *Maturitas* 41, no. 1 (January 30, 2002): 61–68; see also J. D. Hutton, H. S. Jacobs, M. A. F. Murray, and V. H. T. James, "Relations between Plasma Oestrone and Oestradiol and Climacteric Symptoms," *Lancet* 311, no. 8066 (April 1, 1978): 678–81.

6. Robert Freedman and Willane Krell, "Reduced Thermoregulatory Null Zone in Postmenopausal Women with Hot Flashes," *American Journal of Obstetrics and Gynecology* 181, no. 1 (July 1999): 66–70.

7. K. Bruck and E. Zeisberger, "Adaptive Changes in Thermoregulation and Their Neuropharmacological Basis," in E. Schonbaum and P. Lomax, eds., *Thermoregulation: Physiology and Biochemistry* (New York: Pergamon, 1990), 255–307.

8. Ellen B. Gold, Barbara Sternfeld, Jennifer L. Kelsey, Charlotte Brown, Charles Mouton, Nancy Reame, Loran Salamone, and Rebecca Stellato, "Relation of Demographic and Lifestyle Factors to Symptoms in a Multi-Racial/Ethnic Population of Women 40–55 Years of Age," *American Journal of Epidemiology* 152, no. 5 (September 2000): 463–73.

9. Kalpakjian et al.

10. Sudip Chakravarti, William Patrick Collins, John Richard Newton, David Howard Oram, and John William Studd, "Endocrine Changes and Symptomatology after Oophorectomy in Premenopausal Women," *British Journal of Obstetrics and Gynaecology* 84, no. 10 (October 1977): 769–75; see also Donna Kritz-Silverstein, Denise Goldani Von Muhlen, Elizabeth Barrett-Connor, "Prevalence and Clustering of Menopausal Symptoms in Older Women by Hysterectomy and Oophorectomy Status," *Journal of Women's Health and Gender-Based Medicine* 9, no. 7 (September 2000): 747–55; see also National Institutes of Health State-of-the-Science Panel.

11. Nanette F. Santoro, Thomas B. Clarkson, Robert R. Freedman, Adriane J. Fugh-Berman, et al., "Treatment of Menopause-Associated Vasomotor Symptoms: Position Statement of the North American Menopause Society," *Menopause* 11, no. 1 (January 2004): 11–33.

12. Gold et al.

13. Gold et al.

14. Santoro et al.

15. Ibid.

16. Ibid.

17. Ellen W. Freeman, Mary D. Samuel, Hui Lin, Clarisa R. Gracia, Shiv Kapoor, and Tahmina Ferdousi, "The Role of Anxiety and Hormonal Changes in Menopausal Hot Flashes," *Menopause* 12, no. 3 (May/June 2005): 258–66.

18. Leonard M. Germaine and Robert R. Freedman, "Behavioral Treatment of Menopausal Hot Flushes: Evaluation by Objective Method," *Journal of Consulting Clinical Psychology* 52, no. 6 (December 1984): 1072–79; see also Robert R. Freedman and Suzanne Woodward, "Behavioral Treatment of Menopausal Hot Flushes: Evaluation by Ambulatory Monitoring," *American Journal of Obstetrics and Gynecology* 167,

no. 2 (August 1992): 436–39; see also J. H. Irwin, A. D. Domer, C. Clark, et al., "The Effects of Relaxation Response Training on Menopausal Symptoms," *Journal of Psychosomatic Obstetrics and Gynecology* 17, no. 4 (December 1996): 202–7.

19. Ibid.

20. J. A. Sloan, C. L. Loprinzi, P. J. Novotny, D. L. Barton, B. I. Lavasseur, and H. Windschitl, "Methodologic Lessons Learned from Hot Flash Studies," *Journal of Clinical Oncology* 19, no. 23 (2001): 4280–90.

21. H. J. Kang, R. Ansbacher, M. M. Hammoud, "Use of Alternative and Complementary Medicine in Menopause," *International Journal of Gynecology and Obstetrics* 79 (2002): 195–207; see also: F. Kronenberg and A. Fugh-Berman, "Complementary and Alternative Medicine for Menopausal Symptoms: A Review of Randomized, Controlled Trials," *Annals of Internal Medicine* 137, no. 10 (2002): 805–13; J. S. Carpenter and J. G. Neal, "Other Complementary and Alternative Medicine Modalities: Acupuncture, Magnets, Reflexology, and Homeopathy," *American Journal of Medicine* 19, no. 118 (2005): 109–17.

22. R. Upton, ed., *American Herbal Pharmacopoeia and Therapeutic Compendium* (Santa Cruz, CA: American Herbal Pharmacopoeia, 2002), 1–38.

23. Wolfgang Wuttke, Dana Seidlova-Wuttke, and G. Gorkow, "The Cimicifuga Preparation BNO 1055 vs. Conjugated Estrogens in a Double-Blind Placebo-Controlled Study: Effects on Menopause Symptoms and Bone Markers," *Maturitas* 44, Supplement 1 (March 14, 2003): S67–77; see also J. S. Jacobson, A. B. Troxel, J. Evans, et al., "Randomized Trial of Black Cohosh for the Treatment of Hot Flashes among Women with a History of Breast Cancer," *Journal of Clinical Oncology* 19, no. 10 (May 2001): 2739–45; see also W. Stoll, "Phytotherapy Influences Atrophic Vaginal Epithelium Cimicifuga vs. Estrogenic Substances," *Therapeutikon* 1 (1987): 23–31.

24. Alyson Huntley and Edzard Ernst, "A Systematic Review of the Safety of Black Cohosh," *Menopause* 10, no. 1 (January 2003): 58–64.

25. Paula Amato, Sylvie Christophe, and Paula L. Mellon, "Estrogenic Activity of Herbs Commonly Used as Remedies for Menopausal Symptoms," *Menopause* 9, no. 2 (March 2002): 145–50.

26. Erin E. Krebs, Kristine E. Ensrud, Roderick MacDonald, and Timothy J. Wilt, "Phytoestrogens for Treatment of Menopausal Symptoms: A Systematic Review," *Obstetrics and Gynecology* 104 (October 2004): 824–36.

27. Santoro et al.

28. Y. Wyon, R. Lindgren, T. Lundeberg, and M. Hammar, "Effects of Acupuncture on Climacteric Vasomotor Symptoms, Quality of Life, and Urinary Excretion of Neuropeptides among Postmenopausal Women," *Menopause* 2 (1995): 3–12.

29. The American Psychological Association's Division of Psychological Hypnosis, "New Definition: Hypnosis, the Division 30 Definition and Description of Hypnosis," 2005, accessed at www.apa.org/divisions/div30/define_hypnosis.html on May 21, 2005.

30. Alastair H. MacLennan, J. L. Broadbent, S. Lester, and V. Moore, "Oral Oestrogen and Combined Oestrogen/Progestogen Therapy versus Placebo for Hot Flushes," *Cochrane Database Systematic Review,* Issue 4, Art. No. CD002978 (August 17, 2004).

31. Charles L. Loprinzi, John W. Kugler, Jeff A. Sloan, et al., "Venlafaxine in Management of Hot Flashes in Survivors of Breast Cancer: A Randomized Controlled Trial," *Lancet* 356, no. 9247 (December 16, 2000): 2059–63.

32. Santoro et al.

33. Kishan J. Pandya, Gary R. Morrow, Joseph A. Roscoe, Hongwei Zhao, et al., "Gabapentin for Hot Flashes in 420 Women with Breast Cancer: A Randomised Double-Blind Placebo-Controlled Trial," *Lancet* 366, no. 9488 (September 3, 2005): 818–24.

34. Food and Drug Administration, Medwatch, Neurontin, FDA-Approved Labeling Text, February 2005, accessed at www.fda.gov/medwatch/SAFETY/2005/Feb_PI?Neurontin_PI.pdf on October 2, 2005.

35. Santoro et al.

36. FDA Heart Health Online, "Alpha-adrenergic Antagonists," accessed at www.fda.gov/hearthealth/treatments/medications/alphaadrenergicantagonists.html on October 2, 2005.

37. Andrew D. Krystal, Jack Edinger, William Wohlgemuth, Gail R. Marsh, "Sleep in Perimenopausal and Postmenopausal Women," *Sleep Medicine Reviews* 2, no. 4 (November 1998): 243–53; see also von Muhlen et al.

38. Howard Kravitz, Patricia Ganz, Joyce Bromberger, et al., "Sleep Difficulty in Women at Midlife: A Community Survey of Sleep and the Menopausal Transition," *Menopause* 10, no. 1 (January 2003): 19–28.

39. Robert Freedman and Timothy A. Roehrs, "Lack of Sleep Disturbance from Menopausal Hot Flashes," *Fertility and Sterility* 82, no. 1 (July 2004): 138–44.

40. Peter V. Tishler, Emma K. Larkin, Mark D. Schluchter, and Susan Redline, "Incidence of Sleep-Disordered Breathing in an Urban Adult Population," *JAMA* 289, no. 17 (May 7, 2003): 2230–37.

41. Terry Young, Laurel Finn, Diane Austin, and Andrea Peterson, "Menopausal Status and Sleep-Disordered Breathing in the Wisconsin Sleep Cohort Study," *American Journal of Respiratory Critical Care Medicine* 167, no. 9 (May 1, 2003): 1184–85.

42. Meir Kryger, *Can't Sleep, Can't Stay Awake* (Toronto: HarperCollins, 2004), 166.

43. Jerry Avorn, Sebastian Schneeweiss, Lewis Sudarsky, Joshua Benner, et al., "Sudden Uncontrollable Somnolence and Medication Use in Parkinson Disease," *Archives of Neurology* 62, no. 8 (August 2005): 1242–48.

44. Office of Dietary Supplements, Valerian and Chamomile Fact Sheets, 2004, accessed at http://ods.od.nih.gov/factsheets on May 15, 2005.

45. AHRQ Issues New Report on the Safety and Effectiveness of Melatonin Supplements, Press Release, December 8, 2004, accessed at www.ahrq.gov/news/press/pr2004/melatnpr.htm on May 10, 2005.

46. Jennifer Glass et al., "Sedative Hypnotics in Older People with Insomnia: Meta-analysis of Risks and Benefits." *BMJ* 331 (2005): 1169.

47. Marike Lancel, Thomas C. Wetter, Axel Steiger, Stefan Mathias, "Effect of the GABA$_A$ Agonist Gabaxadol on Nocturnal Sleep and Hormone Secretion in Healthy Elderly Subjects," *American Journal of Physiology and Endocrinology Metabolism* 281, no. 1 (July 2001): E130–37.

CHAPTER 6

Vulvovaginal Changes

Throughout our reproductive-age years, many women experience yeast infections and other transient vaginal complaints. For a small percentage of us, the symptoms become chronic and quite severe, but for most, a short course of treatment solves the problem. With menopause, though, the characteristics of vulvovaginal complaints—which affect the vulva (external genitals) and/or vagina (internal pathway)—can differ slightly. Vaginal dryness becomes more common, sometimes interfering with sexual pleasure; itching and irritation may be external rather than internal, and not associated with discharge; or itching may occur primarily at night, resulting in nocturnal scratching. In some women, the vaginal opening slowly becomes less flexible, making penetration uncomfortable.

Like many conditions, vulvovaginal problems affect a large number of women and can become quite debilitating, but they can be effectively treated. Yet, unlike erectile dysfunction and urinary incontinence—subjects that were once discussed only in whispers, if at all, but that now have celebrity spokespersons and enjoy media popularity—vaginal dryness and vulvar itching are still considered taboo topics in polite company. The woman who has these conditions often believes that she is the only person who does and is embarrassed to mention even to her doctor that she has to scratch or that sex is becoming painful.

Vulvar itching can be intense, and many women awaken in the middle of the night scratching furiously. Some of us resort to cold baths and cold, wet washcloths applied to the vulva until the itch goes away. But itching comes back when we wear snug clothes or are warm, such as at night or after a hot bath. And with each scratching episode, changes occur in the skin, which make the condition worse. Many women may feel embarrassed, thinking that the problem is caused by poor hygiene or fearing that it is a sign of cancer (although it is neither). And so we may keep it to ourselves.

I would wake up scratching until I bled. Then I would go into the bathroom and soak in a tub of cold water for an hour. Sometimes I'd be up for hours before I could go back to sleep. None of my friends ever said they had anything like this.

I can talk to my sister about everything. Everything but this.

CAUSES OF ITCHING, BURNING, AND PAIN

Itching, burning, pain, and difficulty with penetration during sex may be caused by infection, thinning of the skin (atrophy), and certain skin conditions, such as lichen sclerosus or lichen simplex chronicus. The following information explains how these causes affect women and how they are evaluated and treated.

INFECTION

Infection is not as common after menopause as it is during the reproductive-age years. Nevertheless, infections of various types may cause itching of the vulva or vagina and, more important, even a mild infection may be the initial cause of the chronic skin condition known as lichen simplex chronicus (see page 96).

Infections of the vagina can be caused by *Candida albicans* (and other yeast species) and *Trichomonas vaginalis*. Another vaginal condition, bacterial vaginosis, is associated with *Gardnerella vaginalis*. These common organisms are frequently the cause of infections in reproductive-age women, as are gonorrhea, chlamydia, syphilis, and herpes. But while women can get infections after menopause, changes in the vaginal pH inhibit the growth of yeast and other bacteria, so infections are less likely to be the cause of vulvovaginal symptoms in older women.[1]

If you are experiencing symptoms, your health care provider can examine your vulva and vagina for infection. Looking at the discharge under a microscope and testing the pH is often enough to determine whether or not there is an infection.[2] Taking a culture for yeast can be helpful.

With menopause, the vaginal lining may become thinner and less protected, a condition called *atrophy*, because of lack of estrogen. Atrophy may affect the pH of the vagina and make you more sensitive to irritation by normal bacteria or yeast, or may encourage an imbalance in the populations of otherwise normal vaginal inhabitants, leading to bad odors or discharge.[3] Vaginal atrophy is discussed in more detail below.

If the cultures are negative, or if you have frequent bouts of itching or irritation, your health care provider should look for other conditions, such as atrophy, lichen sclerosus, or lichen simplex chronicus, that are more common in women after menopause. Self-treatment with over-the-counter remedies or foods such as yogurt, or repeated prescription treatments for presumed yeast infection, can delay the diagnosis of skin conditions, and unnecessary creams can irritate already sensitive skin.[4]

VAGINAL ATROPHY

Vaginal atrophy (thinning of the skin of the vulva and vagina due to fluctuating or low es-

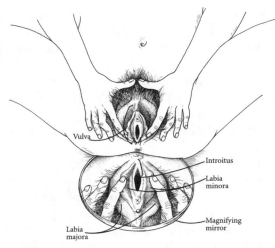

Vulva

Introitus

Labia minora

Magnifying mirror

Labia majora

trogen levels) is a frequent cause of itching and irritation in women during the menopause transition and beyond.

Women who are in the menopause transition may notice vaginal dryness, irritation, or pain with intercourse as the very first sign of the transition. Since many women think that hot flashes are the first sign of menopause, we may not even think "menopause" or "perimenopause" when we begin to experience vaginal dryness. And while some women with atrophy need treatment, the majority of women with low estrogen levels have some degree of atrophy but do not require treatment, especially if we are not having sex that includes vaginal penetration.

What does atrophy mean? The best way to illustrate atrophy is to start with the normal structure of the vulva and the vagina, and then look at what happens when estrogen levels drop.

THE VULVA

The vulva is the part of the female genitals that you can see from the outside. It includes the labia majora (outer lips), the labia minora (small, inner lips), and the introitus (vaginal opening) with its mucus-producing glands.

The Labia Majora
The outer, hair-covered genital lips are called the labia majora. They are mounds of fatty tissue covered by normal, hair-bearing skin. Before puberty the labia majora are hairless and nearly flat. When estrogen, progesterone, and androgens are produced at puberty, the labia majora develop fatty tissue and hair. When hormone levels are low for a prolonged length of time, the labia majora may become flatter, or lax, with less hair. This is a sign of atrophy, or thinning, of the genital tissue.

The Labia Minora
The labia minora are the hairless, thin, inner lips of the vulva. After puberty, estrogen makes them pink and moist. When estrogen levels fall to persistently low levels after menopause, the labia minora become pale and they may actually shrink. Some women develop painful cracks, or fissures, in the delicate skin between the labia majora and the labia minora, or at the very bottom of the vaginal opening.

The Vaginal Opening (Introitus)
The opening to the vagina is called the introitus. Before puberty it may be nearly closed. During the reproductive-age years, and especially after vaginal intercourse, the opening to the vagina is usually wide and stretchy. The stretchiness is due to elastic fibers under the skin that allow it to stretch in all directions. In addition, estrogen causes the mucus-producing glands located at the vaginal opening to secrete mucus on a regular basis, with larger amounts produced during sexual arousal.

Atrophy of the Vulva
When estrogen levels remain low, less moisture comes through the vaginal wall to provide lu-

brication during intercourse. The elastic and collagen fibers that give the opening strength and stretchiness decrease in number, and the skin of the opening becomes thinner and less protective. Sometimes the opening shrinks and becomes quite narrow. The thinning of the skin can make penetration more uncomfortable than pleasurable for some women, and when the vaginal opening narrows, intercourse can be very painful. When a woman stops having vaginal intercourse due to pain, the changes may get worse even faster. In rare, extreme cases, thinning of the tissue may lead to tiny abrasions that cause the sides of the vaginal opening to stick together and the opening may become fused closed in places.

THE VAGINA

The vagina is a stretchy, tube-like structure that extends from the vaginal opening (introitus) to the cervix (the opening of the uterus). In adulthood the vagina is able to stretch in all directions thanks to elastic fibers and small wrinkles in the surface, called *rugae*. Thin, mucous secretions keep it moist.

What Happens in Vaginal Atrophy

When estrogen levels remain low, the rugae flatten and may disappear altogether. Secretions dry up. The vagina becomes shorter, narrower, dryer, and less stretchy. While many women have no symptoms at all, others experience vulvovaginal irritation or dryness. Still others are unable to tolerate vaginal penetration or intercourse. Atrophy is the most common cause of painful intercourse after menopause.

TREATMENT OF ATROPHY OF THE VULVA AND VAGINA

Nonhormonal

Dryness or mild discomfort may be alleviated with vaginal moisturizers or lubricants.

Moisturizers such as Replens or K-Y vaginal moisturizer keep the tissue from cracking; some products are deposited inside the vagina with an applicator, while others may be rubbed into the skin in much the same way hand or body lotion is used.[5] Women should use products specially designed for vaginal use, however, and avoid products that may contain perfumes or alcohol because these may be irritating.

Lubricants are slippery, and are more useful for enhancing sex. Lubricants include water-based products such as Astroglide, Lubrin, Moist Again, and K-Y lubricant, jelly, or Silk-E moisturizer. Some women use oils such as olive oil, but oil-based products may damage diaphragms and condoms and enable bacteria to cling to the vaginal wall, increasing the risk of infection.

Hormonal

For some women with problems related to vaginal atrophy, moisturizers and lubricants do not provide relief because the underlying problem has not been treated. Vulvar and vaginal atrophy respond well to the female hormone estrogen.[6] Estrogen is effective whether administered by pill or patch (both of which are *systemic*, which means that they affect the whole body) or vaginally by tablet, cream, or ring (methods that provide more localized effects in the genital tissues). (For more information on forms of hormone treatment and associated health risks, see Chapter 7, "Hormone Treatment.")

Local estrogen products include creams (Estrace, Premarin, Ogen), a tablet (Vagifem), or a ring (Estring). Very small amounts of estrogen are absorbed from these products. (For more information, see page 110.) Some women use estrogen products more often until the condition improves and then intermittently to maintain healthy vulvovaginal tissue.

I was surprised at how fast that little tiny tablet worked! I felt like I had sandpaper down there, and now it's all slippery again.

A normal effect of estrogen is to thicken the lining of the uterus. Progesterone is the female hormone that keeps the lining from becoming too thick, which can lead to the development of precancerous or cancerous conditions. Women who have not had a hysterectomy and are taking systemic (higher) doses of estrogen must also take progesterone or a progestin to keep the lining thin.[7] The local estrogen preparations can be prescribed in such low doses that the uterine lining may not thicken; however, many health care providers perform ultrasound evaluation of the uterine lining and may administer periodic doses of progesterone to protect the uterus.

LICHEN SCLEROSUS (*LIKEN SKLER-OH-SUS*)

Some women with chronic, intense vulvar itching have a skin condition affecting the vulva that can affect other areas of the body as well. Lichen sclerosus is not necessarily related to low estrogen levels, but is more frequently seen in postmenopausal women or in young girls who have not yet gone through puberty than in reproductive-age women. The condition affects between 1 in 300 and 1 in 1,000 people in the population. It may be hereditary and may increase the risk of cancer of the vulva.

While the cause of lichen sclerosus is still not known, it may be an autoimmune condition. Autoimmune skin conditions result when the body's natural defenses launch an attack against the skin, much as they would toward an infection or foreign substance. The result may be white, parchmentlike skin patches that itch or hurt. The resemblance between the white skin patches and lichen gives the condition its name.

VAGINAL HEALTH AFTER VAGINOPLASTY

Those of us who have had surgery to construct or reconstruct a vagina (called *vaginoplasty*) may wonder if we can expect the same vaginal changes related to menopause as women who have not had surgery. We may have had vaginoplasty as a child or as an adult, because of an intersex condition, sex reassignment surgery, cervical or vaginal cancer, or another reason.

Overall, we can expect to experience many of the same menopausal changes as other women, including shortening of the vagina, atrophy, and dryness. If our vagina is made of a graft of skin, it may not change as much, but if it is mucous membrane, it is more subject to thinning and dryness. Our experiences will vary, just as the experiences of women who haven't had surgery vary.

Ongoing vaginal health care is important and requires follow-up beyond initial postoperative care. (For more information, see "Vaginal Health after Vaginoplasty" at www.our bodiesourselves.org.)

At first, many women who have this condition believe they have a simple yeast infection and use an over-the-counter remedy or get a prescription for a yeast infection medication from a health care provider. This may provide temporary relief because of the cream's soothing effect, but the symptoms come back. Often the woman comes to think she has recurrent or chronic yeast infections and treats herself repeatedly. By the time it is correctly diagnosed, the condition has often been present for a long time and may actually have altered the appearance of the vulva.

APPEARANCE

Lichen sclerosus makes the vulvar skin appear white: not just pale, as in atrophy, but a dull white color. The skin may be very thin, with an appearance similar to parchment or cigarette paper. The condition sometimes occurs in separate patches, but can also be seen affecting the whole vulva, with the white area in a shape resembling a keyhole: wide at the top, around the clitoris, and narrow around the vagina and peri-anal area. If there has been chronic itching and scratching, the skin may appear thickened or scabbed, or it may become infected.

I looked down there and saw this white area and thought, "This ain't right." It was even bruised, and it itched like crazy. I'd dig at it through my clothes when no one was looking.

Without treatment the labia minora (inner lips) may shrink until they disappear, and the vaginal opening may become narrowed and nearly rigid. The clitoris can become buried under the fused clitoral hood. When the skin breaks or fissures form and the vagina becomes narrowed, women often experience pain and have difficulty with sex.

EVALUATION

Self-Examination

Checking yourself with a mirror periodically, when you don't have symptoms, can help you become familiar with what your vulva normally looks like. It will also enable you to detect changes and describe them to your health care provider.

Medical Examination

If you experience symptoms that either keep coming back or never entirely go away, it is very important to receive a thorough physical examination by a doctor or practitioner who is familiar with vulvar conditions and who can have a biopsy performed if abnormal-appearing areas are seen or if symptoms persist after treatment. A very small sample of tissue, about the size of a match head, which can be taken in the office with a little numbing medicine, can be examined under a microscope and can sometimes provide the diagnosis.

TREATMENT

Lichen sclerosus is initially treated with a potent steroid medicine. This is not the type of steroid that causes muscle size to increase. It is an ointment that is used in very small amounts nightly or twice a day until the skin improves, and then is gradually reduced in potency and in number of applications per week. Often, women have to continue to use a mild or moderate-potency steroid ointment long-term to maintain control of the disease.

I felt like I had worms crawling around under my skin. I had never felt anything like it before. Nothing helped until I used the steroid ointment, and then that wormy feeling went away in about a week.

LICHEN SIMPLEX CHRONICUS

This is a noncancerous, intensely itchy skin condition that can occur anywhere on the body and is caused by frequent scratching. The vulva is very prone to benign itching because of its warm, moist environment and the amount of friction it is exposed to daily. A brief infection or irritation may cause the skin to itch. When the skin is rubbed or scratched repeatedly, whether in response to itch or just absentmindedly, a reaction called the itch-scratch-itch cycle is set up in the deeper tissues of the skin. The itching can become intense, often waking a woman up at night.

APPEARANCE

Chronic scratching or rubbing of the skin gives it a thickened, leathery appearance, sometimes reddened or even a little scaly, and may leave visible scratch marks or broken hairs.

EVALUATION

Your health care provider will take a detailed history and do a thorough physical examination checking for infection, allergy-causing agents, irritants, and other conditions that cause itching. Sometimes a tiny biopsy is taken to determine the cause and rule out other conditions.

TREATMENT

Treatment is aimed at removing irritants and stopping the itch. Ice packs and antihistamines can help, as can the use of gentle soaps and avoidance of rough washcloths in bathing. Steroid ointments such as those used for lichen sclerosus are also sometimes useful, and a low-potency ointment may be needed for long-term maintenance. Some women wear clean cotton gloves to bed to cover their fingernails and reduce the effects of unintentional scratching or irritants. It is essential to test and treat for *Candida albicans* (a yeast fungus that can cause infection and may be the source of the irritation).

VULVAR LICHEN PLANUS

Lichen planus is an inflammatory skin disease that most commonly causes an itchy rash of small purplish bumps, often on the arms, legs, or back or inside the mouth. It can also affect the genital area, including the vagina. Many women with vulvar lichen planus also have the disease in the mouth.

The cause of lichen planus is unknown. We know that it is *not* caused by infection, hormonal change, or aging, and is not brought on by things women do or do not do. It is probably autoimmune in origin. Certain medications (such as hydrochlorothiazide) may contribute to the development of the disease.

APPEARANCE

Soreness, burning, and rawness are common symptoms. Superficial layers of the skin break down to form glassy red tender erosions. There may be a white lacy pattern present on the edges of the erosions. These may also occur in the vagina in a patchy or generalized pattern. A sticky, irritating yellow discharge may occur. Scarring can shorten or shut off the vagina.

EVALUATION AND TREATMENT

Diagnosis is made by the characteristic appearance and by biopsy. Treatment involves ultrapotent steroid ointments or oral intramuscular steroids. The disease, like lichen sclerosus, is managed, not cured.

VULVODYNIA

Itching, burning, stinging, rawness, or pain in the vulva in the absence of any known cause is called *vulvodynia*. Symptoms may occur in one site on the vulva or may be experienced all over the vulva; they may last for days, weeks, or even years, then disappear for a time. Tight clothes and sitting often increase the discomfort; sexual intercourse may or may not be painful. The cause of vulvodynia is unknown, but it affects about 8 percent of women. It can be hard to get a proper diagnosis; if your vulva hurts, it is important to find a health care provider who is familiar with vulvodynia.

EVALUATION

Atrophy, infection, and skin disorders must be ruled out with appropriate testing, but there is no clear test for vulvodynia. During a pelvic exam, a provider may lightly touch areas on the vulva with a cotton swab to see where it's sensitive.

TREATMENT

Treatment involves removing any irritants and using gentle local care. Loose clothes and cold packs are helpful. Treatment may also include topical lidocaine (Xylocaine), tricyclic antidepressants, or anticonvulsants such as gabapentin.

CARE FOR YOUR VULVA AND VAGINA

Some simple ways to keep irritants at bay are to avoid tight clothes such as panty hose, tights, or pants with thick seams at the crotch. Wash new underwear before wearing it, and give underwear an extra rinse cycle with plain water every time you wash it. Avoid fabric softeners and dryer sheets.

For washing the genital area, either avoid soaps altogether or use very mild, unscented soaps such as Pears, Basis, or Neutrogena. Once-a-day bathing should be sufficient. Excessive washing can increase the irritation. Soaking with cool tap water or with Aveeno or Domeboro solution can soothe irritated skin. Unless specifically directed by a health care provider, douching is never necessary. Douching and the use of vaginal deodorants can change the normal balance of bacteria in the vagina and lead to infections. Scents used in vaginal deodorants can also cause allergic reactions.

If you experience genital itching or irritation, do not be reluctant to seek help. Itching and irritation are very common and are very rarely a sign of cancer. The cause of these symptoms can be determined in most cases, and successfully treated. Be sure to find a provider with experience in this area if your symptoms persist.

NOTES

1. D. Brown, "Postmenopausal Atrophism, Atrophic Vaginitis, and Other Vaginitides," in R. H. Kaufman, S. Faro, D. Brown, *Benign Diseases of the Vulva and Vagina*, 5th ed. (Philadelphia: Elsevier Mosby, 2005), 391–410.

2. S. Brizzolara, J. Killeen, R. Severino, "Vaginal pH and Parabasal Cells in Postmenopausal Women," *Obstetrics and Gynecology* 94, no. 5 (1999): 700–703.

3. K. Nilsson, B. Risberg, G. Heimer, "The Vaginal Epithelium in the Postmenopause—Cytology, Histology, and pH as Methods of Assessment," *Maturitas* 21 (1995): 51–56.

4. J. Allen-Davis, A. Beck, R. Parker, J. Ellis, D. Polley, "Assessment of Vulvovaginal Complaints: Accuracy of Telephone Triage and In-Office Assessment,"

American Journal of Obstetrics and Gynecology 99, no. 1 (2002): 18–22.

5. M. Bygdeman and M. L. Swahn, "Replens Versus Dienestrol Cream in the Symptomatic Treatment of Vaginal Atrophy in Postmenopausal Women," *Maturitas* 23 (1996): 259–63.

6. Task Force on Hormone Therapy, American College of Obstetricians and Gynecologists, "Genitourinary Tract Changes," *Obstetrics and Gynecology* 104, no. 4 (2004): 56S–61S.

7. E. Wiederpass, J. A. Baron, H. O. Adami, C. Magnussin, A. Lindgren, R. Bergstrom, et al., "Low-Potency Oestrogen and Risk of Endometrial Cancer: A Case-Controlled Study," *Lancet* 353 (1999): 1824–28.

CHAPTER 7

Hormone Treatment

A BRIEF HISTORY OF HORMONE TREATMENT

The two primary sex hormones found in a woman's body are estrogen and progesterone. Testosterone also naturally occurs in women's bodies. "Hormone therapy" is the term that has been used to describe certain drugs that are prescribed to women at menopause. It can refer to the use of estrogen alone or to a combination of estrogen and a progestogen or a combination of estrogen and an androgen (a form of testosterone). (The term *progestogen* refers to a class of substances that includes the natural progesterone in our bodies and synthetic progestins used in hormone treatment.)

Until very recently, this treatment was called "hormone replacement therapy," but the word "replacement" has been dropped. Hormone treatment never literally raised postmenopausal women's hormones to premenopausal levels. Also, medical research has shown that taking estrogen after menopause will not replace the function that estrogen played in the body before menopause and is not necessary for optimal health. Indeed, it confers risk of harm. The concept of estrogen replacement was a clever marketing idea that was never backed up by good evidence. Because the term *therapy* is usually used in medicine when there is a disease or condition that requires therapy and the menopause transition is a normal physiological process, this chapter will use the more neutral term "hormone treatment" instead of "hormone therapy."

WHO SHOULD NOT USE HORMONE SUPPLEMENTS?

In general, you should *not* use hormone supplements if you:

- are pregnant, are planning a pregnancy, or are not protected from pregnancy
- have a history of unexplained vaginal bleeding
- have a history of breast, uterine, or ovarian cancer
- have a history of stroke or heart attack
- have a history of blood clots, such as clots in the lungs or legs
- have a history of liver disease

Estrogen has been used since the 1930s to treat hot flashes and other physical changes that women experience at menopause. But starting in the 1960s, the list of reasons that women were advised to take hormones began to grow. In 1966, the book *Feminine Forever* became a best seller with its claim that "menopause is completely preventable."[1] The book's author, Robert A. Wilson, wrote that because the estrogen level in a woman's body dropped after menopause, postmenopausal women who didn't receive treatment were no longer truly female. Wilson traveled the country, lecturing on this topic and promising that with the help of estrogen therapy, "Every woman alive today has the option to remain feminine forever." But soon after, reporters at *The New Republic* and *The Washington Post* disclosed that Dr. Wilson's lecture tour and work were being supported by a company that manufactured estrogen for hormone treatment.[2] When this issue was raised again in 2002 by Wilson's own son, the company responded that it could not confirm the account because it was so far in the past and the company had no record of any such financial arrangement.[3]

During the decades that followed, drug companies promoted and doctors prescribed hormones to women to prevent and treat an increasingly broad range of ailments and experiences associated with aging, from wrinkles and general aches and pains to Alzheimer's disease, depression, and heart attack. The FDA had initially approved hormone treatment for hot flashes and other problems associated with menopause, not for disease prevention. However, in the late 1980s and the 1990s, several observational studies suggested that hormone treatment might improve women's quality of life and, most significant, protect women against heart disease. In 1986, the FDA reviewed the evidence and found that hormone treatment was effective for treatment of osteoporosis. In 1990, the FDA found that the research done to date was not adequate to support adding heart disease prevention to the list of approved uses. But doctors are allowed to prescribe drugs for uses that are not approved by the FDA. Encouraged by the research suggesting that hormone treatment might be helpful for new uses, as well as by extensive drug company marketing efforts, many health care providers did just that. Such off-label prescribing is common practice in medicine when research to support new claims has not been completed, though in many cases it means that people are taking drugs that haven't been adequately proven to be safe or effective for the purposes for which they are being used.

Some women's health advocates became

concerned that using hormone treatment might actually be harmful to women's health. A few had raised warning flags as early as the 1950s,[4] and the concern grew more intense in the mid-1970s when two studies linked estrogen to endometrial cancer.[5] But researchers soon discovered that adding a progestogen to estrogen ("combined treatment") reduced this risk. After that, doctors began prescribing combined hormone treatment to women who still had a uterus and thus were at risk of endometrial cancer, while women who had undergone hysterectomy continued to take estrogen alone.

In 1977, Barbara Seaman's book *Women and the Crisis in Sex Hormones* alerted women to evidence that taking hormones could cause breast cancer, strokes, and blood clots and warned against the overpromotion of hormones for the treatment of menopause.[6] Like *Feminine Forever,* Seaman's book became a best seller, educating a generation of women about the health risks of hormones. But the effort to sell hormone treatment as a pill to make you healthy, happy, and beautiful continued unabated, supported by multimillion-dollar advertising campaigns. Against a background of seemingly conflicting data, with some research suggesting benefits and other studies indicating dangers,[7] hormone treatment soon became the most prescribed drug in the country.*

The first major study to challenge the theory that hormone treatment was beneficial for heart disease was the HERS study, published in 1998, which found that women with heart disease who used hormone treatment had worse outcomes than those who didn't take hormones.[8] But hormone treatment proponents discounted the HERS results, saying that they didn't apply to healthy women. The widespread use of hormone treatment did not change significantly until 2002, when a large-scale research study of hormone treatment known as the Women's Health Initiative (WHI) revealed evidence that taking hormones did not protect healthy women against heart disease and stroke. In fact, the first publicly released results of the WHI showed that women who took the combination of estrogen and progestin had increased their risk for breast cancer, stroke, heart attack, and blood clots. This led to a swift and significant drop in the number of hormone prescriptions worldwide, as many women stopped taking hormones. Some women later resumed hormone treatment because they were experiencing hot flashes or other menopausal changes that they found problematic, but research has shown that about half the women who stopped taking hormones did not have that problem.[9]

UNDERSTANDING THE WHI RESULTS

There's still debate today about how to interpret the results of the Women's Health Initiative. Because the WHI findings were from a randomized, placebo-controlled trial, they had great credibility and attracted a lot of media attention. After reading about the risks of hormone treatment identified by the study, many women decided to quit or avoid taking these drugs.

The WHI both revealed new risks to hormone treatment and confirmed risks that had previously been suspected. And in 2003, an observational study of 1 million British women

*This overprescription of hormones based on an incomplete and preliminary understanding of their effects underscores the problem with relying on observational studies to guide medical practice. (For more information on different types of research studies, see page 23.) The observational studies of hormone treatment found an association between hormone treatment and lower levels of heart disease, but this type of study cannot prove that a treatment prevents a disease. Still, pharmaceutical companies promoted this sort of evidence, which supported a larger market for their products.

also found an association between use of hormone treatment and an increased risk for breast cancer.[10] Like the WHI, the British study found that the risk of breast cancer increased over time as long as a woman continued taking hormones and that women who took an estrogen-progestin combination had the greatest increased risk but that taking estrogen alone also significantly increased the risk. The effect of estrogen alone on breast cancer risk found by the British study is different from the effect found by the WHI, a difference which has not yet been satisfactorily explained.

It is important to understand the data from the WHI, summarized in the graphs below and on the following page, so that you can make informed decisions for yourself, weighing benefits against risks.

The bar graphs here summarize the results of the WHI. In terms of potentially harmful effects of hormone treatment, they show that taking estrogen plus progestin put women at greater risk for heart attacks, strokes, breast cancer, and blood clots (Figure 1). Women who had hysterectomies and were taking estrogen-only treatment were at a greater risk for strokes (Figure 2). For women older than sixty-five, taking hormones (regardless of whether they were estrogen plus progestin or estrogen only) significantly increased the women's risk for dementia compared to women not taking hormones (Figures 1 and 2).

There were also some beneficial effects of hormone treatment. Women taking estrogen plus progestin were less likely to fracture a hip or develop colon cancer compared to women not taking hormones (Figure 1). Women who had a hysterectomy and were taking estrogen-

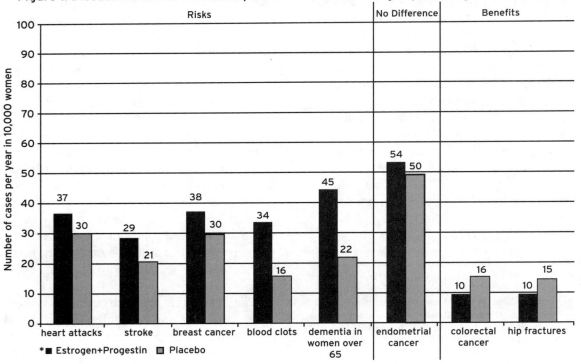

Figure 1: Disease Rates for Postmenopausal Women on Estrogen plus Progestin or Placebo[11]

only treatment were less likely to fracture a hip compared to women not taking hormone treatment (Figure 2).

For some conditions, the difference between the groups was too small to say with certainty whether hormone treatment is beneficial or harmful or neither, when compared to a placebo (Figures 1 and 2).

Each year, for every 10,000 women in the WHI who took estrogen plus progestin treatment,

- 37 women had heart attacks compared to 30 taking placebo pills;
- 29 women had a stroke compared to 21 taking placebo pills;

- 38 women developed breast cancer compared to 30 taking placebo pills;
- 34 women had blood clots in the legs or lungs compared to 16 taking placebo pills;
- 10 women developed colon cancer compared to 16 taking placebo pills;
- 10 women had a hip fracture compared to 15 taking placebo pills;
- and in the age 65+ group, 45 women developed dementia compared to 22 taking placebo pills.[13]

Each year, for every 10,000 women in the WHI who took estrogen-only treatment,

- 44 women had a stroke compared to 32 taking placebo pills;

Figure 2: Disease Rates for Women with Hysterectomy on Estrogen-Only or Placebo[12]

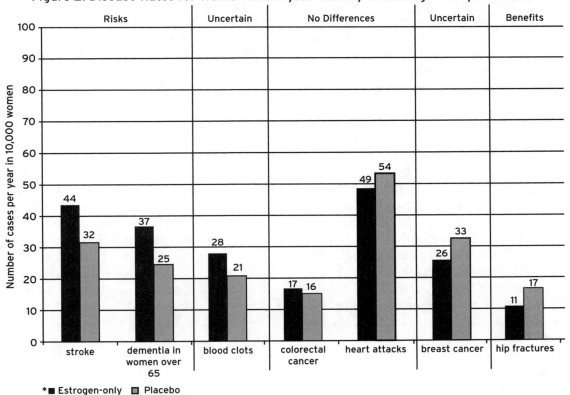

- 11 women had a hip fracture compared to 17 taking placebo pills;
- and in the age 65+ group, 37 women developed dementia compared to 25 taking placebo pills.[14]

Since the results of the WHI were published, critics have raised concerns about the trial design and have argued that recommendations against using hormone treatment based on WHI results have been too broad. They worry that women are being unnecessarily steered away from treatment that might be beneficial. While some of the critics are thoughtful, well-intentioned doctors and researchers, it's important to note that their ideas are frequently disseminated with support from companies that make hormone treatment products and that have an interest in downplaying the significance of the WHI findings.

One of the first points often made by those calling the WHI into question is that the women in the trial were too old—that too many were long past menopause (which occurs, on average, at age fifty-one). In fact, more than 12 percent of the women were between fifty and fifty-four at the beginning of the study. This makes the WHI the largest randomized controlled trial ever done of women in this age group.

Another criticism of the trial is that it did not weigh the benefit that women get from relief of hot flashes and night sweats in its risk-benefit calculation. It is true that hot flash relief was not included in the global measure of risk and benefit that was used to determine whether it was ethical to continue the WHI. The trial was not designed to evaluate the effect of hormone treatment on those problems. But that does not mean that the trial ignored or excluded hot flashes from its assessment. The WHI included some women who had moderate to severe hot flashes (12 percent at the time of enrollment), and those who were assigned to

receive hormone treatment reported getting significant relief in comparison to those in the placebo group. As individual women weigh the risks and benefits of hormone treatment for themselves, relief of hot flashes can clearly be counted on the benefit side. Hormone treatment is currently the only well-studied remedy that has been proven to work in reducing the frequency and intensity of hot flashes.[15] (For more information on hot flashes, see page 75.)

Hormone treatment proponents have also proposed several theories about how variations on the hormone treatment studied in the WHI might turn out to be less harmful and more beneficial to women.

One hypothesis suggests that hormone treatment protects the heart if started immediately at menopause. There is controversy over whether the results from the WHI for women ages fifty to fifty-nine support this theory. Statistical analyses of the WHI data for women with a uterus who were between the ages of fifty and fifty-nine did not indicate significant differences by age in the effect of estrogen and progesterone on the risk of heart disease. In other words, younger women with a uterus were at no less risk nor were they more protected from heart disease compared to older women in the study. But in a controversial analysis of the data on women in the WHI who had undergone hysterectomy, some investigators stated that taking estrogen alone did reduce the risk for some cardiovascular events in women ages 50 to 59. However, the study findings only reached borderline statistical significance, and the way in which the statistical analysis was conducted has been called into question. In any case, even the scientists who developed this analysis agree that there is not adequate evidence to support a recommendation that women should use hormone treatment for this purpose.[16] The current recommendations for hormone treatment issued by the American Heart Association expressly state that hormone treatment should not be used for cardiovascular protection in women at any age.

Others theorize that different doses and methods of administration will give better results. But the bottom line is that all of these ideas are theories that have yet to be tested, and none is yet supported by evidence as strong as that collected in the WHI.

Until there are alternatives *that have been proven* to provide safe and effective relief, some women will continue to face the decision about whether to take hormone treatment.

This chapter provides information for women who are considering hormone treatment because of hot flashes, vaginal dryness, or both that do not respond to other treatments. It discusses the types of hormone treatment available and what is known about their risks, benefits, and side effects.

HORMONE TREATMENT TODAY

PROVEN CLAIMS

There is evidence that taking hormones at menopause reduces hot flashes and night sweats and relieves vaginal dryness.[17] There is also reliable evidence that shows that hormone treatment delays bone density loss and reduces the risk of fractures.[18] The combination of estrogen and progestin has also been shown to reduce the risk of colon cancer.[19]

UNPROVEN CLAIMS

Although health care providers and women have become more cautious, and even skeptical, about unproven claims for hormone treatment, some people continue to believe that hormone treatment has certain benefits even though those beliefs are not backed up by scientific evidence. Women whose health care providers recommend hormone treatment for the following reasons may want to seek other sources of information. Estrogen or combined estrogen and progestogen treatment has *not* been shown to:

- decrease the risk of stroke. (It actually increases the risk.)
- decrease the risk of heart attacks. (Combined estrogen and progestin treatment actually increases the risk.)
- prevent wrinkles or other natural signs of aging.
- reduce urinary incontinence. (It may increase risk of development and exacerbate existing conditions.)[20]
- relieve moodiness or depression.
- improve sexual desire or responsiveness.
- improve overall memory.
- help sleep or increase energy in women who do not have hot flashes.
- prevent Alzheimer's disease or other conditions that cause dementia. (It actually increases risk of dementia in women over age sixty-five.)[21]
- improve overall quality of life.
- relieve joint pain.

For some of these conditions, the research is inconclusive: There are indications that hormone treatment may provide some benefit and indications that it does not. Women's individual experiences raise even more questions, since a variety of responses to hormone treatment have been reported that haven't been confirmed by studies in larger groups of women. There's a lot we still don't know.

DIFFERENT KINDS OF HORMONE TREATMENT

There are a number of different kinds of hormone treatment, as well as varied doses and ways of taking the drugs, and these are each sold under different brand names. Most women who use hormone treatment take either an estrogen-only type or a combination of estrogen plus progestogen. Some women use testosterone (see page 110). Estrogen-only therapies, which are sometimes referred to as "unopposed estrogen," are specifically for women who have had a hysterectomy or do not have a uterus. Women who do have a uterus should not take estrogen-only treatment because estrogen increases the risk of endometrial cancer.[22] A woman with a uterus who decides to take hormone treatment should make sure that she is taking an estrogen-progestogen combination, which will reduce her risk of getting endometrial cancer that is caused by the estrogen part of the treatment.

You may hear hormone treatment referred to as Premarin. This is the brand name of the most commonly prescribed hormone treatment product. Premarin is an estrogen-only product, but the same company also makes a combination product called Prempro that contains both estrogen and progestin. These are the drugs that were tested, at a specific dose, in the Women's Health Initiative.[23] Premarin and Prempro contain a specific kind of estrogen— conjugated equine estrogen—which is made by extracting estrogen from the urine of a pregnant horse (*preg*nant *mar*e's ur*ine*, hence the name).

Other hormone treatment products contain different kinds of estrogen and progestogens, including estrogens extracted from plants and natural progesterone derived from wild yams. Women who are concerned about the commercial use or mistreatment of animals sometimes prefer a product that comes from plants. There is, however, no evidence that one kind of estrogen or progestogen is safer or more effective than another.

ESTROGEN-ONLY AND ESTROGEN PLUS PROGESTOGEN COMBINATIONS

BENEFITS

- fewer and less intense hot flashes
- less frequent and less intense night sweats
- reduced vaginal dryness
- reduced loss in bone density
- reduced risk of bone fractures

Estrogen-only and estrogen plus progestogen combinations both reduce the frequency of hot flashes and night sweats; some women find that they eliminate them altogether.[24] Those of us who are having serious problems with hot flashes and night sweats also often have difficulty sleeping as a result, and the relief that we get from hormone treatment can help us to sleep better.

Estrogen-only and estrogen plus progestogen also relieve the vaginal dryness and thinning of the tissue in the vagina that women may experience after menopause.[25] When our vaginas are dry and the skin there is thin, sexual contact may be uncomfortable or even painful. Hormone treatment can eliminate the discomfort or pain that might prevent some women from enjoying sexual intercourse.[26] Hormone creams or tablets that women apply directly to the vagina may have the same benefits without all of the risks of hormone treatment taken systemically, such as that taken orally or through the skin. (For more information, see page 109.) There are three forms of local estrogen currently available: an estrogen ring, an estrogen tablet, and estrogen creams. These can help relieve vaginal dryness without delivering as much estrogen to the bloodstream as an oral or transdermal hormone treatment does.

Finally, taking estrogen can reduce bone density loss and reduce the risk of breaking or fracturing bones.[27]

NEGATIVE EFFECTS

- bleeding
- bloating
- breast tenderness or enlargement
- headaches
- nausea
- vaginitis and vaginal itching
- leg cramps
- menstrual cramps
- mood changes

Negative effects of hormone treatment vary considerably among women, and the severity and frequency differ as well. Some women have no negative effects; other women experience minor problems, while still others can't take the drugs because the unwanted effects are so strong.

The type of hormone treatment a woman is taking—either estrogen-only or a combination of estrogen plus progestogen—as well as the dose may determine the effects experienced. If you are having problems, it may be helpful to try a lower dose.

RISKS

- blood clots
- heart attack
- stroke
- breast cancer
- gallbladder disease

There are risks to taking any drugs, and we base our decisions about whether to take a particular drug on whether the benefit it can give us is worth the harm it might cause us. It has been known for decades that hormone treatment has some risks. Before we learned the results of the WHI, many health care providers and women believed that the benefits of taking hormone treatment were great enough that they were worth exposing ourselves to the risks. The WHI was a revelation to many people for two reasons: It showed that hormone treatment did not have as many benefits as health care providers had believed it did, and it demonstrated that the risks were greater than had been known. This new information shifted the balance between risk and benefit for many women.

What we now know from the WHI is that using combination estrogen plus progestin hormone treatment can put a woman at greater risk for heart disease, stroke, breast cancer, and blood clots than if she did not use it. Using estrogen-only treatment appears to have fewer risks, although it also increases the chance of experiencing a stroke and uterine cancer. For this reason, estrogen-only treatment is an option solely for women without a uterus.

Long-term estrogen treatment increases a woman's risk for breast cancer. The Nurses Health Study, which followed almost 29,000 women, found a 42 percent increased risk for all types of breast cancer in women who used estrogen alone for twenty or more years.[28] For the type of breast cancer that is hormone sensitive, the study found a 48 percent increased risk after fifteen years of using estrogen alone. A separate study, the Black Women's Health Study of more than 23,000 black women over the age of forty, found an even larger effect.[29] It found that black women who take either combination estrogen-progestin products or estrogen alone for ten years or longer have a 50 percent greater risk of breast cancer.

The WHI researchers also looked at the risk of developing dementia in the group of women in the trial who were older than sixty-five and found that taking hormones—both the estrogen-progestin combination and estrogen only—increased the risk for dementia. Finally, there are indications that taking hormone treatment and then stopping may trigger hot flashes in some women who didn't have them before starting to take hormones.[30]

Studies that have followed women who choose to take hormone treatment at menopause and compared them with women who do not have found that those taking hormones are more likely to get ovarian cancer.[31] This is true for both women taking estrogen alone and those taking an estrogen plus progestogen combination. In 2001, such a study showed that the risk of dying from ovarian cancer doubled with use of estrogen for ten or more years, although ovarian cancer is very rare, so that a doubling of risk still affected a small number of women.[32] A 1998 analysis that pulled together results from previous studies found that staying on hormones for ten or more years may increase risk of getting ovarian cancer by about 30 percent.[33] Neither of these studies was randomized like the WHI. Women taking estrogen plus progestin in the WHI also experienced slightly more ovarian cancer than women taking a placebo, but there were not enough cases of women developing ovarian cancer and women were not followed for a long enough time to draw definite conclusions about the risk.[34] It's not yet possible to make a recommendation based on conclusive scientific data, but women who are concerned about ovarian cancer may choose to avoid hormone treatment or to take it only for a short time.

HOW MUCH AND FOR HOW LONG?

Lowest Possible Dose

The current medical advice is that women who use hormone treatment should take the lowest possible dose.[35] This advice is based on the theory that taking a lower dose may reduce the risks. At this point, however, this is just a theory. There is no conclusive scientific data showing that lower doses are safer than the higher doses that women have taken in the past.

The women who participated in the WHI were prescribed a dose of 0.625 mg estrogen plus 2.5 mg progestin tablets orally. There are a number of different dosage levels available for both estrogen-only and combination estrogen-progestogen treatments. Many health care providers advise women who decide to use hormone treatment to begin with the lowest dose possible and increase only if that dose proves to be ineffective.[36]

Shortest Time Possible

The WHI findings indicate that the longer a woman uses combined estrogen and progestin treatment, the greater her risk for heart disease, stroke, breast cancer, and blood clots, and if she is over sixty-five, the greater her risk for dementia. Therefore, women are advised to take hormone treatment for the shortest time possible and to stop when it is no longer needed for symptom relief.[37] The same recommendation applies to women who take estrogen only, since the risk of stroke increases with longer use, as does the risk for dementia in women over sixty-five. Some health care providers recommend that women using hormone treatment should make regular attempts to taper the dosage to see whether we still need to be using it.

Unfortunately, we don't know how to predict how long an individual woman might continue to experience hot flashes. It is possible that hormone treatment only delays hot flashes (in other words, that women who relieve hot flashes by taking hormone treatment for a period of time will experience the hot flashes later when they stop taking hormones). About half of the women in the WHI who stopped using hormone treatment found that their hot flashes returned.[38]

A sixty-one-year-old woman who stopped using hormone treatment says,

It seems that physicians have such limited knowledge about menopause. I went off the hormones

slowly a year and a half ago. Unfortunately, I am still experiencing hot flashes, and again the night sweats are disturbing my sleep.

Another woman had a different experience when at forty-nine she noticed that she started blushing bright red every time she made a joke in public. She says,

It was unbelievably embarrassing. It never used to happen. Then it dawned on me that I was having these blushes three or four times a day. And it hit me, these must be hot flashes! I tried black cohosh [an herbal supplement; for more information, see page 78] and within two or three weeks my hot flashes disappeared. I took it for two or three months. Then I went on vacation and stopped taking it. The hot flashes never returned.

DELIVERY METHODS

There are many different ways to take hormone treatment: pills, patches, creams, gels, rings, and suppositories. Because pills are the most commonly used form of hormone treatment in the United States, much of what we know about the harms and benefits is based on research using pills.

Oral Tablets: Cyclic or Continuous

Most women using hormone treatment take oral tablets or pills. For women taking an estrogen and progestogen combination, a single pill can include both hormones or they can be in separate pills. There are two ways to take combined hormone treatment: the *cyclic method* (also known as *sequential*) and the *continuous combined method*. With both methods, estrogen is taken every day. In the cyclic method, estrogen is supplemented with a progestogen for ten to fourteen days each month. In the continuous method, a progestogen is included every day. Women taking hormones on the cyclic

method usually experience monthly bleeding, although for some this may decrease over time. Women who have problems with effects from the progestogen (such as headaches, mood swings, and depression) sometimes find the cyclic method easier to tolerate.

Skin Patches and Gels, or Transdermal Administration

Hormone treatment can also be administered through the skin. One way to do this is by using a skin patch, which adheres like a piece of Scotch tape. A woman places the patch on her lower abdomen or buttocks. The patch sticks strongly enough that it will not fall off because of swimming, bathing, and other contact with water. But the strong adhesive may have a downside: some women find that our skin becomes irritated at the place where we apply the patch. There are both estrogen-only and combination hormone patches available.

Two FDA-approved gels called Estrasorb and EstroGel are applied to the skin. The EstroGel label instructs women to apply it on the arm; the Estrasorb instructions suggest application to the legs. There's very little published research on the safety or effectiveness of these products, although one twelve-week study of EstroGel found that it was effective at a 1.25 g daily dose for treating moderate to severe hot flashes.[39]

Transdermal delivery of hormones may have different harms and benefits than oral formulations. Unlike pills, which are processed through the liver, the medication in the skin patch and in gels is absorbed directly into the bloodstream. This may be an advantage for those of us who have a history of liver problems. But there have not been studies that prove that the health risks of the patch or gels are lower than those of the pills. Until there is evidence of that, we have to assume that the risks are the same.

Vaginal Creams, Tablets, and Rings

For women whose only reason for taking hormone treatment is to relieve vaginal dryness or thinning of the vaginal walls, an estrogen cream or tablet that can be applied directly in or around the vagina in very small doses may be effective. Vaginal application of estrogen creams and tablets usually will not relieve hot flashes or night sweats.

The FDA has also approved two vaginal rings that a woman inserts into her vagina and that release estrogen slowly over time. The two rings deliver different doses of estrogen. Femring (the higher dose) is approved for alleviating moderate to severe hot flashes, and unlike other vaginal estrogen products is designed to increase blood levels of estrogen. Estring (which delivers a lower dose) is approved only for relief of vaginal problems associated with menopause, such as dryness and irritation. Some women prefer the ring for vaginal symptom relief because they find it easier to use than other forms of vaginal estrogen.[40]

The risks and benefits of vaginally applied hormone treatment are uncertain. They could be similar to those of oral tablets, but adverse effects are more likely to be localized to the vagina. Even though the amount of estrogen used can be much lower with a vaginal cream or tablet, vaginally applied estrogen does have a measurable effect on blood levels of estrogen.[41] Levels are often in the normal range. The claim that these products don't have a systemic effect is uncertain at best. For this reason, some experts believe it's still necessary for women with a uterus who are using vaginally applied estrogen to take some form of progestogen to reduce the risk of uterine cancer. The most commonly reported negative effects of vaginal creams include vaginal discomfort or pain, breast pain, swelling, burning, itching, and infection.

ADDING TESTOSTERONE TO THE MIX

Estrogen and Testosterone for Hot Flashes

Estratest is a hormone treatment product that combines estrogen and testosterone. It was approved for treatment of hot flashes in women who don't respond to estrogen alone. But the Food and Drug Administration (FDA) has called into question whether there is evidence that it is effective for that purpose. The company that makes Estratest has told the FDA that it will conduct studies to evaluate the product's effectiveness. In the meantime, Estratest remains on the market despite the FDA's statement that it "does not believe there is substantial evidence" that testosterone contributes to the effectiveness of the treatment.[42] Since there are safety concerns about women using testosterone (discussed below), the lack of evidence of effectiveness is particularly worrisome.

Testosterone for Low Sexual Desire

Recently, there has been significant interest in the use of testosterone to treat low sexual desire in women. There is some evidence from clinical trials that postmenopausal women who take testosterone experience increased libido.[43]

A 2003 randomized study on women who had their ovaries removed and were taking estrogen found that using a testosterone skin patch led to some improvement in sexual desire and activity.[44] But in 2004, an FDA advisory committee recommended against approval of a testosterone patch for women because there has not been enough research on the safety of long-term use.[45] Potential safety concerns include increased risk of heart disease and breast cancer.

The limited research that's been done on safety of testosterone use by women is not conclusive, but it raises several concerns. More than one study has shown that women who have higher natural levels of testosterone are more likely to get breast cancer;[46] and among women who have had breast cancer, those with higher testosterone levels are more likely to experience a recurrence.[47] There's also some research indicating that testosterone use may cause an increase in heart disease.[48] Additional research is needed to explore these potential risks.

It is important to note that low levels of natural testosterone before, during, or after menopause are **not** associated with lack of sexual desire or activity.[49] Therefore testing your testosterone level will not tell you whether taking testosterone may improve your low desire.

Women who decide to take testosterone in spite of the fact that evidence for efficacy and harm is inconclusive should be aware that no form of testosterone is approved by the FDA for the treatment of low sexual desire in women. (Estratest, a form of testosterone plus estrogen discussed above, has FDA approval only for the treatment of hot flashes that are unresponsive to estrogen.) However, some health care providers prescribe testosterone products that have been approved for both men and women; some may prescribe Estratest off-label despite the fact that it hasn't been studied for this use; and some prescribe specially compounded testosterone in oral, injectable, or topical form.

Effects may include excessive hair growth on the face, torso, or limbs; clitoral enlargement; acne; frontal hair thinning; deepening of the voice; and menstrual irregularity. Voice changes and hair growth may be irreversible even after testosterone treatment is stopped, especially for women who take high doses.

The causes of women's sexual dissatisfaction are complex, varied, and not fully understood. Our sexual desire and satisfaction may be influenced by our life circumstances, including the quality of our sexual relationships, our emotional and physical health, and our values and thoughts about sexuality, as well as by the aging process and the shifting hormone levels that occur during the menopause transition. (For more information, see "The Medicalization of Female Sexual Desire," page 148.)

NATURAL PRODUCTS: PHYTOESTROGENS AND BIOIDENTICAL HORMONES

Since the release of the findings of the Women's Health Initiative, many companies have taken advantage of the climate of fear surrounding hormone treatment to sell alternative products based on the unproven idea that other forms of estrogen will be safer than the synthetic hormones that were studied in the trial. This idea is based more on the principles of marketing than the principles of science. It's very important to remember that products are not necessarily safe just because they're called "natural." The same questions we ask about drugs need to be answered for any alternative therapy, too. What is the specific reason to take it? Are there well-designed, sufficiently large randomized trials showing that it is effective for the recommended purpose? What are the risks and harms associated with it? Has it been recommended to you by someone who may earn money from its sales?

Phytoestrogens

Phytoestrogens are estrogens in plants. Some women eat specific foods that contain phytoestrogens to get the estrogenic effects. The food most commonly known to contain phytoestrogen is soy, but beans, peas, lentils, and whole grains and seeds, especially flaxseed, rye, and millet, also contain these plant estrogens.

We have relatively little evidence to support claims for the effectiveness of phytoestrogens and even less information about their safety. Alternatives like these are much less likely to be studied in formal research trials than drugs are, but there is some data from both observational and randomized controlled trials. Some studies have shown that eating foods with phytoestrogens provides modest relief of hot flashes,[50] and some studies have found that eating phytoestrogens causes changes in vaginal cells that are similar to the changes caused by taking estrogen and could relieve discomfort.[51]

When it comes to safety, there's even less research to guide us. Women who eat foods containing phytoestrogens may be reassured by the knowledge that people have been eating foods containing phytoestrogens for thousands of years. But the health effects of consuming nonfood phytoestrogens, by taking the phytoestrogen dietary supplements that are now being produced and marketed to women, are not known.

Natural or Bioidentical Estrogen and Progesterone

The kinds of estrogens that we have in our bodies are estriol, estradiol, and estrone. The products that people refer to as "natural" estrogens also contain these hormones. The use of the word "natural" is confusing. Sometimes the term is used because the hormone is plant-derived, but it is misleading to describe these hormone products as natural, because they are synthesized in a laboratory just like the drugs that are called "synthetic" hormones. The real difference is that so-called natural hormones are chemically identical to the estrogens produced in a woman's body, so some people use the term "bioidentical hormones" instead. The terms "natural" and "bioidentical" often are used to describe the same hormones, but "bioidentical" is the more precise name.

The compounding pharmacies that fill prescriptions for bioidentical hormones purchase the hormones that they use from major pharmaceutical companies, and those companies use the same hormones in their own standard drug products. Estradiol, for example, is contained in many pharmaceutical versions of hormone treatment. This means that women who are seeking natural alternatives because they want to avoid the hormones in the drug companies' versions of hormone treatment are in fact using many of the same products when they take so-called natural hormones.

There haven't been large research studies on bioidentical estrogens, but the studies that have been done have shown that they are effective for relieving hot flashes and vaginal dryness.[52] Some alternative medicine proponents claim that they can prevent cardiovascular disease, but there is no valid evidence to support this assertion. There is research, however, showing that bioidentical estrogen may increase the risk of breast cancer, although the evidence is not conclusive.[53] And recent studies have shown that estriol increases the risk of endometrial cancer and the abnormal growth of uterine cells, which can lead to cancer.[54]

Bioidentical progesterone, including micronized progesterone, comes in creams and an under-the-tongue form as well as pills. It is promoted to prevent hot flashes, osteoporosis, and even breast cancer, but the only claim that's supported by evidence is that it relieves hot flashes.[55] The cancer prevention claims are unsupported, and even dangerous. While the oral progestins included in combination estrogen plus progestin hormone treatment protect against endometrial cancer, bioidentical progesterone cream is not well enough absorbed to offer this protection.[56] We also don't know the effect of bioidentical progesterone on risk of breast cancer, but the oral progestin in hormone treatment has been shown to increase breast cancer risk. In the absence of safety data showing that the risks are different, women are probably best served by assuming that the potential harms of bioidentical hormones will be similar to those of conventional hormone treatments.

Regulation of Compounding Pharmacies

Current regulations for the compounding pharmacies that prepare and distribute bioidentical hormones were developed when these companies were small businesses, working with a few health care providers in their communities and serving very few consumers. Today, compounding pharmacies represent a significant and growing industry, and some women's health advocates have pointed out that the old regulations are no longer adequate to protect consumers.

In the fall of 2005, the National Women's Health Network (NWHN) wrote to the FDA documenting significant problems with the way that compounding pharmacies promote and sell compounded hormones, which are often also marketed as bioidentical hormones. The NWHN is a nonprofit public interest group in Washington, D.C., that does not accept any funding from pharmaceutical or medical device companies. It asserted that women are being misled by unsubstantiated safety and efficacy claims about compounded hormones that have not been proven effective or studied for long-term safety. Concerned that the lack of FDA regulation over compounding pharmacies is exposing women to unsafe and ineffective products, the NWHN urged the agency to take steps to make sure that the labels and marketing materials for hormones dispensed by these facilities include the full and accurate information that women need to be able to make an informed decision.

Wyeth, the leading U.S. manufacturer of synthetic hormone treatment, has also written to the FDA. It argued that compounding pharmacies should be subject to the same regulation and oversight as drug companies that sell hormone treatment products. As of spring 2006, both the NWHN and Wyeth were still awaiting FDA action.

OTHER TREATMENTS FOR HEALTHY BONES AND HOT FLASHES

HEALTHY BONES

Nondrug alternatives for making and keeping bones strong include calcium, vitamin D, and regular exercise. Promising interventions focus on reducing the risk of fractures by preventing falls with balance and strength training, making sure that vision prescriptions are up-to-date, checking any prescription drugs for drug interactions that may cause dizziness, eliminating fall-causing hazards in the home, and wearing appropriate shoes. (For more information on getting and keeping healthy bones, see Chapter 16, "Bone Health.")

Some nonhormonal drugs have been shown to reduce the risk of fracture. Both bisphosphonates, like Fosamax, Actonel, and Boniva, and raloxifene (Evista), which is a selective estrogen receptor modulator or SERM, have been approved by the Food and Drug Administration to prevent bone loss and fractures. These drugs seem to have fewer serious risks than hormone treatment, but they are newer and there's little information about how our health will be affected if we take them for more than ten years.

The bisphosphonates have been proven to increase bone density and decrease fractures in women who have osteoporosis.[57] But there is some preliminary and inconclusive evidence that long-term use of these drugs may increase the chance of fracture even while they increase bone density.[58] Long-term use also may make it more difficult for fractures that do occur to heal.[59] These are serious concerns that will take time to resolve as researchers follow women using bisphosphonates over longer periods of time.

Bisphosphonates must be taken first thing in the morning before eating or drinking anything, with a full glass of plain water. The person taking the medication must remain upright without eating or drinking anything else (including other medications) for at least half an hour.

When bisphosphonates first became available, they were prescribed to be taken every day. Because many women found it difficult to fit the multistep process for taking them into a daily morning routine, many experienced problems with the drugs. Now Fosamax and Actonel are available in a formulation that women take weekly, and another bisphosphonate, Boniva, has been approved for monthly use. With less frequent use, most women find it easier to follow the recommended routine.

HOT FLASHES

Scientific research has not demonstrated alternative treatments to be as effective as hormone treatment for hot flashes, but many women find ways to handle hot flashes that don't involve taking hormones. Some women get relief from dietary strategies. Some research shows that paced breathing can decrease the frequency of hot flashes.[60] There is also some promising research on the effectiveness of the herb black cohosh, although it is short-term research, so the safety of using the herb for longer than six months is not known.[61] The National Center for Complementary and Alternative Medicine at the National Institutes of Health is currently conducting research to determine the safety and efficacy of alternative treatments for menopausal symptoms. (For more information on nonhormonal alternatives for menopausal symptoms, see Chapter 5, "Hot Flashes, Night Sweats, and Sleep Disturbances.")

I came up with several coping strategies for hot flashes as alternatives to hormone treatment: avoiding stress, deep breathing, wearing light clothing all year round, avoiding spicy foods, and exercising daily (but not right before bed). Since I've implemented these strategies, I have managed to decrease my hot flash and night sweat frequency and intensity by 50 percent, and things can only get better from this point on. I knew that for women like me, who may no longer have any ovaries, stopping hormone treatment would take a long time. But I also knew that it was doable and, in my view, much better than exposure to the risks.

SURGICALLY AND MEDICALLY INDUCED MENOPAUSE

Some of us experience menopause as a result of surgery or medical treatment. There's less research about the benefits and risks of hormone treatment for women in these circumstances, but we do have some information that can help women decide what to do.

When the ovaries of a woman who has not yet experienced natural menopause are removed, her body produces significantly less estrogen and progesterone. This is known as surgically induced menopause. If a woman has ovarian or uterine cancer, removal of the ovaries is likely to be necessary, but surgeons also commonly remove healthy ovaries when they do a hysterectomy (removal of the uterus). More than half of the more than 600,000 women who have hysterectomies every year also have their ovaries removed in that surgery, even though there is nothing wrong with the ovaries. Some doctors say that this is a cancer prevention strategy, but research has shown that removing healthy ovaries does not offer a clear benefit, and for women under sixty-five whose ovaries are removed, it may increase the risk of dying of heart disease.[62] (The small subset of women with a family history of ovarian cancer may benefit from this prevention strategy, but for most women, it appears to do more harm than good.)

When a woman loses her ovaries, she experiences a sudden drop in hormone levels, which can cause her to experience uncomfortable hot flashes and night sweats. Compared to natural menopause, where hormone levels slowly change and then stabilize over a period of years, surgical menopause forces a woman's body to go through an abrupt withdrawal from hormones. Although there is little scientific data about the severity, frequency, and duration of these physical changes in surgically induced menopause, we do know from women's own reports that surgical menopause can significantly disrupt quality of life.

Medically induced menopause happens when a woman undergoes chemotherapy, radiation, or some other medical treatment that causes her ovaries to stop working. The effect of chemotherapy varies somewhat by age. Younger women (usually under forty) who undergo chemotherapy often—although not always—get normal menstruation back after the treatment ends, but for women over forty, those treatments are likely to trigger the beginning of menopause. There have been some studies testing the use of hormone treatment in women who have had breast cancer, but the WHI finding that the estrogen plus progestin combination increased women's risk of getting breast cancer indicates that taking hormones when one has breast cancer is not a good idea. (For more information on induced menopause, see Chapter 4, "Sudden and Early Menopause." For more information about cancer treatments and menopause, see Chapter 18, "Cancers.")

HORMONE TREATMENT AFTER SURGICAL MENOPAUSE

Many women who take hormone treatment after surgically induced menopause report getting relief similar to that experienced by women who take hormones after natural men-

opause. Specifically, many women report fewer episodes of hot flashes and night sweats. Researchers have also found that younger women who report memory loss after hysterectomies do better on some cognitive tests after beginning to take estrogen, but we don't know whether this is truly an effect of the estrogen or if it might be explained by other factors.[63] For older women, the research evidence is clear: The WHI found that taking estrogen increased the risk for dementia in women over sixty-five who have had hysterectomies.

Little research has examined the health risks of taking hormones for those of us who have had our ovaries removed. The WHI provides some data that is relevant, since all of the women in the estrogen-only part of the study had had hysterectomies, though some of them still had their ovaries. (For a graph summarizing the findings of the WHI for this group, see page 103, Figure 2.) The WHI found that hormone treatment increased the risk of stroke in women who had had hysterectomies. The WHI also indicated there was neither a risk nor a benefit for these women in colorectal cancer or heart attacks, and the effect of hormone treatment on blood clots and breast cancer for these women was uncertain. It is important to note, however, that for women whose ovaries were removed specifically to treat cancer, the risk of either recurrent cancer or other cancers associated with hormone treatment may be greater than for other women.

EARLY NATURAL MENOPAUSE

Sometimes our ovaries stop working before age forty, putting us into what's known as early natural menopause. The medical term for this is *premature ovarian failure.* Just as when it happens later in life, early menopause leads to lower estrogen levels and irregular menstrua-

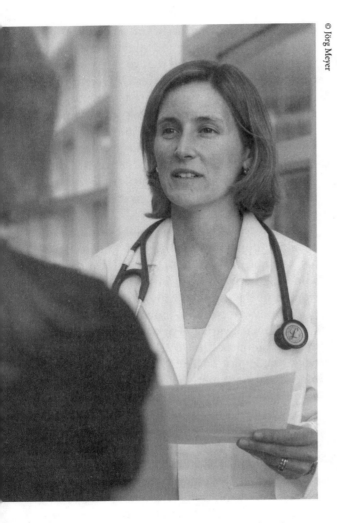

© Jörg Meyer

research evidence showing that the risks are different, women are probably best served by assuming that the risks will be similar.

HORMONES AND TRANSGENDER HEALTH

Hormone treatment is vital for those of us who are transgender and wish to make or maintain (with or without surgery) a physical and psychological transition to a different sex and gender. Hormone treatment allows us to have a body that is more in line with our gender identity, and this can bring a sense of physical and mental well-being; we may therefore be willing to accept health risks that people who are not transgender might consider unacceptable. If we are undergoing hormone treatment related to our gender transition or are considering doing so, we may want to know what that will mean for us in relation to the menopause transition.

For transgender people who are female-to-male (FTM), hormone treatment involving testosterone, or "T," will bring on the cessation of the menstrual cycle, whether permanent or temporary, due to the reduction of estrogen.

For transgender people who are male-to-female (MTF), hormone treatment involves taking estrogen and sometimes antiandrogens. As we age, we experience many of the same health concerns as women who are born female. However, we do not technically experience menopause because we do not have a female reproductive system. The dose of estrogen required for MTF people often is greater than the dose taken by women born female who are taking hormone treatment, which raises concerns about increased risk of adverse effects.

There has been virtually no research done to identify the long-term effects of hormones on transgender people or to understand the men-

tion, which is usually the first sign of early natural menopause that a woman may notice. We don't always know why a woman's ovaries have stopped functioning at an early age, but some causes have been identified and include autoimmune disorders, genetic irregularities/family history, and viral infections. (For more information on early natural menopause, see Chapter 4, "Sudden and Early Menopause.")

At this point, there is not enough scientific data to determine whether women under age forty incur the same risks with hormone treatment as women over age forty. But until there is opause experiences of transgender people. No matter how we use hormones, we may increase the benefits and minimize the risks by working in partnership with a sensitive and competent health care provider, and educating ourselves about our health care risks and concerns. (For more information, see "Hormones and Transgendered Health" at www.ourbodiesour selves.org.)

SHOULD I OR SHOULDN'T I?

I struggle with the flow of information—confusing, contradictory, and not consistent with my experience. All the health professionals I speak to are supportive of my ending hormone treatment . . . but feel I'm fine should I continue to stay on. I wonder whether being on hormones is consistent with being a lifelong feminist. But I feel so good now that it's difficult to consider completely eliminating those little pills.

There is no single answer to the question "Should I or shouldn't I take hormones?" Hormone treatment has been proven to relieve hot flashes and vaginal dryness and to prevent fractures. There are other medicines to prevent fractures, but hormone treatment is the only medicine that is FDA-approved to treat hot flashes and vaginal dryness. Yet it has also been proven to increase the risk of serious illnesses. For the majority of women, who go through the menopause transition without experiencing problems severe enough to interfere with our lives, the risks of hormone treatment outweigh the benefits. It is clear now that the routine use of hormones in healthy women during or after the menopause transition, which was once commonplace, is not recommended. Women who experience severe hot flashes or vaginal dryness may want to consider hormone use, but it is recommended only for the shortest possible time and at the lowest effective dose. Each woman must weigh the risks and benefits to determine whether hormone treatment is appropriate for her.

It is important to know that there is no medical reason to treat menopause. It is a natural and normal stage of our lives. Women who are not experiencing hot flashes or other bothersome physical changes do not need a prescription for hormone treatment, or any other drug, simply because we have reached menopause.

The benefits of hormone treatment in the short term may outweigh the risks for women who are experiencing moderate to severe hot flashes and night sweats and who cannot find relief in another way. If you are considering taking hormones for a purpose other than relief of hot flashes or vaginal dryness or to prevent fractures, you should know that hormone treatment has not been proven to be effective for any other purpose.

If you are considering hormone treatment to help you with one of its proven uses, weigh its benefits against its risks, taking into account your medical history, preferences, and concerns. Consider taking the lowest effective dose for the shortest possible time. If you take hormones, reevaluate your decision regularly in light of changing medical knowledge and your individual situation. Since the research shows that even short-term use of hormones may increase a woman's risk of heart attack, stroke, and blood clots, many women are seeking alternatives to hormones even for those health concerns for which hormones have been proven helpful.

NOTES

1. Robert A. Wilson, *Feminine Forever* (New York: M. Evans, 1966), 19.

2. Gary Null and Barbara Seaman, "Wilson Versus Living Decay," *For Women Only! Your Guide to Health Empowerment* (New York: Seven Stories Press, 1999), 751.

3. Gina Kolata and Melody Petersen, "Hormone Replacement Study: A Shock to the Medical System," *New York Times* (July 10, 2002): A1; see also Amanda Spake, Susan Headden, Katy Kelly, The U.S. News library staff, and Nancy Cohen, "The Menopausal Marketplace," *U.S. News & World Report* 133, no. 19 (November 18, 2002): 42.

4. Madeline Gray, *The Changing Years: What to Do about the Menopause*, 1951, cited in Barbara Seaman, *The Greatest Experiment Ever Performed on Women: Exploding the Estrogen Myth* (New York: Hyperion, 2003), 110.

5. D. C. Smith, R. Prentice, D. J. Thompson, and W. L. Herrmann, "Association of Exogenous Estrogen and Endometrial Carcinoma," *New England Journal of Medicine* 293, no. 23 (December 1975): 1164–67; H. K. Ziel and W. D. Finkle, "Increased Risk of Endometrial Carcinoma among Users of Conjugated Estrogens," *New England Journal of Medicine* 293, no. 23 (December 1975): 1167–70; T. M. Mack, M. C. Pike, B. E. Henderson, R. I. Pfeffer, V. R. Gerkins, M. Arthur, and S. E. Brown, "Estrogens and Endometrial Cancer in a Retirement Community," *New England Journal of Medicine* 294, no. 23 (June 1976): 1262–67.

6. Barbara Seaman and Gideon Seaman, *Women and the Crisis in Sex Hormones* (New York: Bantam, 1977).

7. Nancy Krieger, Ilana Löwy, Robert Aronowitz, Judyann Bigby, Kay Dickersin, Elizabeth Garner, Jean-Paul Gaudillière, Carolina Hinestrosa, Ruth Hubbard, Paula A. Johnson, Stacey A. Missmer, Judy Norsigian, Cynthia Pearson, Charles E. Rosenberg, Lynn Rosenberg, Barbara G. Rosenkrantz, Barbara Seaman, Carlos Sonnenschein, Ana M. Soto, Joe Thornton, George Weisz, "Hormone Replacement Therapy, Cancer, Controversies, and Women's Health: Historical, Epidemiological, Biological, Clinical, and Advocacy Perspectives," *Journal of Epidemiology and Community Health,* 59 (August 2005): 740–48.

8. Stephen Hulley, Deborah Grady, Trudy Bush, Curt Furberg, David Herrington, Betty Riggs, Eric Vittinghoff, for the Heart and Estrogen/Progestin Replacement Study (HERS) Research Group, "Randomized Trial of Estrogen plus Progestin for Secondary Prevention of Coronary Heart Disease in Postmenopausal Women," *JAMA* 280, no. 7 (August 1998): 605–13.

9. Judith K. Ockene, David H. Barad, Barbara B. Cochrane, Joseph C. Larson, Margery Gass, Sylvia Wassertheil-Smoller, JoAnn E. Manson, Vanessa M. Barnabei, Dorothy S. Lane, Robert G. Brzyski, Milagros C. Rosal, Judy Wylie-Rosett, and Jennifer Hays, "Symptom Experience after Discontinuing Use of Estrogen+Progestin," *JAMA* 294, no. 2 (July 2005): 183–93.

10. Million Women Study Collaborators, "Breast Cancer and Hormone-Replacement Therapy in the Million Women Study," *Lancet* 362, no. 9382 (August 2003): 419–27.

11. Writing Group for the Women's Health Initiative Investigators, "Risks and Benefits of Estrogen Plus Progestin in Healthy Postmenopausal Women," *JAMA* 288, no. 3 (July 2002): 321–33; Sally A. Shumaker, Claudine Legault, Stephen R. Rapp, Leon Thal, Robert B. Wallace, Judith K. Ockene, Susan L. Hendrix, Beverly N. Jones III, Annlouise R. Assaf, Rebecca D. Jackson, Jane Morley Kotchen, Sylvia Wassertheil-Smoller, and Jean Wactawski-Wende, for the WHIMS Investigators, "Estrogen Plus Progestin and the Incidence of Dementia and Mild Cognitive Impairment in Postmenopausal Women: The Women's Health Initiative Memory Study: A Randomized Controlled Trial," *JAMA* 289, no. 20 (May 2003): 2651–62.

12. The Women's Health Initiative Steering Committee, "Effects of Conjugated Equine Estrogen in Postmenopausal Women with Hysterectomy," *JAMA* 291, no. 14 (April 2004): 1701–12; Sally A. Shumaker, Claudine Legault, Lewis Kuller, Stephen R. Rapp, Leon Thal, Dorothy S. Lane, Howard Fillit, Marcia L. Stefanick, Susan L. Hendrix, Cora E. Lewis, Kamal Masaki, and Laura H. Coker, for the Women's Health

Initiative Memory Study, "Conjugated Equine Estrogens and Incidence of Probable Dementia and Mild Cognitive Impairment in Postmenopausal Women," *JAMA* 291, no. 24 (June 2004): 2947–58.

13. Writing Group for the Women's Health Initiative Investigators, 321–33. Sally A. Shumaker et al., "Estrogen Plus Progestin," 2651–62.

14. The Women's Health Initiative Steering Committee, 1701–12. Shumaker et al., "Conjugated Equine Estrogens," 2947–58.

15. NIH State of the Science Panel, "National Institutes of Health State-of-the-Science Conference Statement: Management of Menopause-Related Symptoms," *Annals of Internal Medicine* 142, no. 12 (June 2005): 1003–13.

16. J. Hsia et al., "Conjugated Equine Estrogens and Coronary Heart Disease," *Archives of Internal Medicine* 166 (2006): 357–65.

17. Heidi D. Nelson, Elizabeth Haney, Linda Humphrey, Jill Miller, Anne Nedrow, Christina Nicolaidis, Kimberly Vesco, Miranda Walker, Christina Bougatsos, and Peggy Nygren, "Management of Menopause-Related Symptoms," *Evidence Report/Technology Assessment,* Agency of Healthcare Research and Quality, March 2005, accessed at www.ahrq.gov/clinic/epc sums/menosum.pdf on August 8, 2005.

18. U.S. Department of Health and Human Services, *Bone Health and Osteoporosis: A Report of the Surgeon General* (Rockville, MD: U.S. Department of Health and Human Services, Office of the Surgeon General, 2004), 229–30.

19. Writing Group for the Women's Health Initiative Investigators, 321–33.

20. Susan L. Hendrix, Barbara B. Cochrane, Ingrid E. Nygaard, Victoria L. Handa, Vanessa M. Barnabei, Cheryl Iglesia, Aaron Aragaki, Michelle J. Naughton, Robert B. Wallace, and S. Gene McNeeley, "Effects of Estrogen with and without Progestin on Urinary Incontinence," *JAMA* 293, no. 8 (February 2005): 935–48.

21. Mark A. Espeland, Stephen R. Rapp, Sally A. Shumaker, Robert Brunner, JoAnn E. Manson, Barbara B. Sherwin, Judith Hsia, Karen L. Margolis, Patricia E. Hogan, Robert Wallace, Maggie Dailey, Ruth Freeman, and Jennifer Hays, "Conjugated Equine Estrogens and Incidence of Probable Dementia and Mild Cognitive Impairment in Postmenopausal Women: Women's Health Initiative Memory Study," *JAMA* 291, no. 24 (June 2004): 2959–68; see also Shumaker et al., "Estrogen Plus Progestin," 2651–62; Stephen R. Rapp, Mark A. Espeland, Sally A. Shumaker, Victor W. Henderson, Robert L. Brunner, JoAnn E. Manson, Margery L. S. Gass, Marcia L. Stefanick, Dorothy S. Lane, Jennifer Hays, Karen C. Johnson, Laura H. Coker, Maggie Dailey, and Deborah Bowen, "Effect of Estrogen Plus Progestin on Global Cognitive Function in Postmenopausal Women: The Women's Health Initiative Memory Study: A Randomized Controlled Trial," *JAMA* 289, no. 20 (May 2003): 2663–72.

22. Smith et al., 1164–67; Ziel and Finkle, 1167–70.

23. Writing Group for the Women's Health Initiative Investigators, 321–33.

24. NIH State of the Science Panel.

25. Ibid.

26. Ibid.

27. U.S. Department of Health and Human Services.

28. Wendy Y. Chen, JoAnn E. Manson, Susan E. Hankinson, Bernard Rosner, Michelle D. Holmes, Walter C. Willett, and Graham A. Colditz, "Unopposed Estrogen Therapy and the Risk of Invasive Breast Cancer," *Archives of Internal Medicine* 166 (2006): 1,027–32.

29. Lynn Rosenberg, Julie R. Palmer, Lauren A. Wise, and Lucile L. Adams-Campbell, "A Prospective Study of Female Hormone Use and Breast Cancer Among Black Women," *Archives of Internal Medicine* 166 (2006) 760–65.

30. Ockene et al.

31. Garnet L. Anderson, Howard L. Judd, Andrew M. Kaunitz, David H. Barad, Shirley A. A. Beresford, Mary Pettinger, James Liu, S. Gene McNeeley, Ana Maria Lopez, "Effects of Estrogen Plus Progestin on Gynecologic Cancers and Associated Diagnostic Procedures," *JAMA* 290, no. 13 (October 2003): 1739–48.

32. Carmen Rodriguez, Alpa V. Patel, Eugenia E. Calle, Eric J. Jacob, and Michael J. Thun, "Estrogen Replace-

ment Therapy and Ovarian Cancer Mortality in a Large Prospective Study of US Women," *JAMA* 285, no. 11 (March 2001): 1460–65.

33. Pushkal P. Garg, Karla Kerlikowske, Leslee Subak, and Deborah Grady, "Hormone Replacement Therapy and the Risk of Epithelial Ovarian Carcinoma: A Meta-analysis," *Obstetrics and Gynecology* 92, no. 3 (September 1998): 472–79.

34. U.S. Preventive Services Task Force, "Hormone Therapy for the Prevention of Chronic Conditions in Postmenopausal Women: Recommendations from the U.S. Preventive Services Task Force," *Annals of Internal Medicine* 142, no. 10 (May 2005): 855–60.

35. U.S. Food and Drug Administration, "Guidance for Industry: Estrogen and Estrogen/Progestin Drug Products to Treat Vasomotor Symptoms and Vulvar and Vaginal Atrophy Symptoms—Recommendations for Clinical Evaluation," U.S. Department of Health and Human Services Food and Drug Administration Center for Drug Evaluation and Research (CDER), January 2003, accessed at www.fda.gov/cder/guidance/5412dft.pdf on August 8, 2005.

36. Ibid.

37. Ibid.

38. Rodriguez et al.

39. David F. Archer, for the EstroGel Study Group, "Percutaneous 17β-estradiol Gel for the Treatment of Vasomotor Symptoms in Postmenopausal Women," *Menopause* 10, no. 6 (2003): 516–21.

40. N. N. Sarkar, "Low-Dose Intravaginal Estradiol Delivery Using a Silastic Vaginal Ring for Estrogen Replacement Therapy in Postmenopausal Women: A Review," *European Journal of Contraception and Reproductive Health Care* 8, no. 3 (December 2003): 217–24.

41. V. L. Baker, "Alternatives to Oral Estrogen Replacement: Transdermal Patches, Percutaneous Gels, Vaginal Creams and Rings, Implants, Other Methods of Delivery," *Obstetrics and Gynecology Clinics of North America* 21, no. 2 (1994): 271–97.

42. U.S. Food and Drug Administration, "FDA Revises Finding on Estrogen/Androgen Combination Products in the Treatment of Hot Flashes," U.S. Department of Health and Human Services Food and Drug Administration Center for Drug Evaluation and Research (CDER), April 2003, accessed at www.fda.gov/bbs/topics/ANSWERS/2003/ANS01210.html on August 3, 2005.

43. The North American Menopause Society, "The Role of Testosterone Therapy in Postmenopausal Women: Position Statement of the North American Menopause Society," *Menopause* 12, no. 5 (September 1, 2005): 497–511. For a critique of this position paper, see Leonore Tiefer, "Omissions, Biases, and Nondisclosed Conflicts of Interest: Is There a Hidden Agenda in the NAMS Position Statement?" *Contemporary Issues in Ob/Gyn & Women's Health, Medscape General Medicine* 7, no. 3 (September 26, 2005): 59, available at www.medscape.com/viewarticle/513099.

44. U.S. Food and Drug Administration, "Advisory Committee Briefing Document: Intrinsa (testosterone transdermal system) NDA No. 21-769, "Proctor & Gamble Pharmaceuticals, Inc., December 2004, accessed at www.fda/gov/ohrms/dockets/ac/04/briefing/2004-4082B1_01_A-P&G-Intrinsa.pdf on August 8, 2005.

45. U.S. Food and Drug Administration, "Advisory Committee for Reproductive Health Drugs, Meeting Transcript," U.S. Department of Health and Human Services Food and Drug Administration Center for Drug Evaluation and Research (CDER), December 2004, accessed at www.fda.gov/ohrms/dockets/ac/04/transcripts/2004-4082T1.htm on August 8, 2005.

46. Rudolf Kaaks, Franco Berrino, Timothy Key, Sabina Rinaldi, Laure Dossus, Carine Biessy, Giorgio Secreto, Pilar Amiano, Sheila Bingham, Heiner Boeing, H. Bas Bueno de Mesquita, Jenny Chang-Claude, Françoise Clavel-Chapelon, Agnès Fournier, Carla H. van Gils, Carlos A. Gonzalez, Aurelio Barricarte Gurrea, Elena Critselis, Kay Tee Khaw, Vittorio Krogh, Petra H. Lahmann, Gabriele Nagel, Anja Olsen, N. Charlotte Onland-Moret, Kim Overvad, Domenico Palli, Salvatore Panico, Petra Peeters, J. Ramón Quirós, Andrew Roddam, Anne Thiebaut, Anne Tjønneland, Ma Dolores Chirlaque, Antonia Trichopoulou, Dimitrios Trichopoulos, Rosario Tumino, Paolo Vineis, Teresa

Norat, Pietro Ferrari, Nadia Slimani, Elio Riboli, "Serum Sex Steroids in Premenopausal Women and Breast Cancer Risk within the European Prospective Investigation into Cancer and Nutrition (EPIC)," *Journal of the National Cancer Institute* 97, no. 10 (May 2005): 755–65; Stacey A. Missmer, A. Heather Eliassen, Robert L. Barbieri, and Susan E. Hankinson, "Endogenous Estrogen, Androgen, and Progesterone Concentrations and Breast Cancer Risk among Postmenopausal Women," *Journal of the National Cancer Institute* 96, no. 24 (December 2004): 1856–65; Valerie Beral for the Million Women Study Collaborators, "Breast Cancer and Hormone-Replacement Therapy in the Million Women Study," *Lancet* 362, no. 9382 (August 2003): 419–27.

47. L. Holmberg and H. Anderson for the HABITS steering and data monitoring committees, "HABITS (Hormonal Replacement Therapy after Breast Cancer—Is It Safe?), a Randomised Comparison: Trial Stopped," *Lancet* 363, no. 9407 (February 2004): 453–55.

48. Janet R. Guthrie, John R. Taffe, Philippe Lehert, Henry G. Burger, Lorraine Dennerstein, "Association between Hormonal Changes at Menopause and the Risk of a Coronary Event: A Longitudinal Study," *Menopause* 11, no. 3 (May/June 2004): 315–22; Kim Sutton-Tyrrell, Rachel P. Wildman, Karen A. Matthews, Claudia Chae, Bill L. Lasley, Sarah Brockwell, Richard C. Pasternak, Donald Lloyd-Jones, Mary Fran Sowers, Javier I. Torréns, "Sex Hormone-Binding Globulin and the Free Androgen Index Are Related to Cardiovascular Risk Factors in Multiethnic Premenopausal and Perimenopausal Women Enrolled in the Study of Women Across the Nation (SWAN)," *Circulation* 111, no. 10 (March 2005): 1242–49; Gerald B. Phillips, Bruce H. Pinkernell, Tian-Yi Jing, "Relationship between Serum Sex Hormones and Coronary Artery Disease in Postmenopausal Women," *Arteriosclerosis, Thrombosis, and Vascular Biology* 17, no. 4 (April 1997): 695–701.

49. Judith R. Gerber, Julia V. Johnson, Janice Y. Bunn, and Susan L. O'Brien, "A Longitudinal Study of the Effects of Free Testosterone and Other Psychosocial Variables on Sexual Function During the Natural Transverse of Menopause," *Fertility and Sterility* 83, no. 3 (March 2005): 643–48; see also A. Nyunt, G. Stephen, J. Gibbin, L. Durgan, A. M. Fielding, M. Wheeler, and D. E. Price, "Androgen Status in Healthy Premenopausal Women with Loss of Libido," *Journal of Sex and Marital Therapy* 31, no. 1 (January–February 2005): 73–80; and Susan R. Davis, Sonia L. Davison, Susan Donath, and Robin J. Bell, "Circulating Androgen Levels and Self-Reported Sexual Function in Women," *JAMA* 294 (2005): 91–96.

50. Paola Albertazzi, Francesco Pansini, Gloria Bonaccorsi, Laura Zanotti, Elena Forini, and Domenico De Aloysio, "The Effect of Dietary Soy Supplementation on Hot Flushes," *Obstetrics and Gynecology* 91 (January 1998): 6–11; A. Brezinski, H. Adlercreutz, R. Shaoul, et al., "Short-Term Effects of Phytoestrogen-Rich Diet on Postmenopausal Women," *Menopause* 4, no. 2 (1997): 89–94; A. L. Murkies, C. Lombard, B. J. G. Strauss, G. Wilcox, H. G. Burger, and M. S. Morton, "Dietary Flour Supplementation Decreases Postmenopausal Hot Flushes: Effect of Soy and Wheat," *Maturitas* 21, no. 3 (April 1995): 189–95.

51. F. S. Dalais, G. E. Rice, M. L. Dahlquist, M. Grehan, A. L. Murkies, G. Medley, R. Ayton, and B. J. B. Strauss, "Effect of Dietary Phytoestrogens in Postmenopausal Women," *Climacteric* 1 (1998): 124–29; G. Wilcox, M. L. Wahlquist, H. G. Burger, and G. Medley, "Oestrogenic Effects of Plant Foods in Postmenopausal Women," *British Medical Journal* 301 (1990): 905–906.

52. Seth Granberg, Pekka Ylöstalo, Matts Wikland, and Bengt Karlsson, "Endometrial Sonographic and Histologic Findings in Women with and without Hormonal Replacement Therapy Suffering from Postmenopausal Bleeding," *Maturitas* 27, no. 1 (May 1997): 35–40; Elisabete Weiderpass, John A. Baron, Hans-Olov Adami, Cecilia Magnusson, Anders Lindgren, Reinhold Bergström, Nestor Correia, and Ingemar Persson, "Low-Potency Oestrogen and Risk of Endometrial Cancer: A Case-control Study," *Lancet* 353, no. 9167 (May 1999): 1824–28.

53. Helene B. Leonetti, Santo Longo, and James N. Anasti, "Transdermal Progesterone Cream for Vasomotor Symptoms and Postmenopausal Bone Loss," *Obstetrics and Gynecology* 94, no. 2 (August 1999): 225–28.

54. Granberg et al.; Weiderpass et al.

55. B. Leonetti et al.

56. A. Cooper, C. Spencer, M. I. Whitehead, et al., "Systemic Absorption of Progesterone from Progest Cream in Postmenopausal Women," *Lancet* 351 (1998): 1255–56.

57. U.S. Department of Health and Human Services, *Bone Health and Osteoporosis*.

58. Susan M. Ott, "Long-Term Safety of Bisphosphonates (Editorial)," *Journal of Clinical Endocrinology and Metabolism,* 90 (March 2005): 1897–99; Kristine E. Ensrud, Elizabeth L. Barrett-Connor, Ann Schwartz, Arthur C. Santora, Douglas C. Bauer, Shailaja Suryawanshi, Adrianne Feldstein, William L. Haskell, Marc C. Hochberg, James C. Torner, Antonio Lombardi, Dennis M. Black, for the Fracture Intervention Trial Long-Term Extension Research Group, "Randomized Trial of Effect of Alendronate Continuation versus Discontinuation in Women with Low BMD: Results from the Fracture Intervention Trial Long-Term Extension," *Journal of Bone and Mineral Research* 19, no. 8 (August 2004): 1259–69.

59. Ibid.

60. R. R. Freedman and S. Woodward, "Behavioral Treatment of Menopausal Hot Flushes: Evaluation by Ambulatory Monitoring," *American Journal of Obstetrics and Gynecology* 167, no. 2 (1992): 436–39; R. R. Freedman, S. Woodward, B. Brown, J. I. Javaid, and G. N. Pandley, "Biochemical and Thermoregulatory Effects of Behavioral Treatment for Menopausal Hot Flashes," *Menopause* 2 (1995): 211–18.

61. G. Warnecke, "Beeinflussung klimakterischer Beschwerden durch ein Phytotherapeutikum: Erfolgreiche Therapie mit Cimicifuga-Monoextrakt [Influence of Phytotherapy on Menopausal Syndrome: Successful Treatments with Monoextract of Cimicifuga]," *Medizinische Welt* 36 (1985): 871–74; see also W. Stoll, "Phytotherapeutikum beeinflusst Atrophisches Vaginalepithel: Doppelblindversuch Cimicifuga vs. Estrogenpräparat [Phytotherapy Influences Atrophic Vaginal Epithelium—Doubleblind Study—Cimicifuga vs. Estrogenic Substances]," *Therapeutikon* 1 (1987): 23–31; E. Lehmann-Willenbrock and H. Riedel, "Klinische und endokrinologische Untersuchungen zur Therapie ovarieller Ausfallserscheinungen nach Hysterektomie unter Belassung der Adnexe [Clinical and Endocrinological Examinations Concerning Therapy of Climacteric Symptoms Following Hysterectomy with Remaining Ovaries], *Zentralblatt für Gynäkologie* 110 (1988): 611–18.

62. William H. Parker, Michael S. Broder, Zhimei Liu, Donna Shoupe, Cindy Farquhar, and Jonathan S. Berek, "Ovarian Conservation at the Time of Hysterectomy for Benign Disease," *Obstetrics and Gynecology* 106, no. 2 (August 2005): 219–26.

63. Barbara Sherwin, "Surgical Menopause, Estrogen, and Cognitive Function in Women: What Do the Findings Tell Us?" *Annals of New York Academy of Science* 1052 (2005): 3–10.

Changing Selves, Changing Relationships

CHAPTER 8

Body Image

A grown woman should not have to masquerade as a girl in order to remain in the land of the living.[1]

The menopause transition offers us an opportunity to give up the "masquerade" of eternal youth. We need not impersonate the white adolescent girl who is venerated in our culture, especially in the mass media. Rather, we can redefine and embody what it means to be a grown, wise, and beautiful woman. We can change the scripts in new and radical ways for ourselves, our daughters, and future generations. We can "decline to decline"[2] as we grow older and refuse to embrace the culture's rigid definitions of beauty, sexual attractiveness, and importance.

From the time we are little girls, we are judged by our appearance. By adolescence, it becomes clear that our worth as females is often measured by how we look, rather than by our accomplishments. Many of us begin to experience comments about our looks and are the recipients of stares and sexual advances.[3] We often begin to see a relationship between physical attractiveness and dating experiences, job discrimination, educational achievements, and career success.[4] During the teenage years, many of us develop a dislike for our bodies that can last a lifetime.[5]

Our feelings about our bodies can change at midlife. It can be upsetting when our thick hair becomes a bit thinner or the fine lines in our face become more

"Take another look."

MARGARET MORGANROTH GULLETTE

In my youth there was scarcely a part of my body I could look at without critique. But over time I made peace with parts I had disliked for decades. My "broad peasant feet," for instance, began to look shapely. The toes were charming.

Like many women touched by feminism, I was overcoming the self-hatred learned while having had a younger female body in patriarchal, capitalist America. Thank the goddess for no longer being young.

And so in the shower one morning, I made a discovery. As I was twisting to look back down my side, the curves of hip, buttock, thigh, calf, and ankle came into view—startlingly elegant, powerful, and voluptuous. It was a view a painter might love. But had I ever seen an image created from the point of view of a woman looking at her body from above? Never. Certainly no ad had captured those satisfying curves. The assumption of our culture is not just ageist but middle-ageist—that decline starts not in old age but even as early as thirty.

Now, every time I look down at that arrangement of hip and leg I am rewarded. Since I am in my sixties in a culture increasingly obsessed with adolescent bodies, this jolt of pleasure is rare.

The real discovery may be why I can admire these parts of the "aging" corpus: precisely *because* no ad focuses on them. I hadn't learned to hate them. Fortunately for my graceful lower extremities, the frowning eye of the perfection industries has devised no product to improve that view.

Rescued from advertising's mean scrutiny, I offer you the same pleasure. Take another look. Nothing wrong with some healthy narcissism once a day, in a steamy bathroom filled with soothing aromas. Women aging-past-youth can enjoy such a sight for decades. Suppose that every day, just for a minute, every single woman in America loved that much of her body. What a different attitude toward ourselves and others we would carry out into the world.

When friends complain about their bodily "aging," offering a sorry list of what they don't like about their skin, their weight, their hair color, or their muscle tone, my new insight suggests not falling into masochistic empathy. Rather than say, "Yes, I hate mine too," we need to ask, "Isn't that product placement speaking?" or "If the perfection industries didn't make billions on constructing our misery, would we be worrying so much about our hair, our abs, our waists?" Why reinforce women's supposed ugliness in the guise of friendship? Why provide personalized commercials for the commerce in aging?

Focusing instead on what we learn to find lovely, in time we could praise the whole body-mind—its spirit, character, charm, responsiveness. What a taunt to the relentless American cult of youth. It feels good.[6]

pronounced. But many of us discover a new freedom, too, as we leave behind some of our earlier body scrutiny, chronic dieting, and worries about our appearance. While most women consistently wish to be thinner throughout our lives, by midlife some of us worry less about our appearance and weight.[7]

Women after menopause are more likely to accept our bodies than premenopausal women.[8] As one sixty-one-year-old woman put it,

My body image has nothing to do with menopause, it has to do with where I am in my phase of life currently. The reality is I will never run the marathon, be taller, have straight hair, and have unwrinkled skin. It is fine.

EFFECTS OF LOW SELF-ESTEEM

The loss of a youthful appearance, so valued by Western culture, as well as the emotional and social changes that may accompany menopause and aging can hurt our self-esteem. We are also affected by the ageism of our culture. The changes we see at midlife can be disconcerting; sometimes we perceive them as losses. Some research indicates that these changes in body image have a significant impact on our sexual desire and our sexual self-esteem at midlife.[9]

Poor body image and low self-esteem may contribute to problems associated with menopause. For example, several studies have found that a negative attitude about menopause contributes to the severity of depression and headaches; this suggests that when we emphasize the losses rather than the benefits of menopause, severe problems are more likely for some of us.[10] For some of us, negative experiences that appear to be about menopause may be more related to low self-esteem than to the depletion of hormones. Gaining understanding of cultural influences, self-esteem, and the physical and emotional changes associated

with menopause can help us feel empowered during this stage of our lives.[11] (For more information, see Chapter 11, "Emotional Well-Being and Managing Stress.")

ATTITUDES TOWARD AGING

My mirrors at home began to lie to me a few years ago. When I get dressed in the morning and look in a mirror to comb my hair and put on a little makeup, I see a middle-aged woman whose face has just a few lines and whose blond hair has begun to turn gray. This woman is no longer slim, as she used to be, and although her clothes are not as flattering on her body as they were at one time, still she tries to stand tall and do the best she can with what she has. Yet, when I catch sight of myself in a mirror away from home or see a photograph of myself, I am amazed. Do I look like that? Do others see me like that? That woman's face has quite a few lines, her hair is white, and she is much wider around the middle than she realizes.

Our feelings about our bodies are often a result of the attitudes we hold about aging. In recent American culture, the primary discussion of aging in women has centered on menopause as the one defining moment of midlife, and this discussion has often provided us with misleading information that comes from medical models of disease, societal stereotypes, and assumptions. Additionally, our mothers and grandmothers were often silent about their own bodies and their experiences of menopause and aging, or they may have subscribed to a type of false cheerfulness required by a society that restricted us from talking freely with one another about our bodies and our health.[12] One fifty-six-year-old woman says,

I often wonder why my mother and other women of her generation never spoke of the disappoint-

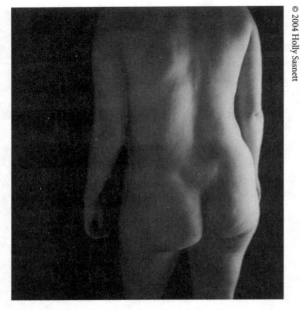

© 2004 Holly Sassett

This photo was taken as part of the ongoing photographic series Body Revisited, a project that helps women with eating disorders gain a different perspective on their bodies.

ments and losses of aging. I believe they were better, stronger, wiser, and less whiny than I. But the silence certainly left me baffled and surprised.

Some of us have come to believe that if we exercise "enough," consume the "right" vitamins, eat the "perfect" foods, and choose the "best" health care provider, we will be assured of total control over our bodies. As a result, we sometimes believe that if we experience hot flashes, wrinkled skin, vaginal dryness, and weight gain, we have somehow failed. When our bodies refuse to perform the way we want, we may feel betrayed. One woman says,

At midlife, I have one word for you—traitor. How could you do this to me? For thirty years, I have taken you to the gym at the ungodly hour of six A.M., where I've stepped, aerobicized, swum, and spun. I've provided you with fresh vegetables,

whole grains, and excellent wines, fed you vitamins and hormones and had sex more times than the national average. And for what? So my waistline could expand into the next clothing size, my breasts look like those of any eighty-eight-year-old, and my butt drop?

SUDDEN AND EARLY MENOPAUSE

Those of us who experience early menopause may feel a more negative effect on our body image and attitudes than women who go through menopause at the usual age.[13] If we have had our ovaries surgically removed, there is no period of gradual physical or emotional adjustment, and we may feel an abrupt sense of loss.

Those of us whose early menopause is due to cancer treatments sometimes report little change in our body images.[14] Still, others of us who are cancer survivors with early menopause talk of the paradox and ambiguity of "experiencing a different body" yet not fitting the description of the average menopausal woman.[15] For some of us, survival issues take precedence over the confrontation of age and menopause.[16]

SOCIAL AND MEDIA INFLUENCES

The idea of physical perfection that dominates Western culture is largely promoted by the mass media. For women, this ideal of perfection is embodied by thin, young, and mostly white women. We are held to rigid standards of appearance and we are subject to sexual objectification that men are not.[17]

Feelings of acceptance and support from significant individuals in our lives can help us resist the media's negative influences.[18] In addition, a woman who is involved in a positive intimate relationship with a partner whom she perceives to be satisfied with her body tends to feel increased

BREAST IMPLANTS

Advertising geared to midlife women is increasing, with many ads featuring opportunities for "body sculpting" and reducing signs of "aging." Not surprising, breast implants are growing in popularity as a means to eliminate "sagging" breasts or to increase breast size. As is the case with much cosmetic surgery promotion, the "before and after" photos do not convey the full range of possible outcomes, some of them quite painful and disfiguring.

Silicone gel breast implants are especially problematic. The largest, best-designed studies suggest increased risk of serious problems and are anything but reassuring.[19] Nonetheless, in the summer of 2005, the FDA expressed its intention to allow silicone implants to be marketed to the general public, if certain conditions could be met. If the FDA approves silicone gel breast implants, it would be in spite of the opposition of its own scientists, who concluded that important safety data were lacking and that more research was needed before general approval of these devices. (Silicone implants had already been available, in poorly conducted clinical trials, to most women seeking reconstruction after mastectomy and to many women whose breasts sagged. FDA approval would make the implants available to everyone, regardless of age or reason for wanting breast implants.)

A more complete picture of the risks of silicone gel implants is available at www.breastimplantinfo.org. In addition, the FDA offers a pamphlet and a booklet that include photographs and describe many of the problems women experience with breast implants (for example, capsular contracture, infection, and necrosis).* The additional problem of silicone's leaking and spreading to other parts of the body, after an implant breaks, needs much further study, especially in terms of immune system problems that may develop.

Many women believe that breast implants will make them feel better about themselves and more satisfied with their lives. Studies do not bear this out, however; in fact, implant makers' own studies show that women tend to have slightly lower self-esteem and less satisfaction with their lives two years after getting breast implants, compared to before.[20] Moreover, many women—especially older women—have to have multiple surgeries before achieving an "acceptable" result.

The marketing of implants reinforces the idea that implants are a safe choice that helps women be the best that we can be. Resisting the idea that implants are the ideal solution to dissatisfactions with our bodies is not easy, especially given the way our culture worships youthfulness and large breasts. But such resistance, accompanied by the ability to appreciate and accept our aging bodies, may help us to preserve our health and well-being—and our good looks—for many years longer.

* These are available online at www.fda.gov/cdrh/breastimplants/indexbip.html and www.fda.gov/cdrh/breastimplants/breast_implants_photos.html.

satisfaction with her body and be buffered from the culture's emphasis on thinness.[21]

But poor body image continues to be a problem, and it's not just young women and girls who suffer from it. Some of us in midlife are vulnerable to disordered eating, anxiety, and depression, particularly if we see our body changes as deficits and sources of shame and guilt. Estimates of the number of women between forty and forty-nine years old who enter eating disorders programs have doubled in the last decade.[22] Some research suggests that approximately 79 percent of deaths related to anorexia occur in women over forty-five years old.[23] Several researchers cite the median age of death for anorexic women to be sixty-nine.[24] However, explanations for these mortality rates are elusive. Some research suggests that there may be a late-onset anorexia or a late reappearance of an anorexia that had been in remission.[25] Societal attitudes and values have changed dramatically in the past thirty years in terms of how we think and feel about our bodies, and the driving force in this change appears to be the emphasis on thinness.[26] Researchers have documented a significant increase in full-body depictions of thin fashion models in the media and suggested that such images may contribute to the increase in eating disorders in American women.[27] We are subjected to approximately 3,000 advertisements a day through newspapers, the Internet, magazines, direct mail, and television.[28] The images reflected in these advertisements almost always feature thinness and youth as measures of our importance, success, and sexuality.

Because of this pervasive imagery, we end up comparing our bodies to those of women who are unusually and sometimes unhealthily thin and often enhanced by cosmetic surgery. The photos of these women are also almost always digitally altered. Many of the older women we see in the media have had cosmetic surgery and other procedures that mask their real age. Natural-looking women over age fifty are virtually nonexistent in the mass media, whether it's in movies or on the evening news.

In our popular culture, we rarely see the bodies and faces of mothers and grandmothers who have nurtured future generations. We rarely see images of those of us who work eighteen hours a day in the care and service of others. We rarely see images of those of us who are ill or have disabilities, those of us who are poor, overweight, or old.

For many of us, the media images confirm our perceived loss of social power and value at midlife. We are no longer reflected in what we read and view. In prime-time network programs between 1993 and 2002, for example, women between the ages of fifty and sixty-four were depicted as elderly rather than middle-aged, and as female characters aged, they became less significant to the story.[29] In prime-time and daytime television, more men at midlife appear than women, and when those of us in our middle years do appear, it is more likely that we will be depicted in more negative ways.[30] Some have described such depictions as reflecting our society's contempt for women who do not measure up to our culture's ideal of beauty, mainly those of us at midlife and in our later years and those of us who are overweight.[31]

The pressure to replicate the media's beauty ideals affects women of all races and socioeconomic groups. One African-American woman describes her struggle with media images:

I want to make peace and accept that my body does not totally define me. I want to rid myself of thoughts that serve to undermine my full potential in life. . . . And yet every day the images projected on the screen and in magazines remind me that I am not among that select group. Even though I know all about the "false" nature of the image, I also know it is used for the basis of comparisons, comparisons that I use against myself.

COSMETIC SURGERY

In the quest for youth and beauty, many women (and increasingly men) turn to cos-

ADVERTISING OUR AGE

"Advertising has always warned women about the dangers of showing any signs of aging, usually by using very young models to hawk products designed to ward off the ravages of time," says Jean Kilbourne, author of *Can't Buy My Love: How Advertising Changes the Way We Think and Feel.* "Oil of Olay avoids this irony and disconnection by not using a model at all. The sexy lingerie spilling out of the drawer is all we need to make us imagine a vibrant, youthful, and completely desirable woman, kept that way through the magic of the product. The copy that says, 'So what if you're not really 28' makes it clear that this is the age one should be aiming for and also that it is never too soon to begin using this product.

"Women are made to be almost as terrified of aging as they are of gaining weight. The stakes are high," Kilbourne says. "A woman who shows up in public with a wrinkled face is an object of pity or contempt. How could she let herself go like that? How dare she remind us that we are all inevitably decaying, that we will one day die? How much better to 'bury the evidence'—as if growing older were a crime."

LIE ABOUT YOUR AGE.
BURY THE EVIDENCE.

total effects

7

Improves appearance of:
1. fine lines and wrinkles
2. age spots
3. texture
4. tone
5. dullness
6. dryness
7. pores

So what if you're not really 28. Your secret's safe with Olay Total Effects Night Firming Cream. Powerfully fights seven signs of aging while you sleep. But your secret is not safe in the medicine cabinet. Curious people can't help but peek. Also try Total Effects 7X— powers out signs of aging all day. Visit Olay.com for a free sample.

OLAY
love the skin you're in

metic surgery. According to the American Society for Aesthetic Plastic Surgery, 10.7 million women had surgical and nonsurgical cosmetic procedures in the United States in 2004.[32] Currently, the most common cosmetic surgery procedures for women are liposuction, breast

MAINTAINING HEALTHY SKIN

To maintain skin health, we need to keep it clean and protected. Here are some other suggestions:

1. Use a sun protector factor (SPF) of at least 15 to 20 even on overcast days. The sunscreen should block both UVA and UVB rays. Wear protective clothing.*
2. Exercise. Staying active is reported to decrease premature aging by providing oxygen to the tissues.[33]
3. Eat well. A diet rich in protein, fruits, vegetables, water, and vitamins C and E maintains healthy skin.
4. Don't smoke. The nicotine from cigarettes prevents blood, oxygen, and nutrients from entering body tissues.
5. Avoid using products that might dry the skin (such as alcohol-based lotions, soaps, and creams; talc powders have been related to yeast infections and ovarian cancer).
6. Avoid cosmetics containing dyes and phthalates. These are chemicals associated with a disruption in hormone function and to rising cases of uterine problems in women.[34]
7. Check your skin for changes on a regular basis. The American Academy of Dermatology recommends skin checks as part of regular physical exams for women and men in midlife.

* There is some controversy about the benefits of using sunscreen all the time, because exposure to the sun helps our bodies synthesize vitamin D. Ten to fifteen minutes of sun exposure without sunscreen at least two times per week is generally recommended to provide adequate vitamin D. If you have limited sun exposure (as do many people in northern climates in the winter) or choose to use sunscreen all the time to protect your skin, include good sources of vitamin D in your diet.

augmentation, eyelid surgery, tummy tuck, and face lift.[35]

The only reasons for cosmetic surgery are to improve the body's appearance and to enhance self-esteem.[36] (This is quite different from reconstructive surgery, which is generally performed in response to trauma, abnormalities, or disease and is intended to improve function or project a normal appearance.)[37] Of course, wanting to look good is a common goal. In many cultures throughout history, people have modified the human body to make it more attractive according to the standards of the day. We tend to see some past modifications—foot binding, for example, and the use of corsets that distorted women's rib cages—as barbaric, yet today's efforts to "improve" the female body also can have harmful physical effects (see "Breast Implants," page 129, for one example). Some plastic surgeons clearly describe their surgical field as "experimental," relatively new, and often marked by an incomplete disclosure of physical harm.[38]

Cosmetic surgical procedures promise us the appearance of ideal youth (which few young people even have). Underlying all of this is the clear message that we are not acceptable as we are. Our midlife and older years, in particular, are to be denied and hidden.

Many of us who came of age during the

1960s and '70s have experienced a sense of power and success as a result of the women's movement for equality. We may find it easier than women who came before us to feel on equal footing with our male friends, colleagues, partners, and lovers. Yet the double standard remains in that we are now expected to be successful *and* young *and* beautiful, in contrast to men, who are often rewarded throughout their lives for success and achievement alone. It is no wonder, therefore, that 90 percent of all cosmetic surgery patients are female.[39]

For some of us, our physical appearance has afforded very real benefits. By midlife we may be aware for the first time that we have depended on this appearance and the benefits that accompanied it. We now find ourselves confronted with a society that no longer rewards us for our appearance. For some of us, cosmetic surgery offers a temporary but welcome relief to this loss of societal rewards. In 2004, Americans spent $12.5 billion for this relief.[40]

Surgery does not come without substantive psychological and physiological risks that are too seldom discussed fully. Many of us subject ourselves to serious medical procedures, spending large sums of money and investing many hours and days for an image that is illusory. The media image of ideal beauty that we pursue is often, in reality, the product of tricks of lighting and photography, unattainable even through cosmetic surgery.

REAL CHANGES TO EXPECT AS WE AGE

We may experience changes in our hair, skin, and body fat distribution at menopause.

THINNING HAIR

Most of us experience some hair loss as we get older, owing to changing hormones, age, and heredity. Some prescription drugs can also

---

APPLE OR PEAR?

Our body shape is determined by the type of fat we carry. Some of us are more prone to an "apple" shape, storing fat around the abdomen. Others of us tend to have a "pear" shape, storing fat around the hips, buttocks, and thighs. However, the distribution of our body fat may change during menopause and midlife. Some of us who were once pear-shaped find ourselves apple-shaped by midlife.

One of the consistent research findings on physiological changes during the menopausal transition is the shift in fat distribution from the thighs to the abdomen without any substantive change in total fat mass.[41] In other words, more women become apple shapes after menopause. Loss of skin elasticity may cause the breasts to droop and flatten, and nipples may become smaller and flatter. Lessening of muscle tone in the abdominal wall can result in a protruding stomach, but regular exercise can counteract much of this particular change.[42]

Being an apple or a pear has certain health implications. Disorders such as heart disease, diabetes, obesity, and breast cancer have been associated with the apple shape. A vulnerability to osteoporosis, varicose veins, and cellulite has been associated with the pear shape. However, diet and exercise can have a significant impact in decreasing our vulnerability to these health risks.

cause hair loss. A small proportion of women experience a pronounced loss of hair at midlife, ranging from thinning and drying of the hair to baldness. Some of us find that thinning and hair loss occur where we part our hair and on the top portion of our heads. Loss of hair can have an impact on our body image, particularly in Western culture, where much value is given to the color, texture, length, and shape of our hair. Hair loss at midlife is usually permanent. It is not reversed with hormone treatment,[43] but some prescription drugs, such as oral minoxidil, have been found to help some women.[44]

SKIN CHANGES

As estrogen levels change, the skin can lose its elasticity and moisture and become dryer, thinner, and more vulnerable to bruising and wrinkling. Some of us describe a crawling sensation or itching of our skin. The wrinkling of our skin is due more to smoking, heredity, and sun exposure than to menopause and aging.[45]

WEIGHT GAIN

The years surrounding menopause are associated with weight gain. However, much research indicates that this gain is associated with aging rather than with menopause. For many of us, this weight gain contributes to a sense of unattractiveness and loss of sexual desire and sexual pleasure. The tendency toward weight gain during midlife is of critical importance because of its relationship to high blood pressure and diabetes. The factor most consistently related to this weight gain is a decrease in physical activity; exercising regularly and eating well may help us reach or maintain a healthy weight.[46] (For more information, see Chapter 12, "Eating Well," and Chapter 13, "Staying Active.")

CELEBRATING US

The traditional definitions of menopause and midlife are often punctuated with the word

---

STRATEGIES FOR ACCEPTANCE AND CELEBRATION

1. Exercise with activities that you find pleasurable and that bring you joy.
2. Eat healthily, sensibly, and with pleasure and enthusiasm.
3. Evaluate unhealthy practices such as smoking and excessive alcohol consumption and find ways to support healthy changes.
4. Seek out new ways of using and knowing your body through sports, dance, yoga, acting, sex, etc.
5. Practice loving the body you have lived in all these years.
6. Practice knowing your inner worth.
7. Support other women through compliments, listening, nurturing, and faithfulness.
8. Self-nurture through massage, hot baths, facials, walks, scented bath lotions, manicures, pedicures, sleep, flowers, candles, etc.
9. Reduce the number of hours you spend on TV programs, movies, and magazines whose images contribute to feelings of inadequacy. Reject the cultural images of "perfect" women and embrace the image in the mirror and in the faces of female friends.
10. Celebrate the life that is uniquely yours.

"decline." The changes in our bodies have been seen as sources of depression and feelings of unattractiveness. Yet many of us are looking forward. We are beginning new careers, returning to school, reevaluating our life choices, and breaking our silences. Many of us feel better than at any other time in our lives, thanks to consciousness about a healthy lifestyle, gratitude for a healthy body or one that has survived illness and other violations, and the wisdom that we have gained over the course of our lives.

One woman honors her body in this way:

I have grown to love, accept, and be inexpressibly grateful for my body. It has served me well. I treat it better than I used to. I have made great friends with my body. While I continue to criticize my body, it's more like the jokey jabs one directs to a close and trusted friend. It reflects intimacy and acceptance rather than the opposite. I don't know whether this is a function of menopause or simply aging, but I thank my great luck to have been given this wonderful body. I am so grateful.

NOTES

1. Germaine Greer, *The Change: Women, Aging, and the Menopause* (New York: Ballantine Books, 1993), 4.

2. Margaret Morganroth Gullette, *Declining to Decline: Cultural Combat and the Politics of Midlife* (Charlottesville: University of Virginia Press, 1997).

3. S. Murnen and L. Smolak, "The Experience of Sexual Harassment among Grade-School Students: Early Socialization of Female Subordination?" *Sex Roles* 43 (2000): 1–17; see also Rachel M. Calogero, "A Test of Objectification Theory: The Effect of the Male Gaze on Appearance Concerns in College Women," *Psychology of Women Quarterly* 28, no. 1 (2004): 16–21.

4. Jennifer J. Daubenmier, "The Relationship of Yoga, Body Awareness, and Body Responsiveness to Self-Objectification and Disordered Eating," *Psychology of Women Quarterly* 29 (2005): 207–8.

5. Ilana Attie and Jeanne Brooks-Gunn, "The Development of Eating Problems in Adolescent Girls: A Longitudinal Study," *Developmental Psychology* 25 (1989): 70–79.

6. An earlier version of this commentary appeared in Women's eNews. It was accessed at www.womens enews.org/article.cfm/dyn/aid/2398/context/archiv e on January 17, 2006. The current version is published with permission of the author.

7. Marika Tiggemann and Jessica E. Lynch, "Body Image across the Life Span in Adult Women: The Role of Self-Objectification," *Developmental Psychology* 37, no. 2 (2001), 243–44.

8. Amanda A. Deeks and Marita P. McCabe, "Menopausal State and Age and Perceptions of Body Image," *Psychology and Health* 16 (2001): 368.

9. Leah Kilger and Deborah Nedelman, *Still Sexy after All These Years: The 9 Unspoken Truths about Women's Desire beyond 50* (New York: Perigee/Penguin, 2006).

10. A. Bloch, "Self-Awareness during the Menopause," *Maturitas* 41 (2002): 65; see also N. E. Avis and S. M. McKinley, "A Longitudinal Analysis of Women's Attitudes toward the Menopause: Results from the Massachusetts Women's Health Study," *Maturitas* 13 (1991): 65–70.

11. Health Information—Health Journey, "Will You Still Love Me When I'm 64?—Menopause, Midlife, and Self-Esteem," Summer 2000, accessed at www.wom health.org.au/healthjourney/menopauseselfesteem. htm on June 29, 2005.

12. Barbara Hillyer, "The Embodiment of Old Women: Silences," *Frontiers* 19, no. 1 (1998): 55.

13. Amanda A. Deeks, "Psychological Aspects of Menopause Management," *Best Practices and Research Clinical Endocrinology and Metabolism* 17, no. 1 (2003): 17–31.

14. Allyson B. Moadel, James S. Ostroff, Lynna A. Lesko, and Daiva R. Bajorunas, "Psychosexual Adjustment among Women Receiving Hormone Replacement Therapy for Premature Menopause Following Cancer Treatment," *Psycho-Oncology* 4 (1995): 278.

15. Maureen A. Broughton, "Premature Menopause: Multiple Disruptions between the Woman's Biologi-

cal Body Experience and Her Lived Body," *Journal of Advanced Nursing* 37, no. 5 (2002): 426.

16. Elaine Anne Pasquali, "The Impact of Premature Menopause on Women's Experience of Self," *Journal of Holistic Nursing* 17, no. 4 (1999): 360.

17. Dalton Conley and Rebecca Glauber, "Gender, Body Mass, and Economic Status," National Bureau of Economic Research Working Paper No. 11343, unpublished (May 2005), accessed at papers.nber.org/papers/w11343 on July 20, 2005.

18. Eric Stice, Diane Spangler, and W. Stewart Agras, "Exposure to Media-Portrayed Thin-Ideal Images Adversely Affects Vulnerable Girls: A Longitudinal Experiment," *Journal of Social and Clinical Psychology* 20, no. 3 (2001): 270–88.

19. Diane Zuckerman. "Are Breast Implants Safe?" *Plastic Surgery Nursing* 22, no. 2 (summer 2002): 66–71.

20. Marcy Oppenheimer, "Safety and Benefits of Mentor Silicone Breast Implants from the April 2005 FDA Analysis and Meeting," Implant Information Project of the National Research Center for Women and Families, accessed at www.breastimplantinfo.org/news/mentor-pma.html on September 27, 2005; see also Marcy Oppenheimer, "Safety and Benefits of Inamed Silicone Breast Implants from the April 2005 FDA Analysis and Meeting," Implant Information Project of the National Research Center for Women and Families, accessed at www.breastimplantinfo.org/news/inamed-pma.html on September 27, 2005.

21. N. Markey, Patrick M. Markey, and Leanna Birch, "Understanding Women's Body Satisfaction: The Role of Husbands," *Sex Roles: A Journal of Research*, August 2004, accessed at www.findarticles.com/p/articles/mi_mi2294/is_3-4/ai_n6212703 on September 16, 2005.

22. Gina Shaw, "Eating Disorders Increasing among Women 35 and Older," *Washington Diplomat* (August 31, 2003), accessed at www.washdiplomat.com on July 7, 2005.

23. Merryl Bear, "Food and Weight Preoccupation during Midlife," Canadian Women's Health Network, July 2004, accessed at www.cwhn.ca/resources/eating_disorders/preoccupation.html on June 24, 2005.

24. Louise Gagnon, "Despite Image, Most Anorexics Are Forty-Five or Older," *Medical Post* 32, no. 34 (1996): 42.

25. Claire Wiseman, Suzanne Sunday, Fern Clapper, Wendy Harris, and Katherine Halmi, "Changing Patterns of Hospitalization in Eating Disorder Patients," *International Journal of Eating Disorders* 30, no. 1 (2001): 69–74; see also Paul Hewitt, S. Coren, and G. D. Steel, "Death from Anorexia Nervosa: Age Span and Sex Differences," *Aging and Mental Health* 5, no. 1 (2001): 41–46.

26. Colette Bouchez, "Eating Disorders as a Midlife Crisis," Health on the Net Foundation, August 31, 2003, accessed at www.hon.ch/News/HSN/514038.html on July 1, 2005.

27. Mia Foley Sypeck, James J. Gray, and Anthony H. Ahrens, "No Longer Just a Pretty Face: Fashion Magazine's Depiction of Ideal Female Beauty from 1959–1999," *International Journal of Eating Disorders* 36, no. 3 (2004): 342–47.

28. Jean Kilbourne, "The Strength to Resist: Media's Impact on Women and Girls," Cambridge Documentary Films, 2005.

29. Nancy Signorielli, "Aging on Television: Messages Relating to Gender, Race, and Occupation in Prime Time," *Journal of Broadcasting and Electronic Media* 48, no. 2 (June 2004): 279–301.

30. Doris G. Bazzini, William D. McIntosh, Steven M. Smith, Sabrina Cook, and Caleigh Harris, "The Aging Woman in Popular Film: Underrepresented, Unattractive, Unfriendly, and Unintelligent," *Sex Roles: A Journal of Research*, April 1997, accessed at www.findarticles.com/p/articles/mi_m2294/is_n7-8_v36/ai_19656786#continue on September 18, 2005.

31. Kilbourne.

32. American Society of Plastic Surgeons, "2004 Cosmetic Gender Distribution (Female)," 2005, accessed at www.plasticsurgery.org/public_education/loader.cfm?url=/commonspot/security/getfile.cfm&PageID=16148 on July 5, 2005.

33. Roy Shephard, "Aging and Exercise," in *Encyclopedia of Sports Medicine and Science*, ed. T. D. Fahey, Inter-

net Society for Sport Science, March 1998, accessed at sportsci.org on September 18, 2005.

34. Campaign for Safe Cosmetics, "Recent Reports on Chemicals in Cosmetics," accessed at www.safe cosmetics.org/about/reports.cfm on September 18, 2005.

35. American Society for Aesthetic Plastic Surgery, "Statistics 2004," accessed at www.surgery.org/press/sta tistics-2004.php on September 16, 2005.

36. Medline Plus, "Reconstructive Surgery," 2005, accessed at www.plasticsurgery.org/public_education/ procedures/ReconstructiveSurgery.cfm on July 5, 2005.

37. American Society of Plastic Surgeons, "What Is the Difference between Cosmetic and Reconstructive Surgery," accessed at www.plasticsurgery.org/ FAQ-What-is-the-difference-between-cosmetic-and-reconstructive-surgery.cfm on September 18, 2005.

38. Robert Goldwyn, "Reality in Plastic Surgery: A Plea for Complete Disclosure of Results," *Plastic and Reconstructive Surgery* 114 (October 2004): 24–27.

39. American Society for Aesthetic Plastic Surgery, "Statistics 2004," accessed at www.surgery.org/press/ statistics-2004.php on September 18, 2005.

40. Cosmetic Surgery.com, "Quick Facts," 2005, accessed at www.cosmeticsurgery.com/quick_facts/default. html on July 7, 2005.

41. Deeks, "Psychological Aspects."

42. Women's Resources Health Center, "Changes to Expect," 2005, accessed at www.healthsquare.com/ fgwh/wh1ch28.htm on July 5, 2005.

43. Nicholas Raine-Fenning, Mark Brincat, and Ives Muscat-Baron, "Skin Aging and Menopause: Implications for Treatment," *American Journal of Clinical Dermatology* 4, no. 6 (2003): 371–78.

44. Vera Price, "Treatment of Hair Loss," *New England Journal of Medicine* 341, no. 13 (1999): 964–73.

45. Health-cares.net, "What Causes Wrinkles," accessed at skin-care.health-cares.net/wrinkles-causes.php on July 25, 2005.

46. Laurey R. Simkin-Silverman and Rena R. Wing, "Weight Gain during Menopause," *Post Graduate Medicine* 108, no. 3 (2000), accessed at www.post gradmed.com/issues/2000/09_00/silverman.htm on July 5, 2005.

CHAPTER 9

Sexuality

Declining sex hormones signal the end of our reproductive capacities, but not the end of our capacities for sexual enjoyment. Despite old stereotypes that women dry up and become nonsexual after menopause, the reality is often quite different.

The women in my family were strong sexual beings. When one of my aunts was seventy-five, I gave her a vibrator. She reacted with shock, but when she died over a decade later, it was in her nightstand, much used.

PHYSICAL CHANGES AND EMOTIONAL REACTIONS

My first signs of perimenopause were extreme fatigue and vaginal dryness. My husband and I fondly described this sexual time as "the Sahara Desert." We had many hysterically laughing moments trying to bring moisture to this dry land! . . . I found I needed to alter my lifestyle, and I stopped working so insanely.

The physical changes that come with menopause may affect our sexuality. Changes in menstrual bleeding patterns are early signals of the menopause transition. Some women's periods just shorten and fade without any fanfare. Other women experience longer and heavier bleeding periods that sometimes may require medical intervention. Anxieties and shame can accompany such heavy bleeding, especially when a woman worries that she will bleed through her clothes. While some women welcome the freedom from menstruation and from the possibility of pregnancy and are more interested in sex, others mourn the loss of fertility and feel less feminine. Sometimes sex can relieve some of the tension; sometimes it is the last thing we want. Hot flashes and night sweats can also dim sexual feelings.

For some women, dryness and thinning of the vagina may be the first noticeable and disturbing experience of the menopause transition. (For more information, see Chapter 6, "Vulvovaginal Changes.") These changes can make sexual activities, especially vaginal penetration, uncomfortable or even painful and can test the resilience of our communication with our partners. A woman in her early sixties describes her experience:

Vaginal dryness and the resulting pain at intercourse not only hurt, they made me mad. I felt resentment that I was always the one responsible for birth control, with the diaphragm, spermicides, the pill, and then the IUD. Now I was back to stuffing the creams into my vagina for lubrication to have sex I'm hardly in the mood for anymore. I decided the only way to deal with my anger was to share it with my husband. I showed him all the creams and made him read the warnings on the packages. It turned out my anger was more about the grief I felt at losing my natural lubrication that I had taken for granted all my sexual life. Sharing this with him was transforming. It was like he had joined the planet I was living on, sharing the grief and loss, and understanding the risks. I was able to cry and feel much closer to him. I'm using the vaginal ring, which only needs changing every three months, but I still need additional lubrication. Now using lubrication is as automatic as using toothpaste when I want to brush my teeth!

Some of us experience changes in our sexual response, including lack of or greatly reduced sexual interest and desire, problems with mental or physical arousal, less lubrication, and less intense orgasms. These changes may happen gradually or suddenly. We may be confused over whether or not to attribute them to aging, menopause, or the weathering of a long-term relationship. A fifty-five-year-old woman says,

I'm in a twenty-year marriage and we've had a wonderful, satisfying sex life. But the sensations suddenly stopped for me. It seemed like it was overnight. My husband has been very accepting and supportive, but not me. I have cried about this many nights. I feel like I've lost a whole part of myself.

Another woman, who has large fibroids and did not take hormones, describes a difficult eight-year menopause transition that started at the age of forty-six:

During the worst of perimenopause I felt old and unattractive, and I was very bad-tempered and insecure, even anxious. However, now that I am almost completely out the other side of what was basically a whole-organism ordeal, I finally feel very good about myself. I was dismayed that I developed pretty severe vaginal atrophy right around when my period stopped. This was so bad without estrogen that fairly rapidly it made intercourse completely impossible. Even after the worst of perimenopause was over, I had lost almost all sensitivity in my genitals, and so it was hard to become aroused. I persevere, and am able to have orgasms using masturbation, thank goodness, but I was very surprised that my sexuality could change so much at menopause! No one ever told me to expect all this!

BODY IMAGE

How we feel about our bodies often influences how we feel about ourselves and our sexuality. Women sometimes stake our sexual happiness on hoped-for weight loss or another such physical "improvement."[1]

As we age, we may not feel attractive and we may fear that we are no longer attractive to our partners. Our partners may worry that it is they who are no longer sexually attractive to us. We may start looking at each other's aging bodies and feel disappointment, disgust, or contempt at the wrinkles, paunches, thinning hair, or sagging breasts. It is normal to have these feelings. It is important to recognize them for what they are: grief at loss and aging and a changing body image.

I still feel sexy, but then I remember that I am "middle-aged" and know that a middle-aged woman is not perceived as sexual.

I'm fifty-four and in a relationship with a woman much younger than me. My being in menopause really brings out our age difference. I'm mortified at having to use lubricants and a vibrator when I used to be so responsive. I wonder how long she's going to find me attractive.

One study found that the more a midlife woman perceived herself as less attractive than when she was ten years younger, the more likely she was to report a decline in sexual response or activity over the past ten years.[2] The sense of being less attractive can come from a variety of sources: the unrealistic, narrow ideals of our ageist and sexist society, a woman's own judgments about the physical markings of aging, or a perceived or real judgment from a partner. (For more information see Chapter 8, "Body Image.")

Physical changes don't have to translate into sexual dissatisfaction. Rather, our feelings about those changes seem to make the difference. Two women who participated in the study voiced their different reactions:

Not being able to achieve significant weight loss has some effect on my self-image. "Matronly" is not a sexy term unless you're Mae West.

I keep gaining weight. . . . The weight doesn't seem to affect my husband's desire and I don't feel less sexy. Hooray![3]

CHANGING RELATIONSHIPS

Our sexuality may be changing physically at menopause, but whether we are distressed about it or not depends to a considerable extent on the status of our relationships, our health, and our past sexual experiences. We can find ourselves in sexual turmoil, filled with new doubts or new passions. Or we may accept the sexual changes we notice as part of our aging. We may want to change old relationships, or end them. We may feel hurled into physical or emotional makeovers by forces either inside or outside us. We may feel more stuck than we have ever felt before. Or we may not feel very different at all.

Our sexuality at menopause is affected by all our earlier emotional and physical experiences of sex, including adolescent sexual identity and experimentation, childbearing and child rearing if we have children, and experiences of sexual abuse or assault. By the time we reach menopause, many of us have experienced several sexual relationships, while some of us have experienced only one, and others none. We may have stayed in a long-term relationship and experienced several distinct stages in its growth or stagnation or both. One sixty-five-year-old woman says,

I've had a lot of sexual relationships, including ones outside of marriage. [I lived in a very] dry and ultimately unloving and unsexual marriage for a long time. I think I shut down my physical side for that period and focused on my children and work. It's the postmenopause and the divorce that I feel reawakened me. In my current relationship, now two years old, I am having a great time with sex.

The endurance or failure of the sexual aspect of a relationship can be influenced by life experiences such as fluctuating finances, trauma, or ill health.

After our daughter died, I didn't know how we could go on living or what would happen to our marriage. When we were able to make love, I knew our marriage would survive.

At age sixty-eight, my husband endured an operation to remove his prostate. The cancer had escaped the boundaries of the prostate gland and it was necessary to then try radiation followed by hormone therapy—essentially castration. It has been hard for him to give up sex. . . . Verbal affection, cuddling, and most of all humor keep our marriage healthy and happy.

We may have had multiple long-term relationships and learned more about ourselves and our choices as we moved along.

When I was divorced, I aggressively sought out partners and was pretty promiscuous for about ten years. But then I found a relationship that I wanted to stay in and I felt really sexual in the first several years. Now that has waned and we have a nice warm relationship. It amazes me

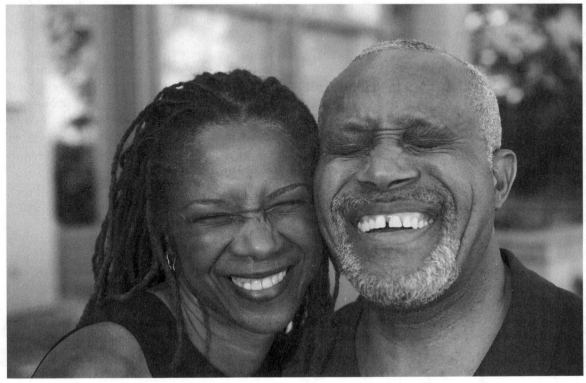

when I think about how I used to be. Too much sex and not enough love. Now we have plenty of love, not much sex.

In a healthy relationship, we feel alive, able to keep growing in self-respect. There is room for spontaneity, and for anger without destruction. We can be joined but not lose ourselves; we can share roles. A sixty-year-old woman says,

I've been in the same monogamous relationship for forty years. It's been wonderful. I was very lucky to meet and marry someone who shared common goals and aspirations. We've always communicated well, which might be the bedrock of a good relationship. Crises seem to have made us closer instead of exerting stress. Our sexual life, like other aspects of our life, has changed and evolved.

By menopause we may have come to feel differently about cultural norms that influenced our earlier lives. A fifty-five-year-old woman who comes from a Catholic background says,

After my four children, the only problem I had sexually was being afraid of getting pregnant, so I would reject my husband. It was very hard on our relationship. After my cancer treatments and menopause, it was like connecting again with being free and not worrying about pregnancy. At one time I believed that sex was for procreation, but now I think that men and women are brought together to love each other and to enjoy each other sexually. I don't know if this is what the church is teaching now, but I know I enjoy it and so does my husband.

The menopause transition often is a wake-up call to examine our relationships. Patterns of relating that felt fine to us when we were younger may no longer work as well. A fifty-five-year-old woman describes her experience:

As I approached fifty, I felt I needed to be away from people much more, and I semi-retired from my job. Once there, I found I needed to be away from my husband as well, and we began a process that resulted in our divorce after a twenty-year marriage. One great current in this process was my realizing I did not want to have sex with him. We stopped, and our marriage unraveled.

We may have unconsciously endured long-term unhealthy relationships. Staying in such relationships "for the sake of" the children, our parents, society, or religious values may have taken a physical and psychological toll on our lives. The transition of menopause or other health changes may inspire us to face truths about what was not working, and to take action.

For half of my twenty-five-year marriage to my husband, I had a secret affair with a woman. It was a loveless, emotionally abusive marriage and I had to end it. But coming out as a lesbian was the hardest thing I ever had to do. I lost custody of my four children for a while. It's been a long struggle, but now my partner and I proudly co-parent with my ex.

THE IMPORTANCE OF COMMUNICATION

If we have not felt safe communicating our needs to our partners throughout a relationship, we may have trouble navigating sexual changes during the menopause transition. Resentments may be expressed indirectly rather than directly. Sex, which might have started out to be the glue that held us together, can become a weapon either partner can use—by demanding or withholding sex. In such an environment we may not express our needs for more or less sex or our desires for or objections to certain activities. We also may not be comfortable discussing feelings about the pace of sexual activity. Only with effective communication can couples reach compromise and accommodation, relax about performance, and experiment with a range of sexual activities to give and receive pleasure and experience intimacy.

RANGE OF SEXUAL EXPRESSIONS

If sex has been mainly a positive experience in our lives, by menopause we have discovered sexually pleasurable activities both alone and with partners. As we have matured within ourselves and in our relationships, our sexual activities may have expanded from being genitally centered to include additional sensual and emotional experiences.

In genitally centered sex, orgasm is often the goal, whether through stimulation of the clitoris or the vagina, with or without vaginal penetration with a finger, tongue, penis, vibrator, or dildo. Orgasms come easily for some women and are more elusive for others. Many women find the most reliable orgasm comes through a combination of clitoral and vaginal stimulation. Some of us can feel judgmental about how we achieve orgasm.

I grew up believing that an orgasm from clitoral stimulation wasn't a real orgasm and that a "real woman" had an orgasm in her vagina only during intercourse.

Some of us experienced orgasms with clitoral masturbation when we were young and were able to incorporate it in our sexual activities with partners. Others, if we masturbate at all, consider it a private activity we would rather do alone. We may have found ourselves in relationships in which we faked an orgasm rather than disappoint our partners. Some of us found satisfying sex without orgasm.

An effect of menopause is that I have enormous difficulty achieving orgasm, but it doesn't usually bother me. It bothers my partner, and it is important to him.

Many of us can achieve orgasms when we masturbate alone but not with a partner. Lonnie Barbach and Betty Dodson offer support and comprehensive guides to women interested in being comfortable with and expanding our skills in masturbating alone or with partners or both.

Many find oral sex (stimulation with the mouth and tongue on the penis and vulva) an important part of foreplay or an enjoyable alternative to intercourse. For some women, saliva may provide just enough lubrication to vaginal tissues to ease vaginal dryness, but most women find the wide selection of over-the-counter lubricants sexy and silky (and some partners like the taste). Some women find anal sex, which can involve licking and penetrating the rectum, very sexually stimulating; for others it's a turn-off.

For some women, *outercourse,* defined as lovemaking without vaginal or anal penetration, provides varied and playful ways to be sexual with a partner when intercourse isn't desired or has to be avoided. The goal may be more about achieving emotional and physical closeness than achieving orgasm. Outercourse activities are limitless: they can include cuddling, kissing, bathing or showering together, reading erotic stories and sharing erotic fantasies with each other, dancing naked, sensual massage, and mutual masturbation.

Some women find that erotica, some of it created by and for women for all sexual tastes and sexual orientations, offers innovative ways to expand pleasure. Erotica includes novels, shorts stories, and videos. Sex-toy parties at which women can learn about and buy vibrators, dildos, and other sex toys, as well as condoms and dental dams, are competing with Tupperware parties, and women gather to write and share erotic fantasies. Over a period of twenty-five years, the Kensington Ladies' Erotica Society wrote and eventually published their stories (see below).[4] (For more information about sexuality and sexual activities, see the chapter in sexuality in the most recent edition of *Our Bodies, Ourselves*.)

We may choose to be celibate for some period of our lives, either in a relationship or not.

I'm forty-nine and never married. I've been celibate for the past fifteen years, initially due to events/lack of opportunity, more recently by choice. I'm becoming a whiz at self-discovery in terms of physical needs and pleasure. I'm looking into buying a vibrator for the first time, just to

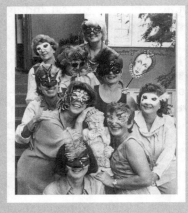

© Jill A. Weinstein

"Our fascination with erotica doesn't fade, even though the body parts do."
THE KENSINGTON LADIES' EROTICA SOCIETY

Menopause might have been breathing down our necks when we started meeting in 1976, but we had no interest in discussing it or anything from our "real" lives. Occasionally at our monthly dinner meetings, we would spot a Lady or two lifting her top and waving it wildly for that blessed breeze, and we would smile indulgently. Although four of us came to erotica from a women's consciousness-raising group that was strictly political, for the most part we were escapists, eager one night each month to abandon our roles as good women and good mothers and to fantasize about what we did and didn't find erotic.

Instead of confiding in each other about hot flashes, we let the stories we wrote suggest more playfully what was happening in our lives and in our bodies. In our early books we wove erotica into our childbirth stories; in our latest we devoted a section to "Flesh in Flux," creating sexy scenes that don't flinch at the physical signs of aging. By concocting our homemade brand of erotica and injecting laughter into the heavy breathing, we freed ourselves of stereotypes and taboos of an ageist society.

Our fascination with erotica doesn't fade, even though the body parts do. Now, pushing seventy and beyond, we agree that we enjoy being the sum of all the ages we've ever been, despite the occasional nudge from a cardiologist or oncologist. We like what a middle-aged friend replied when someone asked her age: twenty-two going on ninety. Though our bodies have started to go their own ways, like most women our age, we feel, on the inside, mischievous and ageless.

try something new and to give my poor fingers a vacation.

BIRTH CONTROL

As we go through the menopause transition (sometimes called perimenopause), our hormones fluctuate and our menstrual cycles may become erratic. Some of us may think that we no longer can get pregnant, but this is not true, as the many unexpected pregnancies experienced by women in our forties prove. Perimenopause can begin as early as our late thirties, but for most begins in our forties—as much as eight years before we reach menopause, which usually happens during our late forties or early fifties. While women are less likely to conceive as we grow older, the age at which an individual woman is no longer able to get pregnant varies. Because ovulation can occur right up to the last menstrual period, women who have sex with men and don't want to become pregnant should use contraception until one year after our last period.

Improved hormonal birth control methods such as low-dose combined oral contraceptive pills, progestin-only pills, implants, and the vaginal ring have fewer negative effects than hormonal contraceptives of the past, but each method has risks as well as benefits. Certain hormones can affect bone density, clotting, and vaginal lubrication for women nearing menopause. Barrier methods such as the diaphragm, the cervical cap, and the male or female condom don't affect your body chemistry but may not be as convenient or effective at preventing pregnancy. Improved IUDs are now considered to be much safer than those available when many of us were first becoming sexually active. Options should be evaluated according to your individual needs and personal and family medical history. For a more complete discussion of

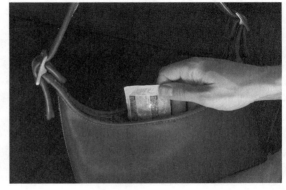

birth control, see the most recent edition of *Our Bodies, Ourselves.*

UNEXPECTED PREGNANCY

This was my third marriage, I was forty, and I had never been able to conceive before, so we didn't use birth control. I was really ambivalent when I found out I was pregnant. I considered an abortion but couldn't go through with it. I love my daughter now, but I still have a lot of guilt about feeling so mixed. . . . I don't come from a family where children are embraced and loved.

While those of us in our late thirties, forties, and early fifties have far fewer pregnancies than younger women, a disproportionately high percentage of our pregnancies are unexpected. Slightly over half of all women forty or over who get pregnant were not intending to conceive.[5] If you did not expect or desire to become pregnant, consider all of your options, which include having an abortion or placing the baby for adoption, as well as bearing and raising a child. Knowing that this may be your last possible pregnancy may make this a particularly difficult decision, so get as much nonjudgmental support as you can.

ABORTION

Abortion is safe and currently legal in the United States, although depending on where you live and what your financial situation is, you may have difficulty finding a clinic or practitioner who will provide one. The safest, easiest, and most affordable time to have an abortion is in the first three months of pregnancy. Approximately one of out every three women in the United States will have an abortion before the age of forty-five.[6] Among women over forty who become pregnant unintentionally, nearly 65 percent have an abortion.[7]

When my youngest child was eight months old, I discovered I was three months pregnant. I took many things into consideration while trying to make this decision. I felt that my husband and I were too old to have another child. I had suffered through postpartum depression with each of my pregnancies. The second pregnancy was worse than the first and required medication. I was terrified of going through it a third time.

Everyone at the clinic was very nice. I cried during the entire "counseling" session, and the nurse asked me if this is what I wanted. It wasn't really, but I had determined that this was the best thing for my family. It was really weird, but the day of the actual abortion, I had this incredible calm inside me.[8]

PLACING A CHILD FOR ADOPTION

Women who do not want an abortion and also do not want to raise a child may choose to place a child with a relative or an adoptive family.

If you plan to place a child with an adoptive family, it is important to create an adoption plan with an adoption counselor and to use a reputable agency. A good agency pays for your legal and counseling services and does not offer you money. It treats you, not the adoptive family, as the client. To avoid a less desirable agency, call your state's office for children for a list of agencies with complaints lodged against them. Most states require adoptive families to undergo an evaluation. If your state does not require one, consider your own requirements for the family.

It is standard practice for the birth mother to choose the adoptive family from a pool of applicants. If you are not offered this opportunity, you may want to choose another agency. Today, increasing numbers of birth mothers are choosing open adoptions, which allow us to have some level of ongoing contact with our children. If you choose closed adoption, consider picking an agency that will keep information about you to give to the child and adoptive family if they request it.

MOTHERHOOD

Some of us who find ourselves unexpectedly pregnant at midlife decide to become mothers. We may already have older children or we may be first-time mothers.

Like so many things in life, being an older mother is a mixed bag. On the one hand I am more patient, and I have a better perspective on what my values are, on what's important. I don't get all worked up over what kind of haircut he has, or if his room is clean. On the other hand . . . it's hard!

SEXUALLY TRANSMITTED INFECTIONS

Even after we are no longer able to become pregnant, we still must protect ourselves from sexually transmitted infections (STIs, also called sexually transmitted diseases or STDs). Protection is particularly important for those of us who have new or multiple partners, but even those of us who are in long-term relationships may benefit from taking precautions, because we may not know the risks to which our partners are exposing us. According to the Centers for Disease Control, nearly 65 million Americans (almost one in four) are living with a lifelong STI.[9]

Our children were grown and had left home. My husband (now ex) had a job that took him away for days at a time. I suspected nothing until I went for my routine Pap smear. It turned out I had the high-risk form of HPV (human papillomavirus), which can be a precursor to cervical cancer. I felt so outraged and betrayed. It took me a year to appreciate what a friend said to me at that time, "Thank God that's all he gave you."

Only condoms protect you against certain STIs, such as HIV (the virus that causes AIDS), which are transmitted by semen, vaginal secretions, and blood. Condoms may not completely safeguard against genital ulcer diseases such as genital herpes or human papillomavirus (HPV), but they do reduce your exposure as they cut down on skin-to-skin contact. Genital herpes can be transmissible even when there are no outward symptoms, so communication with your partner about your sexual histories and practices is essential for prevention. Safer sex practices for oral sex include using a condom with a man and using dental dams or a heavy plastic wrap placed over the vulva during oral sex with a woman. (For more information about sexually transmitted infections and safer sex, see the most recent edition of *Our Bodies, Ourselves.*)

CHANGING DESIRE

Our libido, or sexual energy, fluctuates throughout our lives. There is no agreement about whether sexual interest declines chiefly because of declining hormones, other aspects of aging such as poor circulation, or the influence of other life circumstances, such as the quality of a woman's sexual relationship, her overall emotional and physical health, financial stability, and family and cultural values. Furthermore, researchers report that even if our libidos decline, we can find satisfaction with our sexual lives once we have adjusted to this change.[10]

For me libido is about juiciness . . . about how close to the surface my sexual being is, and how readily she takes over my psyche. It is exuding pheromones, feeling sex in every pore of my being, the gut-wrenching electricity of an exchanged look, getting creamy from a fantasy or an unexpected thought. I am still able to have any of these responses, but far less frequently than I used to, and that's okay!

To me libido is a sexually energetic drive promoted by hormones. It has definitely changed and I miss the strong pulsing rush of sexual energy. I occasionally feel a sexual pulse but it isn't very strong. My sexual self must be maturing, because physical (sexual) intimacy that included orgasm used to be very important; now, it isn't nearly as important. The emotional intimacy in my relationship sustains the effect of orgasm without physical orgasm.

How we experience sexual desire or lusty libido may have more to do with our life circumstances and whether or not we have partners than our hormone levels. Sometimes not being in a relationship can heighten desire.

I still want sex a lot but don't act on my impulses because I'm not in a committed relationship and I don't want flings or one-night stands. I just masturbate when I'm horny.

A fifty-year-old woman says,

I feel that in menopause I'm cycling back to when I was newly married, only better. My husband and I are already talking about the freedoms we will regain, including intimacy at will when our two kids leave home. It will be better than it was when we were newlyweds because behind our lovemaking will be years of experience together and deepening love.

At sixty-four, I find myself in a new relationship, and it has been very important in expanding my sexual self. I have more fun, feel less inhibited—more ready to take on different personae for sexual activity—and am generally ready for sex on a regular basis. It's probably the most open relationship sexually I have ever had.

I used to feel very sexy, but I believe my asexual feelings are related to being married, not to menopause. I believe I am a passionate sexual and earthy woman that others find attractive, but in order not to act on my feelings, I neutralize them to stay faithful—weird, but true. I also believe that my libido has stabilized, in that it does not push me around but allows me to experience warm feelings and passion when I wish to.

Researcher Rosemary Basson reports that emotions and thoughts have a stronger impact on a woman's assessment of whether she is aroused than does blood flow to the genitals.[11] John Bancroft of the Kinsey Institute has suggested that a reduction in sexual desire or response may be an adaptive response to a woman's relationship or life problems rather than a disorder.[12] For example, her libido might decline because of a partner's illness or death.

I just don't find myself thinking about sex or having sexual feelings like I did in my younger days. The lack of interest in sex doesn't bother me since I found out that my friends and colleagues feel that way too. If it doesn't have a bad effect on my

marriage, it is okay. My husband says that he also notes less sexual desire than he had when we were young, which is probably good, since at sixty-three I don't think I could keep up with the sex drive of a healthy young man. I'm still orgasmic unless I'm quite tired, so all in all, life is good, and we are both happy with our sex life.

THE MEDICALIZATION OF FEMALE SEXUAL DESIRE

The medical and pharmaceutical establishments claim that there are natural and normal levels of sexual feelings, physical arousal, and orgasm. Based on these claims, psychiatric and medical manuals use such terms as "disorders" and "dysfunctions" to describe our sexual feelings and responses when they differ from these norms.

In the late 1960s, sex researchers William Masters and Virginia Johnson identified phases in a sexual response cycle, which became the framework for psychiatric and medical measurement of sexual response. Failures to "achieve" at any of these levels or phases were considered sexual disorders, or "female sexual dysfunction" (FSD). FSD was further broken down into "hypoactive (below the norm) sexual desire disorder" (low or no interest in sex); "FSAD, female sexual arousal disorder (difficulty or failure to achieve arousal, during which vaginal tissues fill with blood and secrete liquids that constitute our juiciness or "getting wet"); and "female orgasmic disorder," the failure to achieve orgasm. Another sexual "dysfunction" is *dyspareunia,* or genital pain associated with sexual intercourse.

Pharmaceutical companies have a financial interest in defining low desire and arousal as medical problems. If a Viagra-type drug or a testosterone preparation could do for women what such treatments have done for men, it might become another multibillion-dollar blockbuster for the drug companies.

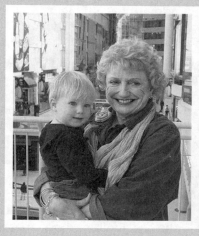

"You never know the sexual history of anybody but yourself."

JANE PECINOVSKY FOWLER

When I was fifty-five years old, I was stunned to learn that I was infected with HIV (after being denied new health insurance because of the results of a routine blood test). That was in 1991. It turned out I had been living with the virus since 1986.

As a woman newly divorced in 1983, after twenty-four years of marriage, I had not been on the dating circuit for a quarter century. I never dreamed that a man I began seeing—he'd been a close friend my entire adult life—would be HIV-positive. It never occurred to me to ask, or demand, that a condom be used during sex. Why should I? I knew I couldn't get pregnant. And I knew little about HIV at that time—only that it was some mysterious ailment affecting the gay community. What did heterosexuals have to fear?

In the beginning I told only my parents, son, and close friends, who were compassionate and supportive. I lived in semi-isolation because I did not have the confidence to put myself in public situations where I might experience discrimination or rejection. Then, after four uneasy years, I realized that my silence was not helping me or anyone else. Suddenly I was inspired to say, "Look at this old, wrinkled, jowly face. This is another face of HIV." I found a voice in me I didn't know I had.

In 1995 I was among the organizers of the National Association on HIV Over Fifty, and I started speaking out: at local, state, regional, national, and international meetings and conferences. Seven years later I founded HIV Wisdom for Older Women (www.hivwisdom.org), a national program dedicated to the prevention of HIV infection in mid-aged and elder females and to life enrichment for those who are aging with the virus. Because older women are an isolated and ignored group at risk for HIV and other STIs, I also want to raise the consciousness of the health care community, as well as the public, about today's sexual realities.

I'm now seventy years old and healthy. Since the antiretroviral drug "cocktail" was introduced in 1996, and I started taking the combination therapy, the amount of virus in my blood has decreased to a nearly undetectable level. Of course I still have HIV, because there is no cure. But I'm lucky. I have not progressed to full-blown AIDS.

Today I remind women in the menopausal transition, "You never know the sexual history of anybody but yourself." I tell women that if you are not in a *mutually* monogamous relationship in which neither of you is STI-infected, you must understand the necessity of practicing safer sex. If a partner won't use protection, find another partner. And to older men using meds to correct erectile dysfunction, I say, "And now if you can get it up, cover it up."

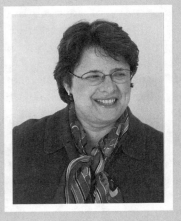

© Dan Hallman

"I believe that sexuality is not primarily about biology."

LEONORE TIEFER

When I sit in my sex therapist chair, I hear from women and men whose sexual concerns reflect their worries about money, their relationship problems, and other realities of their lives more than their biological conditions. For example, I recently met with a woman who had lost her sexual desire for her beloved boyfriend of nine months. In our conversation it became clear that she desperately wanted to please her fella so he would propose marriage, and this pressure was affecting her enjoyment of sex. Sounds simple, but this college-educated, much-traveled, high-earning woman had, until seeing me, been convinced that she had abnormal hormones, and the hardest part of the hour was persuading her to tell me some things about herself and her relationship instead of obsessing about her biology.

I believe that sexuality is not primarily about biology but is first and foremost a reflection of the social, political, and cultural climate of its time. Unfortunately, some people who study sexuality think it's all (or mostly) about biology.

In 2000, I organized the New View campaign to respond to the medicalization of female sexuality and resist the avalanche of drugs the pharmaceutical companies are marshaling to treat "female sexual dysfunction." The researchers, educators, and activists of the campaign have testified, written books and articles, and gone toe-to-toe with industry-sponsored promoters of pills and patches as solutions to women's sexual problems. While some women may have sexual problems that could benefit from such medical interventions, we believe that most women would benefit more from an approach that considered other aspects of their lives.

Women's sexuality starts with the culture. Mass media have shifted gears such that now if a woman has "low desire" or "low libido," she is considered to have a disorder that requires medical intervention. "I have to have a strong sexual desire" may soon be part of our culture, just like "I have to be thin."

But this model for understanding women's sexuality and women's sexual problems is inadequate. It suggests that if you tell your health care provider about a low interest in sex, your provider may simply prescribe a pill without taking the time to investigate the circumstances of your life or relationship. (Although well-trained providers will do both.)

Psychologist and sexologist Leonore Tiefer challenged this medicalization of women's sexual problems with the New View campaign (www.fsd-alert.org). The campaign's "manifesto" proposes a new set of nonmedicalizing, nonstigmatizing classifications. It holds that sexual functioning is about much more than the physical functioning of our sex organs. The New View classification defines sexual problems as "discontent or dissatisfaction with any emotional, physical, or relational aspect of sexual functioning, arising in the following aspects of women's sexual lives: socio-cultural, political or economic factors; partner and relationship factors; psychological factors; and medical factors."[13]

Drug companies have experienced some setbacks in their search for a pharmaceutical "fix" for women's sexual problems. In 2004, Pfizer abandoned eight years of searching for a "female Viagra." The company concluded that while Viagra can cause arousal in vaginal tissues, women did not report much increase in desire to have sex.[14] Proctor and Gamble's application for a testosterone patch for women was turned down by the Food and Drug Administration in December 2004 for the lack of long-term safety data.[15] The company is planning to resubmit the application with new study results.

The claim that the most influential sex organ in both men and women is the brain is not a joke. But "it's all in your head" has different meanings for different groups. To sex therapists like Tiefer, how a woman thinks and feels about herself as a sexual person affects her sexual functioning. To medical researchers, a drug targeted at brain chemicals that affect women's feelings and behaviors may be the blockbuster they seek. One company is developing a nasal spray that will stimulate the production of dopamine, a chemical in the brain associated with feelings of pleasure.

We do not need to rely on sexual desire to motivate us to have and enjoy sex. Desire for physical and emotional closeness, tenderness, appreciation and confirmation of her attractiveness, relief from tension, help getting to sleep, and confidence in her ability to have an enjoyable experience are only a few of the motives a woman may have for sex. Once involved in sexual activity, many women will feel sexually aroused enough to continue. In some cases, this cycle may not work, especially if women are feeling pressure to have sex in order to accommodate a partner or fulfill a societal expectation. Some researchers believe that, first, a woman's attitudes about her sexual experiences when she was younger and, second, her relationship with her sexual partner are the most powerful predictors of sexual interest in later life. One study reported that the "lack of frequent desire does not appear to preclude emotional satisfaction and physical pleasure with relationships."[16] Other researchers found that in spite of diminished desire, orgasm, enjoyment, and frequency of sexual activity, the vast majority of midlife women in their study felt sexually satisfied, both physically and emotionally, in their relationships.[17]

Many of us who do not experience strong sexual desire have found ways to integrate sexual activity into our lives. A woman who has been married for thirty-seven years says,

I know that a healthy sex life is important in my marriage and just plan to make love regularly and not let too much time go by. Saying no to my

TESTOSTERONE

There is increasing interest in using testosterone to treat low sexual desire in women. Some evidence suggests that it can improve sexual function in postmenopausal women, but not enough research has been conducted to understand its effectiveness or long-term risks. (For more information, see "Testosterone for Low Sexual Desire," page 110.)

husband often would hurt him, and I don't want to do that because [wanting him to be happy] is part of having a love relationship. It's not that I don't enjoy sex; it just doesn't go through my thoughts as it used to do. It's almost like, "Yes, I remember what that was like, it was nice, but I don't think unbidden about sex."

There are those who mourn the loss for many reasons: It was an integral part of our identity and we don't want to give it up. A fifty-five-year-old woman who uses hormone treatment to relieve vaginal discomfort says,

My sexual desire and response is certainly not what it used to be, but I no longer feel like my switch is stuck in the off position. I recently had days of old-fashioned horniness. I am not the kind of person who takes lots of medication. I do wish there would be recognition that for some women, their relationships are not the problem, and that taking hormones may in fact be the appropriate solution.

ILLNESS, DISABILITIES, AND SEXUALITY

The older we grow, the more likely we are to experience illness and conditions connected with aging. For example, between the ages of forty-four and fifty-four, incidence of most cancers doubles. Many of us and our partners may have chronic physical conditions like diabetes, multiple sclerosis, high blood pressure, vascular problems, heart and lung disease, and mental health conditions such as anxiety and depression.

These conditions, their symptoms, and medications to treat them can have a profound effect on our or our partners' sexuality. Commonly used medications can affect desire, arousal, and quality of orgasms. These include blood pressure and heart medications such as

digoxin and Inderal; the cancer medication tamoxifen; tranquilizers such as Ativan, Valium, and Xanax; and some antidepressants, antihistamines, and decongestants.[18] If you suspect that any of these medications may be affecting your sexual responses, you may want to research alternatives and talk with your health care provider about ways to reduce the dose or switch to a drug with fewer adverse effects.

The possibility that antidepressants can reduce sexual responses puts women in a bind. Low libido is often a symptom of depression, yet it also can be an effect of the very medications intended to improve the condition. The popular antidepressants Paxil and Prozac and Zoloft can affect sexual responses in some people.[19] Some experts recommend switching to the antidepressants Celexa, Wellbutrin, Serzone, and Desyrel, which seem to have less of a negative effect.[20] Another alternative you may want to consider is a "drug holiday," a brief period of not taking a daily drug in order to minimize undesired effects. For example, skipping weekend doses of an antidepressant when one might want to have sex may revive sexual responses.[21] It is important to learn about the effects of changing or stopping the medication and to work with a knowledgeable provider. (For a detailed description of ten chronic diseases or disabilities, their effects on sexuality, special implications, and coping strategies, see the chapter "Sexuality" in *Our Bodies, Ourselves.*)

Experiencing cancer and its treatments can have a devastating effect on a woman's entire life. Women's self-esteem, body image, and sexuality can be irrevocably changed by breast cancer surgery and other treatments.

A lesbian in a twenty-year relationship describes her experience:

Cancer and cancer treatment created a really rough time in our relationship. Chemo and radi-

ation threw me into a premature menopause. Every time we had sex, I would get an infection. Then I would be on antibiotics for a couple of weeks and the cycle would repeat. We both began to hold back and avoid sex. A deeper expression of emotional intimacy is the bridge we created to come back together.

A fifty-five-year-old, never-married woman who survived cancer still struggles with depression and its effects:

After treatment for breast cancer, I started on tamoxifen. After two years, the lining of my vagina started to thin, but I couldn't use any estrogen cream because of the tamoxifen. I had renewed a relationship with an old lover, but intercourse was excruciating. My vagina narrowed, and I tried stretching devices but suffered more tears. A vibrator worked better in stretching my vagina. Intercourse still hurt but less and less so. I was on Prozac, which inhibited orgasm. I tried changing the antidepressant but nothing has been good, so I'm back on Prozac. It keeps me in a good place, but still no sex with a partner and even orgasms with masturbation are not as good. I feel something vital has been taken from me. I feel almost castrated.

After my surgery for cervical cancer, I was apprehensive about feeling inside and having orgasms, but that went away as soon as I found myself to be the same. The pain and tightness for the first month after surgery and again during radiation got better each time we had intercourse. It really helped to have had a loving and sexually pleasurable marriage for the thirty years before my cancer.

We may have accepted uneasy truces with uterine fibroids or with excessive bleeding throughout our menstruating years. Or we may have had such difficulties with fibroids and bleeding,

especially in perimenopause, that we've settled on hysterectomies.

I went to six doctors before I was comfortable with the hysterectomy. The deciding one was a doctor who advocated saving my cervix to keep sexual sensations. I really appreciated that and didn't lose sexual feeling. He told me my cervix would probably bleed. It does and I don't mind because I kept my ovaries, so I'm still ovulating. What's funny now (four years later) is that he's telling me that the latest research recommends against keeping the cervix. What to believe!

We may have had to learn how to accommodate our partner's medical condition and its effect on our sexual experiences. One fifty-eight-year-old woman reports,

My partner's prostate surgery left him completely unable to have an erection. He learned how to inject his penis right before intercourse. Sex feels more mechanical now. Sex is still good but I miss how the sexy feeling of an aroused penis in response to me used to ignite my own arousal.

Multiple sclerosis often exacerbates what menopausal women experience.

I was diagnosed with MS at age forty-six, right when my marriage was breaking up. I also got breast cancer then. After chemo and tamoxifen, my periods didn't come back. I was still pretty sexually active until I started using a wheelchair about fifteen years ago. That's when I started to feel sexually invisible. I actually found some dates on the Internet, but I got either men who thought they were defective and could be with me, or those with perverse interests. I had great sex with a sweet man, but he saw himself as defective, as not very bright. I masturbated very successfully with a vibrator and even ejaculated. My vagina has never dried up, not even with all the drugs for

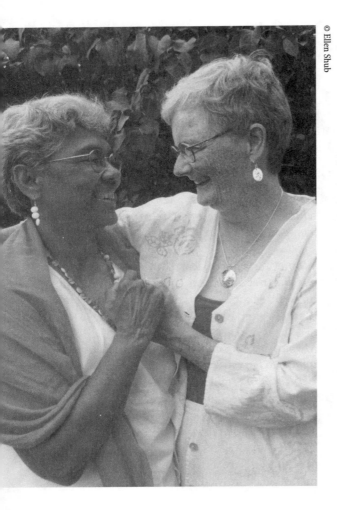
© Ellen Shub

MS. But now I'm pretty numb. I can still feel sexual with my first boyfriend, with whom I'm still friends, because he remembers me from before.

STRATEGIES AND APPROACHES

As we consider how changes related to menopause, medical conditions, and emotional realities affect our sexuality, we face a vast range of options. We may choose to change our habits, take medication, or go for individual or couples counseling. We may not know which, if any, of these options to try first. If we're not comfortable canvassing our friends and relatives, we may try our health care providers. Sometimes we already know how we feel and just need to find support for a decision we've already made.

It took a bit of time to understand that the reason sex was not comfortable was the dryness. I found saliva did not work as well as a lubricant and used Astroglide. Replens also makes sex much more enjoyable. I've used black cohosh, evening primrose oil, and vitamin E to help with hot flashes. I also cut out caffeine and try to walk regularly.

I had frequent yeast infections and soreness. Six months of Diflucan got rid of the yeast infections, and with HT [hormone treatment] and Estring, no more soreness. My sex life is better than ever. I struggle with the confusing flow of information regarding HT; my health professionals are supportive of my ending it but say I'm fine should I continue it. I'm staying on HT and taking a "wait and see" attitude. I feel healthy and strong, happy to be at this stage of life with more time for work, fun, and my partner.

I've used progest cream, vaginal estrogen, and topical testosterone. While they help a bit, I can't stand having to remember the varying schedules. I also feel the bedtime rituals get too long when I'm so tired at the end of the day, and then start moisturizing my face, lips, heels, and then have to inject and rub hormone creams on as well. I've just started with Vagifem, an estrogen pill suppository, which seems much easier. In the meantime, I'm working to grab life and stay connected to the people I love.

Searching for intimacy often intensifies as physical changes take hold. Emotional intimacy has sometimes been the way into physical intimacy with a partner. How well we have succeeded at it may predict how well our ability to keep and increase that intimacy will sustain us through the physical changes of the menopause transition.

If sex diminishes, is intimacy also diminished? How can we find, or increase, intimacy in ways that are nongenital? We have to start with being comfortable and intimate with ourselves. Self-intimacy is knowing ways to love, be honest, and have fun with ourselves, and being able to hold on to ourselves while still being in an active relationship with another. It can include enjoying eating, playing, reading, gardening, hiking, biking, walking, and playing with pets. It includes being sensual, feeling alive with all our senses: enjoying a warm bath, feeling smooth materials next to our skin, listening to music that moves us, dancing, massaging, and masturbating. The greater our ability to be intimate with and for ourselves, the greater will be our ability to share intimacy with another person. Physical and emotional intimacy with a partner can come from cuddling while watching TV, long hugs before getting up in the morning, singing together, and sweating together from physical activities.

One woman found renewed sexual energy when she took up belly dancing at age forty:

When I first started belly dancing, I hated what I saw in the mirror. Then the moves started to change my shape and my posture. I connected with muscles I didn't know existed. The pelvic and spinal undulations opened my breath and changed my thoughts. I felt the return of sexual energy that I thought I had abandoned when I became a mother.

Many women feel ambivalent about our partners' using Viagra and other erection-enhancing drugs. The use of such drugs can affect sexual dynamics by emphasizing the achievement of erections over other aspects of the sexual experience, such as emotional closeness. It's important to share our concerns with our partners and be willing to explore sexual activities that are not so dependent on an erect penis.

My partner has turned to Viagra sometimes in the past two years. It does make a difference, although it is not essential to the pleasure of the act. I am generally nervous about taking almost anything, which extends to my partner's taking anything too, although the Viagra seems to have for him only limited side effects, which are not pleasant but are not lasting.

The ads for Viagra for men and women leave me cold. Who needs to **** like bunny rabbits at this age? We can savor the relationship, the mood, and the partner.

By the time we've reached midlife, all of us have experienced change and loss. Weathering these transitions, we can discover unexpected resilience. Many of us feel more confident than ever before. One fifty-nine-year-old woman says,

Four years ago I ended a thirty-one-year marriage. I was convinced my sex life was over. I am delighted to share that I have a wonderful partner and the most fulfilling sex of my life. Although I take no hormones or antidepressants, I do not have a problem with vaginal dryness and have a very active libido.

So much has changed in these four years. Besides ending my marriage, I lost my mother, moved from my home, and watched helplessly as my son's marriage fell apart. Yet I have never felt more in control of my life or more excited by it. I find freedom in my sexual life, not just because I no longer worry about pregnancy, but because I know who I am and I really like what I know about myself. I am a grandma, a mom, a friend, and a lover, and I've never been more me!

NOTES

1. Sallie Foley, Sally Kope, and Dennis Sugrue, *Sex Matters for Women* (New York: Guilford Press, 2002), 131.

2. P. B. Koch, P. K. Mansfield, et al., " 'Feeling Frumpy': The Relationships between Body Image and Sexual Response Changes in Midlife Women," *Journal of Sex Research* 42, no. 3 (2005): 215–23.

3. Ibid., 219–20.

4. Kensington Ladies' Erotica Society, *Sex, Death, and Other Distractions* (Berkeley, CA: Ten Speed Press, 2002).

5. Stanley Henshaw, "Unintended Pregnancy in the United States," *Family Planning Perspectives* 30, no. 1, accessed at www.agi-usa.org/pubs/journals/3002498.html on October 14, 2005.

6. "State Facts about Abortion," Alan Guttmacher Institute, accessed at www.guttmacher.org/pubs/sfaa/alabama.html on October 12, 2005.

7. Henshaw.

8. Feminist Women's Health Clinic, "Many Voices, Many Choices: Personal Stories about Abortion," accessed at www.fwhc.org/stories/perso.htm on October 14, 2005.

9. Centers for Disease Control and Prevention Report, "Tracking the Hidden Epidemics: Trends in STDs in the United States," 2000, accessed at www.cdc.gov/nchstp/dstd/Stats_Trends/Trends2000.pdf on October 14, 2005.

10. Virginia S. Cain, et al., "Sexual Functioning and Practices in a Multi-Ethnic Study of Midlife Women: Baseline Results from SWAN," as reported in Rosemary Basson, "Recent Advances in Women's Sexual Function and Dysfunction," Part 2 of 2, *Menopause* 11, no. 6 (2004): 720.

11. Basson, 716.

12. J. Bancroft, J. Loftus, and S. Long, "Distress about Sex: A National Survey of Women in Heterosexual Relationships," *Archives of Sexual Behavior* 32, no. 3 (2003): 193–208, as reported in "Women's Sexual Health in Midlife and Beyond," *Association of Reproductive Health Professionals Clinical Proceedings,* May 2005, 8.

13. Ellyn Kaschak and Leonore Tiefer, eds., *A New View of Women's Sexual Problems* (Binghamton, NY: Haworth Press, 2001).

14. Gardiner Harris, "Pfizer Gives Up Testing Viagra on Women," *New York Times,* February 28, 2004.

15. Katherine Hobson, "A Drug for Arousal," accessed at www.usnews.com/usnews/health/articles/050124/24sex.htm on July 14, 2005.

16. Cain et. al.

17. Koch et al., 219.

18. Foley et al., 268, 284.

19. Ibid.

20. Sandra Leiblum and Judith Sachs, *Getting the Sex You Want* (New York: ASJA Press, 2002), 176–77.

21. Ibid., 177.

CHAPTER 10

Family Life and the Workplace

We are social beings and the quality of our relationships—at home, at work, or in social settings—plays an important role in our well-being. Shifting relationships, new expectations, and competing responsibilities can affect our emotions and physical health as we go through the menopause transition. Understanding our own social circumstances, the ways they affect us, and the fact that we are not alone in the hurdles we face can bring a sense of relief. It may also help us determine if we need to make changes or ask for help.

Around the time of menopause, we may have completed our intensive child-rearing years. Or we may be in the midst of raising young children, teenagers, or grandchildren. If we had hoped to bear children but have not done so, we may be mourning the loss. Our parents, grandparents, in-laws, and elderly relatives, if they are still alive, may become more dependent on us. We face caregiving and eventual bereavement, as well as our own aging. On top of that, most of us are working and planning for retirement, if we can afford to think about stopping work at all. How we experience these events varies. This can be a productive time of growth, development, and new dreams.

When I anticipated menopause, I thought it would feel like a loss, but I don't feel that way. It coincides with my second and last daughter finishing high school, which is more of the big change. I went back to school six years ago and started a new career of

physician assistant, which is great, stimulating and energizing, and I'm sure that has helped with this transition in my life. I'm really okay with it.

This may also be a time of new burdens, fears, losses, and grief. We may assess and renew our values, relationships, and sense of ourselves.

At age fifty-four, I feel the clock is ticking and I'm more aware of the passage of time. My mother died last year, as did a close fifty-two-year-old friend. I want to use my time well and feel I am leaving a legacy. Who are the people I care most about? What are the values that I hold dear and what do I stand for?

Since my father died last year, there's no one in my life who I know really loves me and stands behind me. I'm a single mother, so I'm always busy, but I'm so lonely! Where am I supposed to meet somebody at this age?

THE FAMILY: A CLUB-SANDWICH GENERATION

A sense of family connection is important to many of us, however we define family. At the same time that we are going through the menopause transition, many of us face changes in our family roles and relationships. We may be "sandwiched" between the needs of two, three, or four generations.

BECOMING A MOTHER

More and more women are raising children in midlife. Some of us are becoming pregnant without the assistance of reproductive technologies; some of us are using technologies such as in-vitro fertilization, either with our own or with a donor's eggs, to conceive; and some of us are adopting.

Midlife women may experience motherhood differently than younger mothers do. As older women, we are more likely to be financially and emotionally prepared to raise a child and bring a wealth of life experiences to our mothering. Those of us who delayed childbearing for a long time or struggled with infertility often particularly savor our parenting experiences. On the flip side, we may have less energy to bring to the physical and emotional labor of raising children, and we may have very high standards for ourselves and our children that are difficult to live up to. We also may find ourselves coping with the menopause transition or caring for our elderly parents at a time when we are still changing diapers.

*Our first child was pretty mellow. But our second child—born when I was 51—is fiery and passionate and not at all easygoing. And I'm **always** tired. What else can I say? Life has not been the same.*

(For more information on whether and how to become a midlife mother, see "Considering Parenting" and "Infertility and Assisted Reproduction" in *Our Bodies, Ourselves*.)

LAUNCHING CHILDREN

Mothers whose children are ready to leave home may feel a sense of loss and loosening of family bonds as we face the "empty nest."

I had my kids late. I'm fifty-five, my younger son is fourteen, and the oldest is going to college next year. I don't know what to expect. My older son is making his leave-taking a bit easier by getting obnoxious. . . . I do feel a sense of sadness; I loved being a mom of young kids.

Transitioning into our new roles can feel like a drastic change after years of daily intimacy and contact. A postmenopausal woman recalls,

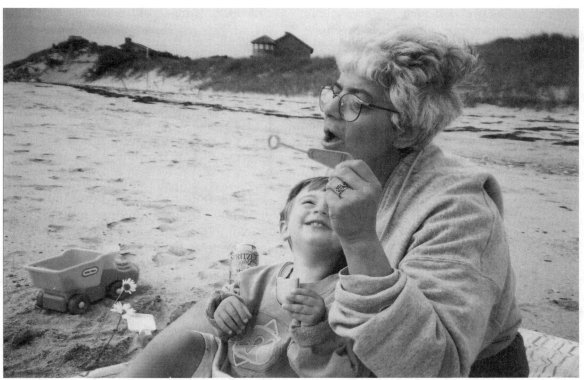

I remember how profound it was for me to accept that my childbearing days were over. It had nothing to do with wanting more children. I had ended that phase of my life. I just needed to grieve the loss of this time of life. Women need to be given the opportunity to do this and not just feel pressure to "move on."

Life after kids depends on where we are in our marital status, work, relationships, health of our parents, and age. We may choose to shift focus to other parts of our lives, to start new careers, go back to school, or take up new hobbies. It can feel like a power surge: "It's finally a time for *me*." "What do I want?" "How can I make it happen?"

Sometimes our life after kids becomes life with our kids once again. If children "boomerang" in their twenties and thirties and move back home to live because of a job loss, divorce, or other change of circumstance, our family dynamics change. This is particularly true when our children bring children of their own with them.

CARING FOR AGING PARENTS

The typical caregiver in the United States is a forty-six-year-old female who has some college education, works, and is spending more than twenty hours a week caring for her mother, in addition to providing housekeeping for a spouse or partner and primary care for children or grandchildren.[1] Given her age, the typical caregiver is also likely to be going through the menopause transition.

My husband had just had spinal cord surgery and my mom, breast cancer surgery, and they were both here. I was really about at the end of my rope because I didn't have the wherewithal to cope.

Many of us struggle to balance raising children or grandchildren, caring for aging or disabled loved ones, maintaining a household, and working full-time or part-time. Although men are more involved with caregiving now than in previous generations, women still do the majority of it. While we reap the benefits, we also shoulder the problems: emotional stress, risk to our health, reduced wages and job security, and diminished retirement guarantees. Without social and economic policies that support, affirm, value, and supplement the caregiving that we do, we're facing an impossible task. Our society may sentimentalize motherhood and caretaking, but it does little to support the concrete needs of mothers and other caretakers. We need affordable, accessible, high-quality, comprehensive long-term care services to support our work at home, and paid leave from our jobs to do it.

If you are a caregiver—whether it's a labor of love, a duty, or some combination of the two—give yourself credit and feel proud. You are doing important work. Providing continuity of love, care, and connection across the generations is of great value.

When my mother came home from the hospital, she was happiest when I drove down every other weekend to spend time with her. The minute we were alone together, we felt liberated. I called her friends and invited them over, cooked, paid bills, and generally kept her normal life going. She kept telling me how relieved she was that I was there. I thought, Finally, here's one thing in my life that I am doing right.

Many of us may be worried about not having time for our spouse or partner or for our children, missing work, or not saving enough for a secure retirement. When the physical or emotional demands upon us increase, we are more likely to feel burdened by our caretaking responsibilities and less likely to take care of ourselves.

I was not putting myself first. I was putting my husband's needs, my children, my job, and everything else first. My health was suffering and my quality of life was really in bad shape.

Take time to do good things for yourself. It is important to acknowledge your feelings, monitor and learn to manage your stress, and take care of your own health.

Also, recognize that caring for elderly family members is a responsibility that is difficult if not impossible to manage alone. Whenever possible, enlist help from others—whether your siblings, partner, children, other relatives, family friends, or paid professionals. Ask those who live far away to contribute financially or to provide you with occasional breaks. Organizations in your community may also offer help, such as free meal delivery and respite care. If you are financially able, consider hiring someone to help with cleaning or provide other assistance.

Caregiving can bring us closer to family, but sometimes it causes strain in family relationships. If conflicts arise on health care decisions, financial and living arrangements, or communication problems, help is available. The National Family Caregiver Support Program, created in 2001, is the first universal federal program providing information, support, counseling, respite, and other services to caregivers. (For information in your local area, call Eldercare Locator at 1-800-677-1116.) You may also be able to find a support group in your community. If you live far from your older relatives, geriatric care managers can help organize needed services and solve problems.

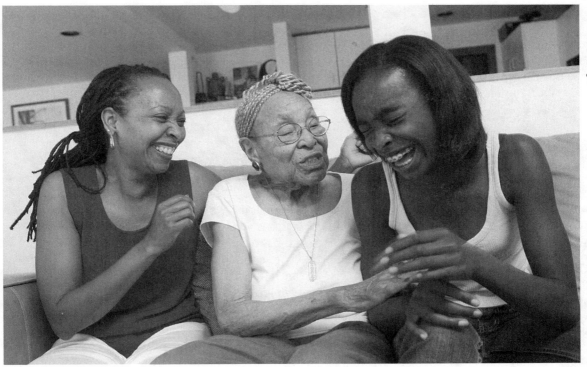
© ColorBlind Images

Try to avoid potential problems by preparing in advance. Find out if your parents have drawn up a will, a health care proxy, and an advance directive or living will with instructions for emergency care and end-of-life decisions; if they haven't, ask them to consider doing so. Make sure you and other important people in their lives have copies. Know where to look for Social Security cards, financial account information (pensions, checkbooks, savings passbooks, stock certificates, bonds, and trusts), health insurance (Medicare, co-insurance, Medicaid, long-term care), home insurance, and other legal documents. Having a power of attorney or signature on an account enables you to take care of bills and transactions if this becomes necessary. Find out what kind of living situation your parents want if they can no longer live independently. As we take care of others, it's also important to think about our own aging and anticipate our own long-term care needs.

THE WORKPLACE

Although menopause marks the end of our reproductive lives, it's not the end of our productive lives. Work can give us a sense of accomplishment, increased self-esteem, financial security, increased independence, and communities of new friends and coworkers. However, many of us may find ourselves in low-level jobs, laid off, or frozen out of the workforce by age discrimination, just when we ought to be at the peak of our earning power. Choices for work may narrow, and we may find change difficult. Fortunately, we don't have to struggle alone;

ABUSE

Violence against women is pervasive in the United States and around the globe. We continue to be at risk for physical, sexual, emotional, and financial abuse. Exposure to violence not only can cause immediate harm; over a lifetime, it puts us at greater risk for depression, anxiety, obesity, and other health problems.[2]

Some of us who have been in long-term abusive relationships may feel freer to leave if our children are now leaving home. But abusive relationships may be hard to end, particularly if we lack financial independence. If we are divorced, widowed, or single, we may find ourselves in a new relationship that is abusive. Or we may find ourselves needing to care for a parent who is abusive to us.

Over the past thirty-five years, advocates for combating violence against women have developed laws, policies, and services to help those of us who encounter violence and abuse. If you are in an abusive relationship, you can take steps to plan for your safety. Find someone to tell about the abuse, whether it is a supportive friend, appropriate service provider, or your health care practitioner. Help is available. Call the National Domestic Violence Hotline: 1-800-799-SAFE. Ask if your area has a local domestic violence hotline. If you are in an emergency situation, call 911.

Abuse may be a factor in depression. Counseling may help you deal with the feelings.

there are lots of us, and we're starting to have some clout.

FINDING OR CHANGING JOBS

At this time, many of us decide to go back to school to earn a degree, take classes in continuing education or certificate programs, or obtain special training for employment. Even if we've spent years at home, we have abilities that can be transferred to the workplace. Some of us want to change jobs or negotiate improvements in our current situations.

Research your options. Talk to other women, build a support network, and find out about programs in your state, city, or community. Women Work! The National Network for Women's Employment, a nonprofit organization, provides services for women entering or reentering the workforce (1-202-467-6346,

or www.womenwork.org). Employment counselors and life coaches also can be helpful.

WORK-FAMILY BALANCE

Many of us are balancing work with raising children or grandchildren, caring for aging or disabled family members, or both. These multiple responsibilities can be both gratifying and stressful. Sixty-five percent of working women who are caregivers report having to make workplace adjustments; these include having to go in late to work, leave early, take time off, request unpaid leave, go from full-time to part-time (which usually means losing benefits), turn down promotions, or quit working entirely.[3]

We need to develop workplace survival skills. These may include planning ahead and gathering phone numbers of neighbors, friends, and community services to call if an emergency comes up, or hiring a professional geriatric care manager to handle a crisis. You may want to form a support group at work, talk to your employer about alternative ways of getting a job done, or find a workplace that offers good work-family polices and use it as a role model in talking to your employer. Remember to take care of yourself, too; sometimes, taking ten minutes to meditate or go for a walk in the middle of a challenging day can help.

Both women and men need support in balancing work and family roles. We need employers to develop family-friendly policies, including flextime, compressed hours, telecommuting, part-time work with benefits, job sharing, access to counseling, and paid family leave and sick leave.

PLANNING FOR RETIREMENT

This is also a time to think about our later years. Money is crucial to aging well and healthfully. Because women live longer and earn less than men, we face extra challenges in saving funds for our retirement years. Unfortunately, traditional sources of retirement income are less stable than before. Far fewer people receive defined-benefit pensions, and the current level of Social Security payments is not guaranteed forever. Although some of us can expect retirement income from husbands or partners, most women receive nothing other than Social Security. Even those who were promised continued benefits after retirement may be denied pensions or health insurance when former employers merge, are bought out by other companies, or go bankrupt.

Take time to plan for your financial security in retirement: Make a long-term budget, check your pension benefits if you have them, find out what your Social Security benefits will be, increase your savings, start an IRA account, and consult a financial planner. Seminars and courses in financial planning are offered at adult education centers and community colleges.

NEW VISIONS FOR LIFE AFTER MENOPAUSE

The image of postmenopausal women is changing. We're looking at more active years than our mothers did and can explore options, discover strengths, and enjoy life on our own terms. We need a new blueprint for these years, one that allows for changes in family structures, work patterns, and our roles as caregivers, as well as new definitions of retirement, and the possibility of many healthy postretirement years. The menopausal transition is a change, but it can be a time of great enrichment.

NOTES

1. National Alliance for Caregiving and AARP, *Caregiving in the U.S.: Findings from the National Caregiver Survey* (Maryland: 2004); see also Families and Work Institute, *Generation and Gender in the Workplace* (New York: 2005).
2. S. R. Dube, R. F. Anda, C. L. Whitfield, D. W. Brown, V. J. Felitte, M. Dong, and W. H. Giles, "Long-Term Consequences of Childhood Sexual Abuse by Gender of Victim," *American Journal of Preventative Medicine* 5 (June 28, 2005): 430–38.
3. National Alliance for Caregiving and AARP; also unpublished analysis of survey data by Les Plooster, program associate for National Alliance for Caregiving.

Taking Care of Ourselves

CHAPTER 11

Emotional Well-Being and Managing Stress

Emotions surrounding menopause vary and evolve. We may feel like celebrating the transition, we may barely notice it, or we may be concerned or upset about changes. How we feel about menopause is linked to our physical experience and overall health. But it is also deeply connected to our financial circumstances, our work and family life, our social networks, our coping skills, the messages we hear from our culture, and our own perceptions.

In a study on menopause and psychological development, researchers found that the menopausal transition is a positive period for most women. Even if we start out with negative emotions, these often become more positive as we go through the transition.[1] Many of us note improvements in our family or home life, our sense of personal fulfillment, and our ability to focus on new interests and friends.[2] One woman says,

This has been one of the most liberating times in my life. I travel by myself all over the world; I'm not so concerned about what people think about me anymore. My self-esteem has gotten a boost and I've gotten a lot closer to my girlfriends.

Research shows that, in general, factors that most accurately predict feelings of well-being in our postmenopause years include good health, adequate income, social support, and a positive outlook about our health and our ability to handle stress.[3] While some of these factors are beyond our personal control, others may be responsive to changes we can make. We can take active steps to embrace good health habits, build supportive social networks, and learn ways to cope better with stress.

If we are coping with problems associated with menopause or other health concerns, balancing caregiving and work, struggling to get by on too little money, or facing abuse or discrimination, we are likely to feel overwhelmed and exhausted at times. Finding ways to take care of ourselves can help foster the resiliency we need to make changes in our lives and cope with challenges.

STRESS

Many factors can contribute to how much stress we experience. Having too many demands upon us can generate stress, as can many of life's daily hassles, the inequities of our lives, and ageist or negative attitudes about aging. *Stress* can be defined as a state or condition caused by our body's automatic response to a perceived or real threat. While the thoughts and realities that trigger stress are processed in our minds, stress ultimately affects the whole body in a physical way. Sometimes we can reduce or eliminate the causes of our stress; when that's not possible, we may be able to find ways of better managing stress.

THE STRESS RESPONSE

The stress response is designed to protect us from danger. Back in early human existence, the response allowed us to sense danger and mount an instantaneous, automatic response to increase our chances of survival. Called the *fight-or-flight response,* it relies on a complex relay of chemicals in the body to mobilize key systems. Our heart rate increases, our blood pressure increases, muscles tense in preparation for action, and adrenaline pumps through our body. As critical systems are activated, the redirection of hormones and blood flow dampens other systems like the digestive and reproductive systems, which are not essential for a quick escape.

Triggered occasionally, the stress response serves us well. We can be more productive with a certain level of stress. Unfortunately, in an era when "threats" come from all directions (blaring car alarms, long traffic jams, demanding employers, financial problems, rude people), we tend to overactivate the response, and stress becomes *distress.*

What makes this response more complex is that the threat does not even have to be real. Perceived threats or even expectations, like anticipation of a hot flash during a speaking engagement or anxiety about a pending deadline, can trigger the same physiologic response. Over time, stress hormones pulsing through our bodies can affect our health, although their influence is not fully understood. It may involve many factors, including the way we manage stress.

THE FINE ART OF EFFECTIVE COPING

While there are many conditions in our lives over which we have little to no control, finding coping skills and using stress management techniques can help us change our reactions to these circumstances, find more balance in our lives, and become more resilient. We take care of our emotional well-being in many ways: We may call a friend, go for a walk, cry, go to church, take karate lessons, make love, garden, seek spiritual guidance, watch a funny movie, protest an injustice, or cook.

STRESS AND HEALTH

Stress has a clear impact on our bodies. When we are scared or tense, our hearts race and our breathing becomes shallow. When our lives are particularly stressful, many of us experience headaches, digestive problems, insomnia, and a host of other discomforts. Some research provides evidence that chronic stress can make us more prone to anxiety and depression and put us at higher risk of experiencing intense hot flashes and insomnia.[4]

It is important to recognize the physical effects of stress. Yet stress is not a simple phenomenon. People sometimes assume that stress alone is responsible for a wide range of physical, psychological, and behavioral problems that may in fact stem from other causes. Some research does not make clear the difference between **correlation** and **cause and effect**; many conditions correlated with stress are not necessarily caused by stress, although stress may be a factor. For example, a research study concluding that stress puts women at higher risk of experiencing intense hot flashes and insomnia may not examine the possibility that women who experience hot flashes and insomnia are more likely to feel distressed by the experience, and therefore report higher stress levels.

Health problems that are little understood are often blamed on the catchall "stress." Women are particularly vulnerable to having our ailments dismissed as the results of stress. For example, before the cause of multiple sclerosis—an illness that disproportionately affects women—was known, women who experienced its symptoms were often considered to have a mental impairment and diagnosed with "hysteria."[5] Similarly, researchers have tried to link stressful life events or certain personality traits to an increased likelihood of developing or having a recurrence of breast cancer, but there is no evidence to back this up.[6]

The ways that stress affects our bodies and minds are complex, not fully understood, and correlated with many other factors, such as our access to resources, our family histories, and the toxicity of our local environment. For this reason, it is vital that we consider the broader context of our lives at the same time that we learn how stress may affect us. When we focus on stress alone as the cause of most or all health problems, we run the risk of ignoring multiple social, political, and genetic determinants of health.

I go swimming for twenty minutes and it's like I'm addicted. It totally clears my head and it changes my breathing pattern. It just slows everything right down. I feel exhilarated when I'm done.

Women have practiced calming rituals such as prayer, meditation, yoga, drumming, dance, and tai chi for thousands of years. These practices continue to offer us wonderful ways to release emotion, connect to our minds, bodies, and spirituality, and reach a state of relaxation.

I think yoga is my meditation practice. It's the one thing I can do that takes a hundred percent of my mind, so that it really is a timeout from life and it also strengthens me. I'm certainly more flexible and I'm certainly stronger.

Playing the rhythmic patterns of the drum, whether alone or in community, functions as a spiritual practice, fostering meditative experiences . . . and it's just plain fun. Through my drumming, I've also met a variety of spiritually

WAYS TO TAKE CARE OF OUR EMOTIONAL WELL-BEING

- Pay attention to what you think and feel. Identifying and understanding the sources of stress in our lives is a first step toward coping.
- Eat well, get enough rest, and be physically active. These wellness strategies can help us feel calm and more resilient. Exercise and regular movement in particular can help us release the pain of anger, grief, fear, or depression.
- Stay connected to people you care about; develop and nurture your relationships. Consider joining a support or common-interest group; reach out to neighbors; volunteer.
- Cultivate peace of mind and relaxation. Some of us find meaning and comfort in meditation, prayer, or participation in a religious community. Others relax through activities such as singing, painting, reading, or gardening. Engage in activities that foster your gratitude, appreciation, and compassion.
- Work for social/political change. When the stressors in our lives are too big and powerful to tackle on our own, working with friends, neighbors, or colleagues to change the conditions that make our lives difficult can give us a sense of purpose and help us see our individual concerns within a larger societal context.

oriented women, many of whom are older than I, who talk passionately and with conviction about those traditions or societies that value aging.

ACKNOWLEDGING OUR FEELINGS

Many of us learned at an early age that we're not supposed to be angry or aggressive or want or need "too much." When we repeatedly suppress these "negative" feelings, we may eventually be less aware of what we feel. Yet many of us have much to be angry about, from the pervasiveness of racism, sexism, and other injustices that affect our lives to the individual losses we have suffered. Learning to know what we feel and why we may feel as we do, and learning how to release or express our feelings in appropriate and constructive ways, can free us to feel better about our lives. Keeping a journal, making art, seeing a therapist, crying with friends,

or exercising vigorously can all be helpful ways of releasing and addressing emotions.

I find it helpful to write out my thoughts. By journaling, I feel more clarity about what I'm feeling and why I'm angry. I feel more control.

When my teenagers are pushing my buttons, I say I need time out and I do short bursts of running. I find it a really great way to get rid of tension. It just dissipates.

PROBLEM SOLVING

I joined a local Paid Sick Leave Coalition to channel my frustrations about the lack of good work/family policies that are desperately needed.

Knowing when to take action is an important part of effective coping. Although we can't control all of the external circumstances of our lives, if we can focus on solutions to specific problems, we are more apt to take the actions that will ultimately benefit us. The action we choose may involve changing jobs, reassessing a relationship, seeking out advice or support, fighting for a cause, or simply changing a schedule.

Part of my stress was my commute. So I did negotiate working one day a week from home.

I have ended a few friendships because they were not healthy for me. I realized that I had been attracted to needy friends who complained to me about the same problems over and over and yet never took any "advice." When I tried to change the basis for the relationships, it just didn't work. In that case, the only thing to do is to move on. I choose now to be around positive people.

When our relationships are a source of stress, learning effective communication styles can be extremely helpful. Positive communications may involve setting boundaries, saying no, carving time for ourselves, or recognizing and addressing the sources of our anger or frustration. An eighty-year-old woman recalls entering midlife while trying to take care of a son with a disability. Finding it difficult to get good care for him, she started a business that addresses the needs of the developmentally challenged.

The best part of midlife for me was starting a new business. I started my business in 1982 with $80,000, 6 clients, 4 staff. Today the business has $5 million revenue, 350 clients, and 156 staff. This all started twenty-three years ago when I was fifty-seven. There have been major changes in my life since then—death of husband, new business—but my outlook is basically the same. I am essentially an optimistic person and see the glass half full. And believe that change is possible

and there is always a way around an obstacle; you just have to keep looking for it. Sometimes it is the least obvious way.

RETHINKING OUR THOUGHTS

Our perceptions and interpretations affect our experiences. Sometimes we react automatically to things that happen to us with negative thoughts. Learning to be aware of our thought patterns and developing skills to reframe our thoughts may help us cope better. Reversing pessimistic thoughts may start with asking yourself some basic questions: Does this thought contribute to my stress? Is this a logical thought? Is thinking this way helpful to me? Is this thought true? (For more information about "restructuring" thoughts, see *The Feeling Good Handbook* by David Burns.)

Studies show correlations between negative perceptions of menopause and women's experience of this transition.[7] While it's not entirely clear how perceptions and experience interact, in cultures in which aging women are given elevated status or in which menopause is viewed as a normal stage of the life cycle, women report menopause as being less problematic.[8]

If we develop skills to reframe our thoughts with a more positive twist, we may sometimes be able to shift from recoiling from "threats" to rising to "challenges." Listening to our thoughts can help in identifying defeatist ideas.

THE RELAXATION RESPONSE

In the late 1960s, members of a group that practiced transcendental meditation walked into Harvard Medical School claiming that they could reduce their blood pressure using meditation alone. Though skeptical, cardiologist Dr. Herbert Benson agreed to study them. Fascinated by the striking physiologic changes he noted—a decrease in heart rate, breathing rate, blood pressure, and metabolic rate—he coined the term *relaxation response* to describe the phenomenon.[9] Today, studies continue to replicate these early findings.[10]

The relaxation response is the exact opposite of the stress response. Achieving this state has a rejuvenating effect on the mind and body. In scientific studies, daily elicitation of the relaxation response (RR) has been shown to decrease hot flashes, improve sleep, lessen PMS, and improve energy.[11] Women who participated in a ten-week program that combined RR with cognitive techniques have reported improved interpersonal relationships, spiritual growth, and better stress management; they were also more apt to engage in health-promoting behaviors such as exercising and eating a nutritious diet.[12]

Eliciting the Relaxation Response

We can learn to evoke the relaxation response using many techniques. These include meditation, prayer, deep breathing, yoga, tai chi, and a variety of other techniques, such as mindfulness, imagery, or progressive muscle relaxation. (See the Mind/Body Medical Institute, www.mbmi.org, for more information.) All techniques have two basic components. First is the **focusing of attention** through repetition of a word, prayer, phrase, or physical activity; and the second is the **passive disregard of everyday thoughts** when they occur and the return to the repetition. The common denominator in all of these methods is that they attempt to break the train of everyday thought and disengage the stress response.

It's like learning to ride a bike. It can take a lot of repeated tries before all of a sudden, oh, that's how you do it. It took me a while. Once you figure it out, you've got it.

I do meditate now, and I know how to get into the state. And it makes me feel really good. I know that it's a tool, that if I need it, it's there for me and works. I'm always in a hurry. I'm always busy. So, a situation that would create anxiety in the past—now it doesn't have that kind of effect on me.

If RR is evoked regularly, the effects tend to carry over. The same stressors no longer have the same impact on us. Some women refer to RR as "rolling with the punches." A regular RR practice of twenty minutes a day is required to achieve maximum benefits.

Mini Breaks and Mindfulness

Relaxation breaks can be worked into even the busiest schedule. "Mini" relaxation responses are helpful, especially during times of stress. These breaks involve taking a few deep breaths, creating a soothing image to focus on (like swimming in a cool pool), or doing gentle stretches to relieve tension. Some women find these breaks can help short-circuit hot flashes.[13]

I use them when I'm feeling stressed. In traffic it's just about sitting back and taking a few deep breaths. If too much is going on at work and I feel overwhelmed and I'm feeling stretched, it just becomes a part of you. You say, okay, I'm not responding well to what's going on. I need to take a few steps back.

It is also helpful to be mindful when you can. The concept of mindfulness has roots in Buddhism and other traditions that place great importance on conscious awareness and attention. *Mindfulness* is focused awareness on the present moment, the *opposite* of multitasking. It elicits the RR by focusing the senses (sight, smell, touch, etc.) on the moment. It allows us to let go of the future (often fraught with anxiety) and let go of the past (often fraught with regret). Try it while reading to a child, walking your dog, eating a piece of chocolate, listening to music, or watching a sunset. It's a powerful way to move into relaxation.

As a mother, you're multitasking all the time. Mindfulness made me realize it's okay to focus on one thing at a time. There is so much pressure in our society to do more than that.

I find myself finding ways to "self-nurture" and being mindful to live in the present and not dream off about what may or may not ever be.

I look outside and reflect on what is going on outside with the sky, clouds, sun, rain, or snow. Nature is amazing to me and can always make me feel good.

CONTEMPLATION

Some women use a form of meditation called *contemplation* to help cultivate personal insight or desirable emotional states such as tolerance, loving kindness, peace, and serenity. In the stillness of meditation (see sidebar, page 174), you can pose a question and wait for an answer to come to you. If you are stressed or angry, you can contemplate positive emotions such as forgiveness, gratitude, or acceptance. Imagine yourself filled with the emotion or repeat the word.

I picked "gratitude" and I closed my eyes and focused on my breathing. . . . Within seconds of starting to reflect about what in life I should be most grateful for, the word "myself" came shouting out at me. For my own mind to say "myself" was something so far out of the blue that it was like a personal epiphany. . . . I needed to work on taking better care of myself. I have been able to get so much insight just by tapping into my "inner self." The answers are right there if I take the time to ask the right questions and give myself the chance to hear the answers.

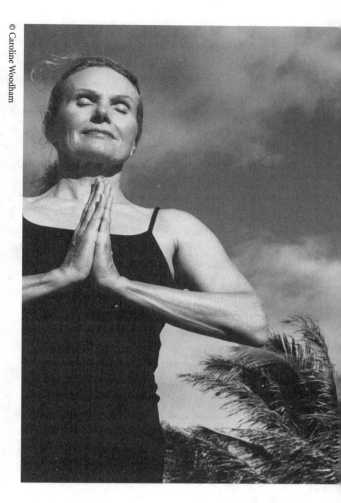

© Caroline Woodham

SPIRITUALITY

Spirituality means many things to many women. It is often linked to formal religion but does not have to be. Spirituality is about creating connection and finding meaning in something larger than ourselves. Embracing spirituality can be a transforming, transcendent experience.

Spirituality is the most important thing for me. It is my peace, my love nucleus, my energy, my breath, hope . . . really my lifeline.

MEDITATION

1. Assume a comfortable position and close your eyes.
2. Take a few deep breaths to calm your mind and body. Inhale deeply, expanding your stomach. As you exhale, imagine that you are blowing out a candle.
3. Then concentrate on a mental focus, such as a word or sound or phrase or prayer that you repeat silently to yourself in rhythm with your breath.
4. If your thoughts or something from the outside world distracts you, take a deep breath and return to your mental focus. Instead of getting caught up in an internal dialogue, gently redirect your attention to your out-breath, focus word, or phrase. You will find that with time and practice, this redirection becomes easier.
5. Continue for 10-20 minutes. (Place a clock nearby, so that when you feel your time is up, you can take a quick look and then choose to continue or stop.)
6. Take a few slow, deep breaths, stretch, and slowly open your eyes.

There are many paths to spirituality. Many women have a sense of spirituality related to a church, synagogue, or temple; for some of us, our spirituality is grounded in nature. Many of us also find spiritual connection as we bond with other women and men.

We may encounter spirituality in unexpected ways. One woman recalls,

I had a house fire and lost most of my belongings on Christmas Eve six years ago. It was a religious experience. You learn to get right to the basics: love.

Whatever our path, many of us believe that we are connected to ourselves and to others on a profound level, and that life has meaning and purpose. Sometimes during our darkest moments, this belief helps us find an open door. It can help us discover a sense of peace even when our lives are out of control.

Our spiritual journeys may start with finding our own voices. We may begin by asking questions: What am I most passionate about? What do I believe most in? What is my purpose? What is my legacy? For many of us, the path to spirituality is a gift in itself. It's an opportunity for personal growth, awareness, the rekindling of old passions, and the embracing of new possibilities.

I love midlife. I have learned that and I am being brave enough to attempt things I haven't before. I feel like there is nothing I cannot do.

MOVING TO ACCEPTANCE

Certain things in life we cannot change or solve. When we are faced with the death of a loved one, an illness, the loss of a job, or any other major crisis, effective coping requires acceptance. This is one of the most difficult tasks we face.

A fifty-five-year-old woman says,

I was nowhere near menopause when I went through chemo-induced menopause ten years ago. It was like being slammed into a brick wall at warp speed and has left me with nuclear-level hot flashes day and night. From sleeping on flannel sheets to sleeping in a T-shirt and briefs, from waist-long straight hair to short curls, from nor-

• *Deep breathing techniques can reduce the intensity of hot flashes.*

Reality. Researchers have found relaxation techniques involving progressive muscle relaxation and deep-breathing exercises reduced self-reported hot flashes by about 50 percent.[14] Objective skin temperature measurements were used to help demonstrate that the women who learned and practiced breathing techniques were most effectively able to reduce the number of hot flashes. (For more information, see "Cool Off!" page 78.)

mal body hair to almost none, and of course the loss of a breast: It was an overwhelming load of issues to deal with. My life has been threatened and changed and my personal philosophy has changed with it.

As a cancer survivor, this woman went on to face another hurdle:

An art teacher for thirty-seven years, I was devastated when my job was eliminated two years ago due to enrollment declines. I hadn't come out the other side of the menopause tunnel yet. Then I reclaimed at least part of my essential life. I had time and energy to pour into my artwork and within a short period of time had achieved spectacular results. My work is flowing, and recognition and sales of it are booming.

Many of us find that accepting that which we cannot control allows us to move forward with greater ease. We may need to seek out support and cultivate appreciation for what we have, or recognize positive changes resulting from difficult circumstances.

SOCIAL CONNECTIONS

Boosting our social supports during and after the menopause transition is important on many levels. Positive connections can serve as a

buffer to stress and anger.[15] When we are socially isolated, we are at greater risk for heart disease and depression.[16] When we feel committed to work, family, friends, home life, and community, we become more resilient.[17] Reaching out to friends can dramatically affect our moods and our lives. As one fifty-seven-year-old woman notes,

I think women's relationships with other women are absolutely essential for survival in this culture. There is a serious negative attitude about aging and it's so important to relate to peers who understand the issues and can support each other. Finding others who share interests is also key. Women don't always have to do things selflessly for others. We must nurture ourselves, too.

Taking care of ourselves is key. There is a difference between selfishness and self-care. Self-care means moving away from the belief that your needs come last. It means caring enough about yourself to prioritize those activities that will promote your own health: taking time for socializing, for relaxation, and for embracing what is meaningful to you. Many of us lead busy lives, and the hours of the day evaporate. We reap many benefits when we realize that scheduling time for ourselves is essential to our health.

I now find myself considering what I would like to do and seeing to it that I do it . . . little things like taking time to enjoy my garden and a quiet cup of tea out there in the mornings before the day begins.

I get coffee every Saturday with a group of my friends. I have a social network. I built that into my life.

I had friends in my book club who were going through the same thing at the same time. We shared so much and laughed a lot. It was great to hear that we all had such similar issues. We shared solutions and our own research. It was a lifesaver for me.

I started to ask older women what was going on. The stories began to pour out, and I got the best advice possible: "Recognize the moments and learn to laugh."

Many of us are learning to laugh and finding joy in the menopause experience. Groups heralding midlife are gaining members. And there is a push to do more. One woman sums it up,

Yes, I'm menopausal in a midlife transition, but other than talking to friends, I don't feel I have any cultural support as I face my "empty nest." At other stages of life there are rites of passage, and we need to develop some for midlife.

Rituals have long been used to help people move through transitions (birth, death, coming of age). Rituals bind us to community and support us through change. Until now, menopause in our culture has been taboo. That is changing. We are talking about it and some women are beginning to create rituals for menopause. One woman who participated in a ritual to honor the life stage of the "crone" or "wise woman" says,

I was personally having a difficult time at letting go of my childbearing/rearing time, a wonderful part of my life, and this ritual, in a circle of friends, helped me move into this new phase with hope, joy, and meaning.

The idea behind these rituals is to recognize where we've been and where we're going; to celebrate womanhood; to renew our bonds; and to discover meaning and purpose. As the idea catches on in the United States, we may see these rituals go mainstream. The goal is to join other cultures in paying homage to wisdom and new beginnings.

EMOTIONAL WELL-BEING AND SOCIAL CHANGE

As we go through the menopause transition, we may work as individuals and in groups to change what we can, whether it is the outside circumstances that are contributing to stress in our lives or our own reactions to those circumstances. Coping skills and stress management techniques can help us manage the stress of our demanding day-to-day lives, but they alone can not alleviate known health predictors such as poverty, homelessness, racism, and other oppressive conditions. For that, we need to work together for social change and justice.

NOTES

1. H. Bush, A. S. Barth-Olofsson, S. Rosenhagen, and A. Collins, "Menopausal Transition and Psychological Development," *Menopause* 10, no. 2 (2003): 179–87.

2. North American Menopause Society 1998 Menopause Survey. *Menopause: The Journal of the North American Menopause Society,* Volume 7, Issue 2.

3. N. A. Woods, et al., "Patterns of Depressed Mood Across the Menopause Transition: Approaches to Studying Patterns in Longitudinal Data," *Acta Obstet Gynec Scand* 81 (2002): 623–32.

4. E. W. Freeman, M. D. Sammel, H. Lin, C. R. Gracia, S. Kapoor, T. Ferdousi, "The Role of Anxiety and Hormonal Changes in Menopausal Hot Flashes," *Menopause* 12, no. 3 (May/June 2005): 258–66.

5. Collin Lee Talley, "The Emergence of Multiple Sclerosis, 1870–1950: A Puzzle of Historical Epidemiology," *Perspectives in Biology and Medicine* 48, no. 3 (summer 2005): 383–95.

6. Susan Love, "Keeping Emotions Bottled Up," accessed at susanlovernd.com/community/questions/question 010525.htm on August 29, 2005.

7. H. Bush, A. S. Barth-Olofsson, S. Rosenhagen, and A. Collins, "Menopausal Transition and Psychological Development," *Menopause* 10, no. 2 (2003): 179–87.

8. R. Formanek, *The Meanings of Menopause* (Hillsdale, NJ: Analytic Press, 1990), 161, 167.

9. Herbert Benson, *The Relaxation Response* (New York: Avon Books, 1975), 83.

10. R. H. Schneider and C. N. Alexander, "Long-Term Effects of Stress Reduction on Mortality in Persons > or = 55 Years of Age with Systemic Hypertension," *American Journal of Cardiology* 95, no. 9 (May 1, 2005): 1060–64.

11. Leslee Kagan, Bruce Kessel, and Herbert Benson, *Mind over Menopause: The Complete Mind/Body Approach to Coping with Menopause* (New York: Free Press, 2004), 195–218.

12. Leslee Kagan, Eileen O'Connell, et al., "The Impact of Group Cognitive-Behavioral Therapy on Menopausal Symptoms," abstract presented at the North American Menopause Society (NAMS) Meeting, 1999.

13. Robert R. Freedman, "Hot Flash Etiology: New Directions for Research," *Menopause Management* 11, no. 4 (July/August 2002): 8–14.

14. R. R. Freedman et al., "Behavioral Treatment of Menopausal Hot Flushes: Evaluation by Ambulatory Monitoring," *American Journal of Obstetrics and Gynecology* 167 (1992): 436–39.

15. Alice D. Domar and Henry Dreher, *Healing Mind, Healthy Woman* (New York: Bantam Doubleday Dell, 1996), 134.

16. B. H. Brummett, J. C. Barefoot, and I. C. Siegler, "Characteristics of Socially Isolated Patients with Coronary Artery Disease Who Are at Elevated Risk for Mortality," *Psychosomatic Medicine* 63, no. 2 (March–April, 2001): 267–72.

17. Kagan, et al., *Mind over Menopause,* 287–88.

CHAPTER 12

Eating Well

Although the basic principles of healthy eating apply throughout our lives, we have particular reasons to choose a healthy diet in the years before and after menopause. Changes in our diets at this time may help relieve problems associated with the menopause transition, reduce our risks of developing chronic diseases, and make us feel healthier and stronger. Eating well and staying active can improve the odds that the rest of our years will be healthy ones.

WHAT IS A HEALTHY DIET?

"Eat a low-fat diet." "Stay away from carbs." "Don't eat for three hours before going to bed." Advice about what to eat and what not to eat is abundant and often conflicting, and it is sometimes tempting to stop paying attention and simply eat whatever we want.

Yet beneath the latest headlines, fads, and advertising, researchers and nutritionists actually agree on many basic principles of healthy eating. The following recommendations are gathered from sources that include the 2005 federal dietary guidelines, the American Heart Association's dietary guidelines, and the Harvard School of Public Health's Department of Nutrition, where investigations by Dr. Walter Willett and others have generated much scientific knowledge on how diet and nutrition affect women's health.

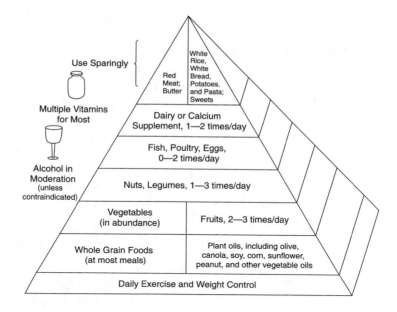

Source: *Eat, Drink, and Be Healthy,* by Walter C. Willett, M.D. (New York: Simon & Schuster, 2001)

The Healthy Eating Pyramid, developed by nutritionists at the Harvard School of Public Health, summarizes the latest evidence on good nutrition. To find out more about the Healthy Eating Pyramid, see *Eat, Drink, and Be Healthy* by Walter Willett, and the Nutrition Source website at www.hsph.harvard.edu/nutritionsource/.

EAT WHOLE GRAINS

As much as possible, eat your grains in minimally processed whole-grain form. Try eating more whole grains such as brown rice, oats, or barley, and foods made with whole grains, such as whole-wheat pasta or whole-grain breads. Limit highly processed grains such as white bread, white pasta, and refined cereals. Whole-grain foods have numerous health benefits and reduce our risk of developing various conditions, including heart disease, diabetes, diverticular disease, and constipation.

EAT PLENTY OF VEGETABLES AND FRUITS

These staples of a healthy diet help prevent heart disease, stroke, and some types of cancer; reduce the incidence of cataracts and macular degeneration, two common age-related causes of vision loss;[1] and help maintain good bowel health. Choose vegetables and fruits from a wide range of colors—from the deep blue/purple of eggplants and blueberries to the dark green of spinach and broccoli to the bright red of tomatoes and strawberries—to ensure that you get adequate fiber and a wide range of vitamins, minerals, and phytochemicals.

CHOOSE HEALTHY FATS

For years fat has gotten a bad rap. Americans have repeatedly been told to eat a diet low in fat, but this common nutritional advice fails to take into account that different kinds of fat affect our bodies in differing ways. There are two major types of natural fats—saturated and unsaturated. (Unsaturated fats can be further classified as either monounsaturated or polyunsaturated.) A third type of fat, trans fat, is created in the manufacturing process of many commercially prepared foods.

Unsaturated fats—the kind in olives, nuts, avocados, fish, and vegetable oils—are "good" fats that help our bodies absorb the nutrients in our foods and lower the risk of heart disease.

Saturated fats are found in foods such as whole milk, butter, cheese, red meats, and coconut. Standard nutritional advice recommends limiting saturated fats in our diets, as they are believed to contribute to high blood cholesterol levels, which are linked to heart disease. While there is some controversy about how important it is to limit saturated fat,[2] most nutritionists suggest substituting low-fat dairy for full-fat products and limiting our intake of fatty meats.

Trans fats, on the other hand, are clearly "bad" fats. These fats, also known as hydrogenated fats, are found in many commercially prepared baked goods, margarines, snack foods, and processed foods. All foods that list partially hydrogenated oils in the ingredient list contain trans fats. New government regulations mandate that trans fats be listed on all food labels. Trans fats contribute to heart disease and should be eliminated from our diet wherever possible.

CHOOSE HEALTHY PROTEIN SOURCES

Choose nuts, beans, tofu and other soy-based products, chicken, fish, and lean cuts of meat to meet your body's need for protein. These foods are high in protein and other nutrients but low in saturated fats.

WHY EAT LOCALLY GROWN FOOD?

What we eat and where our food comes from have changed dramatically over the last century. The large corporations that produce, process, and distribute the vast majority of our foods aim to produce as much food as they can for the lowest possible cost, regardless of the consequences to our health or to the health of the environment. Agribusiness regularly wastes enormous quantities of resources, creates pollution, raises animals under unsanitary and inhumane conditions, produces inadequately tested genetically modified foods, and heavily advertises the most processed, least healthful foods.*

In response, many of us are turning to locally grown, often organic foods. Some of us are growing our own food, shopping at local farmers' markets, or joining community-supported agriculture groups (CSAs), which allow members to pay a yearly fee to support a farm in exchange for a weekly share of fruits, vegetables, and other farm products.

Choosing foods that are locally grown and organic is beneficial for all: We get fresh, nutritious food, and our food dollars support environmentally sustainable farming practices, local farmers, and the local economy. To find out where you can find locally grown organic foods near you, visit the Local Harvest website at www.localharvest.org.

* To find out more about how the food industry affects our health, see *Food Politics: How the Food Industry Influences Nutrition and Health* by Marion Nestle, and *Fast Food Nation: The Dark Side of the All-American Meal* by Eric Schlosser.

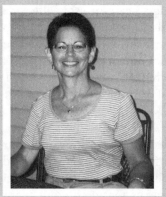

"I made it my mantra to change my lifestyle."

DEBRA WALFIELD

I used to be a closet eater. I figured if no one was looking, I didn't eat it. Although I hid it well, I was thirty pounds overweight. I used to stay up late at night reading and eating junk food like chips—I craved the salt—and chocolate.

Then I found out I had prediabetes, which means my blood sugars were high and I was on my way to getting diabetes. Both my parents have diabetes, so I know how serious it is. That was the incentive I needed to lose the weight. I volunteered to be in the Diabetes Prevention Program and was randomized to the lifestyles group. The program is great. I received coaching about making diet and exercise changes and behavior modification. That and having a support network were key.

I made it my mantra to change my lifestyle. Changing my eating habits was the hardest part, but within a few months I met my goal of losing eleven pounds and over the next year took off the whole thirty pounds.

I changed my method of cooking and now eat more vegetarian-style. I keep my portion sizes small. I don't deny myself, but if I have chocolate, I let it melt in my mouth and really taste it. I don't keep foods I used to binge on in the house anymore, like M&M's. And walking regularly is as much for my emotional well-being as it is for my physical.

I no longer have prediabetes. But I have to keep trying to push the diabetes back. Menopause was a challenge in terms of keeping the weight off. And I just went through some stressful times and put some weight back on. But I'm committed, and now I know I can put the brakes on the gain.

CUT DOWN ON "EMPTY CALORIES"

As much as possible, avoid eating highly processed sugary snacks, sodas, and sports drinks. These foods contain lots of calories but little if any nutrients; they also make your blood sugar and insulin levels shoot up and then crash, which can contribute to health problems and weight gain.

REMEMBER THAT SIZE MATTERS

It is easy to eat more than you need in our "supersize" culture, with its big portions and abundant, inexpensive junk food. Aim to balance your food intake with your activity level and keep your portion size moderate.

REDUCING HEALTH RISKS

The foods we eat can help us decrease our risk of developing illnesses or manage the ones we have.

HEART DISEASE AND STROKE

Coronary heart disease is much more likely after menopause than before.[3] Heart disease is the leading cause of death of American women;

cardiovascular disease (including stroke) kills twice as many women as all forms of cancers combined, including breast cancer.[4] (For more information, see Chapter 17, "Heart Health.")

We can reduce our likelihood of developing cardiovascular disease by participating in regular physical activity, quitting smoking or not starting to smoke, maintaining a healthy weight, and eating a "heart-healthy" diet. Such a diet includes plenty of dietary fiber, minimizes trans fats and saturated fats, and replaces these "bad" fats with unsaturated fats from fish and plant sources such as most vegetable oils, nuts, and seeds. The long-term Nurse's Health Study found that women who increased their intake of unsaturated fats lowered their risk for heart disease by about 30 to 40 percent.[5]

Cholesterol

Women in the perimenopausal and post-menopausal years tend to experience a change in cholesterols: Our so-called "bad" LDL (low-density lipoprotein) cholesterol increases and our "good" HDL (high-density lipoprotein) cholesterol goes down a bit. If LDL cholesterol is high and HDL is low, our risk of heart disease may increase. (There is some controversy about the effect of cholesterol on heart disease risk.)

While decreasing the amount of cholesterol we eat in foods may have a modest effect on blood cholesterol, the biggest dietary influence on cholesterol is the mix of fats in our diet. Certain types of fat—again, unsaturated fats from fish and from plant sources such as most vegetable oils, seeds, and nuts—are clearly good for cholesterol levels. Other types of fats—particularly trans fats but also saturated fats—are bad. Consuming less saturated fat and cholesterol in our diets can reduce the rise in LDL, according to findings from the Women's Healthy Lifestyle Project, a clinical research trial that followed 535 women for five years, starting at age forty-four to fifty.[6] (The study did not con-sider trans fats as a separate category of fats.) Women who made "heart-healthy" lifestyle changes in diet and exercise also were able to keep their perimenopausal weight gain in check. Women in the control group, who didn't make any lifestyle changes, on the other hand, gained an average of 5.2 pounds.

Soy

There is some evidence that adding soy to our diets, in the form of tofu and other soy-based foods, can lower cholesterol levels. Soy is an isoflavone, which means that it contains plant estrogens (phytoestrogens). Isoflavones have a similar chemical structure to estrogen and can exert a weak estrogenlike effect on the body. In 1999, the U.S. Food and Drug Administration approved the health claim that 25 grams per day of soy protein—as part of a diet low in saturated fat and cholesterol—may reduce the risk of heart disease. There are some concerns, however, that supplements containing soy protein or soy extracts are not as beneficial or as safe as food sources, particularly for women who have had breast cancer or are at high risk for it.[7]

Flaxseed

Flaxseed is another source of phytoestrogens that is increasingly in the spotlight. It also has a promising role in heart protection, largely because it contains alpha-linolenic acid (ALA), an essential fatty acid that the body cannot produce on its own.[8] ALA is a precursor of the heart-protective omega-3 fatty acids found in heart-healthy foods such as salmon and other fatty fish. (Although the mercury content of certain fish such as swordfish, shark, and tuna is a health concern for fetuses and young children whose nervous systems are still developing, for women past childbearing years, the benefits may outweigh the risks. Women who may still get pregnant should avoid eating fish that may contain high levels of mercury.)[9]

Alcohol

Much research has shown that moderate drinking—which is generally considered to be one drink a day for women—can lower our risk of cardiovascular disease. Recommending that women drink moderately, however, is problematic, given that many of us have difficulty controlling the amount of alcohol we drink, and heavy drinking has severe negative health consequences. Moderate drinking is also associated with an increased risk of breast cancer. Before deciding whether or not to drink alcohol, it is best to consider your individual risk factors. Women who have a personal or family history of addiction or breast cancer may want to consider avoiding alcohol; however, women with no such history who do not drink may want to consider adding a daily drink.

DIABETES

Type 2 diabetes (which used to be called adult-onset diabetes) is epidemic in the United States. As we age, we are at increased risk for diabetes, which now affects over 18 million adults in America—more than half of whom are women.[10] (For more information, see page 284.) While genetics may play a role in who develops diabetes, research data from the long-term Nurses' Health Study suggests that 90 percent of type 2 diabetes in women is attributable to behavioral and lifestyle factors such as excess weight, lack of exercise, and an unhealthy diet.[11]

But that's good news in terms of prevention. The Diabetes Prevention Program, a national clinical trial, found that just thirty minutes a day of moderate-intensity physical activity and a 5 percent to 10 percent loss in body weight will reduce the risk of a person's developing diabetes by more than one half.[12] Two-thirds of the participants in this study were women, of all ages and ethnic groups. In the study, every-body was told to eat less fat and exercise more, but one group received intensive training in how to diet, exercise, and change other behaviors (for example, how to shop for and cook healthier meals and overcome personal obstacles to losing weight). The results were so dramatic—coinciding as well with the findings of several other large-scale international studies—that the study was stopped one year early so the results could be reported to the public in 2002.

These are the most important dietary changes you can make to help prevent diabetes:

- Balance how many calories you eat with how active you are. Limiting portion sizes was one of the major ways that participants in the Diabetes Prevention Program were able to lose weight and reduce their risk for diabetes.
- Eat whole grains and whole-grain products rather than highly processed carbohydrates.
- Eat less saturated fat and avoid trans fats. Learn how to read food labels and become a "fat detective"; foods that contain hydrogenated or partially hydrogenated oils contain trans fats.

CANCER

As we age, we are also at greater risk of certain cancers (endometrial or colon, for example). In the early 1980s, research seemed to indicate that a low-fat diet was beneficial in reducing the risk of some cancers, particularly breast cancer, but further research has failed to confirm that *total* fat intake is a risk factor for cancer. However, new research indicates that certain *types* of fat may increase our risk of certain kinds of cancer. For example, the Nurses' Health Study found that women who consumed large amounts of trans fats had higher rates of non-Hodgkin's lymphoma, and women whose diets were high in saturated fat had an increased risk for endometrial cancer.[13] Such research suggests that avoiding foods that contain trans fats and limiting our intake of saturated fats is good not only for preventing cardiovascular disease but also possibly for reducing our chances of developing some types of cancer.

Maintaining a healthy body weight also appears to be protective against some kinds of cancer: Women who are overweight have a greater chance of developing colon, kidney, endometrial, and breast cancer.[14]

Evidence suggests that foods containing antioxidants (such as fruits and vegetables) have a cancer-protective as well as heart-protective effect. These same foods also tend to contain fiber, which can help prevent colon cancer and type 2 diabetes and ease constipation.

Research also shows that drinking alcohol increases women's risk of breast cancer. (For more information on alcohol and health, see page 282.)

OSTEOPOROSIS

The rapid decline of estrogen at menopause escalates the natural bone thinning that occurs as we grow older and increases our risk of developing osteoporosis. In addition to engaging in regular, weight-bearing exercise, there are several dietary guidelines we can follow to help minimize bone loss. These include:

- **Consume enough calcium.** Foods high in calcium include milk, cheese, and other dairy products, dark leafy greens, beans, and foods such as orange juice that are fortified with calcium.
- **Get adequate vitamin D, either through your diet, exposure to sunshine, or supplements.**
- **Get enough vitamin K.** Foods high in vitamin K include broccoli, brussels sprouts, dark green lettuce, collard greens, and kale. Vitamin K is also made by the bacteria that line the gastrointestinal tract.
- **Get vitamin A in your diet, but don't consume too much.**
- **Avoid eating substantial amounts of protein every day.** When you eat protein, your body releases acids into the bloodstream, which are then neutralized by drawing calcium from your bones. Protein from meats and animal products seem to pull more calcium from the bones than protein from vegetables and legumes.[15]

(For more extensive information on dietary needs and osteoporosis, see Chapter 16, "Bone Health.")

RELIEF FOR MENOPAUSE-RELATED PROBLEMS

Many women are trying dietary changes to reduce problems associated with the menopause transition, either as a substitute for or a supplement to hormone treatment. Our understanding of how food can affect our experiences of menopause is still evolving.

For the last thirty years, I have had increasingly healthy habits, and when I found out my perimenopause was a really strong one, I increased the healthiness of my diet and my exercise level in an attempt to override some of the symptoms. This did not actually work, but it meant I came out of perimenopause in really superb shape, which was nice.

SOY

Soy, which contains plant estrogens known as phytoestrogens, has a similar chemical structure to estrogen and can exert a weak estrogen-

Vitamins play a role in preventing heart disease, cancer, osteoporosis, and other chronic disease. It is best to get these nutrients from the foods we eat, but this is sometimes difficult. Therefore, taking a daily multivitamin may make sense for some people. Avoid excessive supplementation with "megadose" pills. It is generally advisable to discuss taking supplements with a person knowledgeable about them, who can help you choose the right supplement for your needs. Even if you take a multivitamin regularly, eating a balanced, healthy diet is important for your well-being.

like effect on the body. Therefore, it has been investigated as a treatment for hot flashes and other problems that may accompany menopause. However, recent research has failed to show a decrease in frequency or intensity of hot flashes in women who consumed soy.[16]

Some women who experience mild hot flashes say that soy and flaxseed help. Some women also find that soy helps with vaginal dryness, although current scientific evidence doesn't back this up. (Soy and flaxseed are both considered beneficial for our hearts; for more information, see page 182.) More research in this area is ongoing.

Certain foods seem to trigger hot flashes. But if I don't eat foods such as red meat, chocolate, or an occasional margarita, I am fine. Diet seems key in making me feel good.

Some women report that alcohol, caffeine, and cayenne or other spicy foods trigger hot flashes or make them worse. (Alcohol intake affects how hormone supplements are metabolized.) Try not eating or drinking a suspected offender and see if hot flashes subside. Warm skim milk at bedtime may help sleeping *and* provide calcium.

I found that flaxseed oil helped with my dry eye, although not my hot flashes. I've even lost a little weight since I started taking it three months ago, which is great.

(For more information about hot flashes, see Chapter 5. For more information on dry eye, see page 290.)

CHALLENGES TO EATING WELL

Making changes in how we eat and eating well can be challenging. Obstacles abound. Many of us are responsible not only for the food we eat but for the food eaten by our families, who may resist our efforts at change. Finding the time to prepare fresh, healthy meals amid our other commitments is often difficult. Junk foods are cheap and available everywhere, while healthy foods like fruits and vegetables and whole grains are often less available and more expensive. In addition, food represents comfort for many of us, so cutting out certain foods may make us feel deprived and can lead to backlash bingeing.

Despite such challenges, we can adopt healthy eating habits. If you are looking for ways to get fresh, local produce, try starting your own garden (even a few herbs on the windowsill can make a difference), shop at farmers' markets or food co-ops, or join a community-supported agriculture farm (CSA). If cooking every day seems exhausting, set aside one day a week when you can prepare some of your favorite dishes in quantity and freeze portions to be reheated later. Or form a supper club with friends and neighbors or a lunch group with coworkers, in which members rotate cooking and cleaning responsibilities. If you have children at home, try involving them in meal planning and preparation; teaching them to cook may help give them a healthier relationship with food.

You may want to start with changes in certain meals rather than your whole diet. For example, try eating a substantial breakfast, choosing from whole-grain breads and cereals, eggs, fruit, and yogurt. Or substitute nutritious snacks such as carrots or apples with nut butter for the baked goods, candy bars, or coffee that may be your habitual pick-me-ups. When choosing to eat more healthy foods, you may find it helpful not to forbid yourself other foods entirely. Try thinking of them as a rare treat to be savored.

EATING WELL ON A LIMITED BUDGET

Living on a tight budget can present a challenge for eating well. Low-cost, easily available foods are often low in nutrients and high in calories. One strategy for coping with this challenge is to buy fewer food items but make each one higher in nutrients. For example, whole-grain breads and pastas are filling and have more nutrients than French fries or potatoes.

Also, use high-cost meats sparingly. Stir-fry

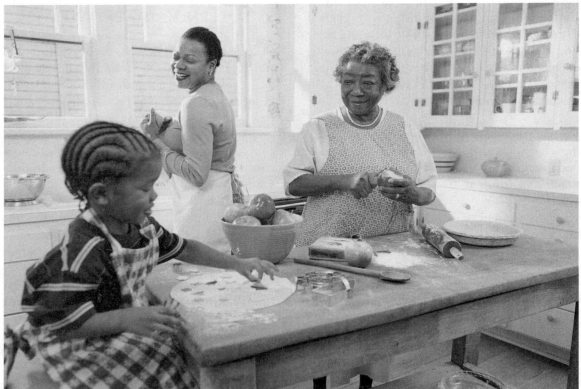

© Donna Day

small bits of meat with vegetables or cut meat up into casseroles to make it stretch. Consider low-cost protein alternatives, such as beans or tofu.

It also helps to plan meals ahead of time. Preparing foods ourselves is often less expensive than ordering takeout and healthier. Keep a list of favorite recipes that are quick and easy to prepare to avoid resorting to highly processed "fast foods" when short of time. Keep basic ingredients on hand that don't go bad, such as pasta, rice, canned light tuna, canned tomatoes, and frozen vegetables.

Use coupons to plan the shopping list and stick to that list when in the store. Buy store brands rather than the heavily advertised, more expensive national brands.

All women can also benefit from the federal government's WISEWOMAN program, geared to women with low incomes who don't have sufficient health insurance. The WISEWOMAN program (www.cdc.gov/wisewoman or call toll-free 1-888-232-4674) offers information and local services to lower risks of cardiovascular and other diseases through changes in diet and physical activity.

A HEALTHY WEIGHT

WEIGHT GAIN IN THE MENOPAUSAL TRANSITION

By the time I had gone three months without my period, I felt as if I had instantly gained weight. I could almost feel the extra pounds on my stomach and rear end. It was a wake-up call to take a look at all those bagels and cookies I've been eating.

It's not just our imagination. There is a tendency to gain weight at this time in our lives, particularly around the waist. Although many of us find our appetite has increased, the weight gain may occur even if we are eating the same way we always did. Although menopause is not strictly speaking the cause of this gain, it is true that estrogen has a role in body fat distribution. Women of childbearing age tend to store fat in the hips and thighs, while postmenopausal women store fat around the abdomen, more as men do.

Weight gain is probably related to changes in metabolism that occur with age. Our body's metabolism slows and we tend to lose muscles and replace them with fat. Muscles burn more calories than fat, so we need fewer calories than before. We also tend to be less active as we grow older. On average, women gain about a pound a year during the perimenopausal and postmenopausal years.[17]

My job is more sedentary, I'm on a new medication, and there seems to be more junk food around. It's all conspired against me and I've gained five pounds. I don't care if I'm as slender as I was in my thirties. I just want to be more fit and, sure, drop some pounds I've gained. I used to eat more healthily, but it's hard to get "back on the wagon."

OUR BODY WEIGHT, OURSELVES

Why can't we be happy the way we are, the way we look?

For many women, weight is a complicated, emotionally fraught issue. Many of us feel stuck between our knowledge of the importance of healthy eating and our desire to accept ourselves.

I spent so many years endlessly dieting and trying to be skinny, skinny, skinny. It was so freeing to fi-

nally stop *and accept my body. As I reach middle age, I know I should eat better, but as soon as I put any restrictions on what I can eat, I feel deprived and instantly crave the very foods that are bad for me.*

While there are clear health risks to being overweight or obese, the solution most often proposed—for individuals to diet and lose weight—oversimplifies complex realities. We live in a world where highly processed, refined foods are cheap and readily available. Processed foods are far more profitable to the food industry than whole, unprocessed foods, and ads incessantly push fast food, soft drinks, and other high-calorie, low-quality products. The government subsidizes the production of grains including corn and wheat, which are used primarily to make corn sweeteners and refined carbohydrates, but not far healthier foods such as fruits, vegetables, beans, and nuts, thereby

BODY WEIGHT AND HEALTH

Research on body weight and health often fails to tease apart the intertwined yet distinct risk factors of overweight, poor nutrition, and low levels of fitness. The assumption seems to be that people who are overweight also eat poorly and don't exercise. In real life, these factors vary from person to person: We all know thin people who eat tons of junk and never exercise and overweight people who eat well and are active. Our genetic makeup and metabolism, as well as our diet and activity levels, help determine our body shape and size.

Studies have linked being overweight with an increased likelihood of developing heart disease, diabetes, and certain cancers. But it's important to remember that weight alone is not the sole or best predictor of health. Research that categorizes risk by fitness levels instead of by body weight shows clearly that both exercise and weight independently affect our risk of certain health problems.[18] More research is needed, particularly to measure the impact of healthy eating and regular physical activity on people of all weights.

For now, it is clear that positive changes in any one of these areas—improving our eating habits, exercising regularly, or maintaining a healthy weight—will increase our chances of good health. The combined strategy of healthy eating and regular physical activity has yielded health benefits in numerous studies. One without the other doesn't seem to work as well as the two together.

DISORDERED EATING

It is well known that eating disorders are widespread among teenagers and young women. But disordered eating and preoccupation with weight affect women at midlife and later, too. The menopause transition, like adolescence, is a vulnerable time for women as we deal with physical changes and struggle to redefine ourselves in a world that values youth.

Eating disorders (anorexia, bulimia, and binge eating disorder) represent the dangerous extremes of unhealthy eating. Whether because earlier treatments didn't work, treatment was never sought, or it's a new pattern, eating disorders around the time of menopause are a serious problem. It is well worth seeking help because much more is known these days about how to treat eating disorders. Treatment may include counseling, medication, and the involvement of one's partner, spouse, or other friends, family, or support group.

creating artificially low prices for the foods that are worst for us.

In addition, people's exercise and activity levels have radically declined. Changing technologies and lifestyles mean that fewer people engage in sustained physical activities. Television, computers, the lack of public safety in cities, suburban sprawl, and cuts in physical education programs in schools mean that many of us spend the vast majority of our days sitting. This is in stark contrast to only fifty years ago, when most labor was manual and the chores of everyday living demanded that people moved their bodies throughout the day. These factors, along with other economic realities and food politics, have translated into greater numbers of overweight or obese people. In 1980, just under half of U.S. adults were overweight; by 2000, this figure had jumped to 64.5 percent.[19]

Dieting is a big industry in North America, with estimated annual revenues of $35 to $50 billion.[20] Many of us struggle endlessly with our weight. Yet this chronic dieting has not slowed the rise in the number of Americans classified as overweight or obese.[21] Dieting is notoriously unsuccessful at producing substantial long-term weight loss: The majority of people who

lose weight regain it within five years.[22] In addition, preoccupation with thinness and dieting are risk factors for the development of serious eating disorders.[23]

Given this dismal reality, what can we do?

- Focus on a healthy diet, not dieting. "Dieting" implies deprivation. Instead, we need to adopt lasting ways to meet the needs of our changing bodies.
- Learn to tune in to your body's cues. Paying attention to what we feel can help us learn to eat when we're hungry and stop when we're full.
- Increase exercise and movement. Add short periods of activity to your day.
- Make small changes in your diet, like substituting a whole-grain cereal for processed breakfast cereal or tofu or beans for red meat in a main dish.
- Don't let your weight determine your self-esteem. The number on the scale tells you one thing: how much you weigh. It says nothing about your value as a person or your chances of happiness.
- Aim for healthy habits—choosing healthy foods and exercising regularly—and let your weight stabilize where it will.

- Learn to accept and even appreciate your body. Body shape is not as changeable as we are led to believe. Genetics plays a strong role: Most of us will never look like supermodels, no matter what we eat or how much we exercise.
- Advocate for changes in our food system. Join your local food co-op. Become involved in community-supported agriculture. Get your local Y or school to substitute healthy foods for the junk food in the vending machines. Educate yourself and your community about nutrition and the politics of food.

NOTES

1. B. J. Lyle, J. A. Mares-Perlman, B. E. Klein, R. Klein, and J. L. Greger, "Antioxidant Intake and Risk of Incident Age-Related Nuclear Cataracts in the Beaver Dam Eye Study," *American Journal of Epidemiology* 149, no. 9 (1999): 801–809; see also L. Brown, E. B. Rimm, J. M. Seddon, et al., "A Prospective Study of Carotenoid Intake and Risk of Cataract Extraction in US Men," *American Journal of Clinical Nutrition* 70, no. 4 (1999): 517–24; P. F. Jacques, L. T. Chylack Jr., S. E. Hankinson, et al., "Long-Term Nutrient Intake and Early Age-Related Nuclear Lens Opacities," *Archives of Ophthalmology* 119, no. 7 (2001): 1009–19; D. A. Cooper, A. L. Eldridge, and J. C. Peters, "Dietary Carotenoids and Certain Cancers, Heart Disease, and Age-Related Macular Degeneration: A Review of Recent Research," *Nutrition Reviews* 57, no. 7 (1999): 201–14; J. A. Mares-Perlman, A. E. Millen, T. L. Ficek, and S. E. Hankinson, "The Body of Evidence to Support a Protective Role for Lutein and Zeaxanthin in Delaying Chronic Disease. Overview," *Journal of Nutrition* 132, no. 3 (2002): 518S–24S; J. M. Seddon, U. A. Ajani, R. D. Sperduto, et al., "Dietary Carotenoids, Vitamins A, C, and E, and Advanced Age-Related Macular Degeneration. Eye Disease Case-Control Study Group," *JAMA* 272, no. 18 (1994): 1413–20; E. L. Snellen, A. L. Verbeek, G. W. Van Den Hoogen, J. R. Cruysberg, and C. B. Hoyng, "Neovascular Age-Related Macular Degeneration and Its Relationship to Antioxidant Intake," *Acta Ophthalmologica Scandinavica* 80, no. 4 (2002): 368–71.

2. Bruce J. German and Cora J. Dillard, "Saturated Fats: What Dietary Intake?" *American Journal of Clinical Nutrition* 80, no. 3 (September 2004): 550–59, accessed at www.ajcn.org/cgi/content/full/80/3/550 on August 9, 2005.

3. American Heart Association, "Menopause and the Risk of Heart Disease and Stroke," accessed at www.americanheart.org/presenter.jhtml?identifier= 4658 on August 9, 2005.

4. American Heart Association, "Women, Heart Disease, and Stroke," accessed at www.americanheart .org/presenter.jhtml?identifier=4786 on August 9, 2005; see also National Women's Health Information Center, "Heart and Cardiovascular Disease," November 2002, accessed at www.4woman.gov/faq/heart dis.htm on August 9, 2005.

5. F. B. Hu, J. E. Manson, and W. C. Willett, "Types of Dietary Fat and Risk of Coronary Heart Disease: A Critical Review," *Journal of the American College of Nutrition* 20 (2001): 5–19.

6. Lewis H. Kuller et al., "Women's Healthy Lifestyle Project: A Randomized Clinical Trial, Results at 54 Months," *Circulation* 103, no. 1 (January 2001): 32–37.

7. "The Role of Isoflavones in Menopausal Health: Consensus Opinion of the North American Menopause Society," *Menopause* 4, no. 4 (July–August 2000): 215–29.

8. Cleveland Clinic Heart Center, "The Scoop on Flax," January 2002, accessed at www.clevelandclinic.org/ heartcenter/pub/guide/prevention/nutrition/flax1_0 2.htm on May 10, 2005.

9. U.S. Department of Health and Human Services and U.S. Environmental Protection Agency, "2004 EPA and FDA Advice for: Women Who Might Become Pregnant, Women Who Are Pregnant, Nursing Mothers, Young Children," March 2004, EPA-823-R-04-005.

10. Centers for Disease Control and Prevention,

"National Diabetes Fact Sheet," U.S. Department of Health and Human Services, Centers for Disease Control and Prevention, 2004, accessed at www.cdc.gov/diabetes/pubs/pdf/ndfs_2003.pdf on June 14, 2005.

11. Frank B. Hu, Joann E. Manson, Meir J. Stampfer, et al., "Diet, Lifestyle, and the Risk of Type 2 Diabetes Mellitus in Women," *New England Journal of Medicine* 345 (2001): 790–97.

12. Diabetes Prevention Program Research Group, "Reduction in the Incidence of Type 2 Diabetes with Lifestyle Intervention or Metformin," *New England Journal of Medicine* 346 (February 7, 2002): 393.

13. Harvard School of Public Health, "Nutrition Source: Fats and Cholesterol," accessed at www.hsph.harvard.edu/nutritionsource/fats.html on August 9, 2005.

14. Harvard School of Public Health, "Nutrition Source: Healthy Weight," accessed at www.hsph.harvard.edu/nutritionsource/healthy_weight.html on August 9, 2005.

15. D. Feskanich, W. C. Willett, M. J. Stampfer, G. A. Colditz, "Milk, Dietary Calcium, and Bone Fractures in Women: A 12-year Prospective Study," *American Journal of Public Health* 87 (1997): 992–97.

16. Erin E. Krebs, Kristine E. Ensrud, Roderick Mac-Donald, and Timothy J. Wilt, "Phytoestrogens for Treatment of Menopausal Symptoms: A Systematic Review," *Obstetrics and Gynecology* 104 (2004): 824–36; see also Fredi Kronenberg and Adriane Fugh-Berman, "Complementary and Alternative Medicine for Menopausal Symptoms: A Review of Randomized, Controlled Trials," *Annals of Internal Medicine* 137 (2002): 805–13.

17. Laurey R. Simkin-Silverman and Rena R. Wing, "Weight Gain during Menopause. Is It Inevitable or Can It Be Prevented?" *Postgraduate Medicine* 108, no. 3 (September 1, 2000): 47.

18. Marion Olmsted and Traci McFarlane, "Body Weight and Body Image," from *Women's Health Surveillance Report: A Multidimensional Look at the Health of Canadian Women,* BMC Women's Health 4, suppl. 1 (2004): S5, accessed at www.biomedcentral.com/1472-6874/4/S1/S5 on June 14, 2005.

19. Craig Lambert, "The Way We Eat Now," *Harvard Magazine,* May–June 2004, accessed at www.harvardmagazine.com/on-line/050465.html on June 14, 2005.

20. Olmsted and McFarlane.

21. Lambert.

22. Wayne C. Miller, "Fitness and Fatness in Relation to Health: Implications for a Paradigm Shift," *Journal of Social Issues* 2 (1999): 207–19.

23. Kelly M. Vitousek, "The Current Status of Cognitive-Behavioural Models of Anorexia and Bulimia Nervosa," in *Frontiers of Cognitive Therapy* ed. Paul M. Salkovskis (New York: Guilford Press, 1996), 383–418.

CHAPTER 13

Staying Active

There is no medicine as powerful as physical activity. Our bodies are meant to move; when they don't, we become susceptible to numerous health problems. When we do stay active, on the other hand, we help keep our heart, bones, and muscles strong. Staying active, together with eating a healthy diet, is the best known prescription for health and well-being. It also can be fun.

I have exercised every year of my life. I ran competitively through high school and college, and swam five miles a week during each of my pregnancies. Exercise is as important to me as breathing and eating. I love the social part of it. Running with my friends is like going to therapy.

Those of us who already have an exercise routine entering perimenopause have a head start. Irritability, depression, sleep problems, and weight gain are reduced and confidence and well-being are increased by physical activity. Some women who exercise even report fewer and less severe hot flashes, although there isn't enough scientific data to back up this claim conclusively.[1] In addition, physical activity *has* been demonstrated repeatedly to have an instrumental role in heading off numerous diseases for which we are otherwise at greater risk. (See sidebar, page 194.)

I started exercising more in my forties than ever before in my life. It helps with my hot flashes, and with the stress and anger I sometimes feel after not sleeping well.

As we approach menopause, our metabolism slows and we lose muscle mass—that is, *if* we don't stay physically active. These are not solely age-related changes, contrary to popular belief. These changes are mainly related to inactivity and poor eating habits. Women tend to become less active over time, particularly after age fifty. While we may have more physical limitations as we age and need to modify our activities, it is important for all of us to find safe, enjoyable ways of moving our bodies. If we don't stay active and use our muscles, we may gain weight and get flabby. Studies have shown that strength can be maintained and perhaps increased at any age—even in your eighties and beyond.

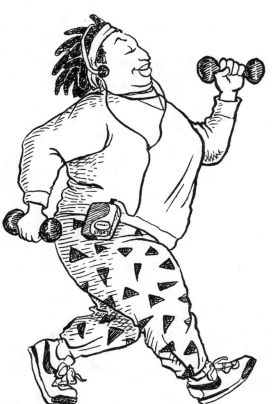

© Alison Bechdel

IT'S NEVER TOO LATE

Those of us who are among the approximately 60 percent of women ages forty-five to sixty-five who don't exercise at the level recommended by the Centers for Disease Control[2] shouldn't despair. It's never too late to start and to reap the benefits. If you used to exercise but don't now, think back to how good it felt. If you've never exercised, the menopause transition is a great time to get moving.

If you are not comfortable with the thought of exercise or are unfamiliar with it, you may need to take a leap of faith to start. Believe in your power to make a positive change. Being more active may feel good starting from day one, and you may find that you start to both feel and look better over time. If it doesn't, you may find that over time it becomes more enjoyable—especially when you find an exercise that is comfortable and fits well into your day.

I used to walk all the time, but now I have a knee problem. I feel better when I exercise, but it's a matter of getting it ingrained into my life again. When I did yoga regularly, it became a habit and I loved it.

MAKING THE COMMITMENT

ASSESS YOUR ACTIVITY LEVEL

Each of us falls into one of three general levels of activity. There are those who are physically active for at least thirty minutes on most days of the week—the time that is recommended by the Centers for Disease Control and the American College of Sports Medicine. Being physically active includes doing housework, gardening, walking, weight lifting, yoga, and swimming. Another variation of this category are people who do more physical activity at one

THE BENEFITS OF EXERCISE

The current recommendation is that we exercise moderately (walk briskly, bike, swim, lift weights) for thirty minutes on most days of the week. Although the intensity and duration of the workout for optimal benefit is still being debated, it is clear that even this minimum amount has enormous health benefits. And less than this has some benefits, too.

DISEASE RISK REDUCTION

Regular moderate exercise:

- reduces high blood pressure.
- controls weight.
- lowers risk for heart disease. (Physically inactive people are twice as likely to develop heart disease as people who are regularly active.)[3]
- lowers risk for colon cancer and breast cancer.
- keeps bones, muscles, and joints healthy, easing arthritis and reducing frailty and incidence of falls and osteoporosis.
- lowers blood glucose and risk for type 2 diabetes.

QUALITY OF LIFE

It also:

- improves mood and sleep.
- relieves stress, anxiety, and depression.
- boosts energy.
- improves self-confidence.
- makes you look and feel better.

time but on fewer days per week, say sixty minutes three times a week. If you are in this category, you are already reaping the health benefits of regular activity but may want to look at your mix of activities. Many women do just one type of activity. Consider doing upper-body strength training and stretching exercises for flexibility, as well as balance training, if you're not already.

In the next category are those who may be active at least ten minutes a day but not long enough to meet the recommended amount of time that will bring health benefits. About 44 percent of women of all ages fall into this category.

Then there are those who are physically inactive. For all the many benefits of exercise, the inverse is true if you are physically inactive. A sedentary lifestyle puts you at risk of premature death from causes that might otherwise be preventable.

If you are in the second or third category,

know that getting started is often the hardest part. It requires some changes in thinking and changes in habits. Change isn't easy, but there are methods many women have used successfully to make it happen. Step by step, you can gradually introduce physical activity into your life.

ARE YOU READY FOR CHANGE?

Even to resolve to become more active is a major hurdle. You have to translate knowledge that exercise would be good for you into resolve to do something about it. It is much easier to do nothing and brush aside the knowledge about the benefits.

I hate to exercise. I go out of my way to avoid it. Intellectually, I understand how important it is. I cringe when I hear a news report about some new disease-fighting benefit of it. I even exercised diligently at one time in my life, running two miles most days of the week. Then I got pregnant, gained fifty-seven pounds, and pretty much never exercised again.

Many of us have a negative voice that plays in our heads. If you climb a set of stairs and start breathing heavily, that voice might say, "What a slug I am." Don't let that voice beat you down. Being winded doesn't mean you're lazy. It means you're out of shape. It doesn't mean you will never be able to exercise. It means you need to start exercising.

Remember how it feels to be winded. Within three weeks of starting a regular exercise program, you will likely feel a big difference. You won't be winded by a set of stairs. You won't be winded by two sets of stairs.

It helps to identify the factors in our life that are associated with positive behaviors so we can tap into them. To want to remain healthy for our children and grandchildren is one such positive force. Positive goals are incentives for change and can fuel the determination needed to make a change, to get started, and to stick with it.

A positive force might be that you've had breast cancer and don't want it to return. There is a growing body of evidence linking increased physical activity to decreased odds of recurrence.[4] Doing something to boost your mood is another positive goal. Or wanting to look good. If we exercise regularly, we often feel more in control of our bodies. We feel stronger and in fact, our heart, lungs, and bones *are* stronger.

Most of us have obstacles in our lives that make change difficult, however. Some obstacles are due to life circumstances (we're providing care for a sick family member, going through a divorce, or living in a neighborhood where it's unsafe to walk), but others we create for ourselves. We need to first identify our personal obstacles so we know which are controllable. Then we can do something about them one by one.

THE TOP FIVE EXCUSES NOT TO EXERCISE

I Don't Have Time
Once you decide to proceed with an exercise program, you will need to find the time. Make it a priority, and schedule it as you would a meeting or appointment. Start by finding at least two times during the week when you can set aside thirty minutes, perhaps during a lunch break or before or after work, or when the rest of your family is busy with a favorite television show. Although you can concentrate and focus better if not watching television, sometimes exercising in front of the news or a particular show can get you in the habit of doing it regularly at a certain time.

Take a hard look at your schedule. Perhaps something else you're doing can be cut out or

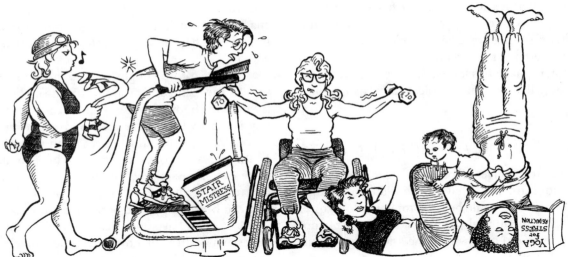

shifted to someone else to do. Work up to a goal of exercising or being physically active for thirty minutes most days of the week.

I Am Too Tired

That's probably true. But here's one of those places where a leap of faith is necessary. If you start exercising (and eating well), you will likely have more energy and sleep better. Try to plan exercise at a time during the day when you're not usually tired. At the beginning, you may have to force yourself to get up and do it, but eventually, you may look forward to it. Keep focusing on the reasons you're doing this.

I Am Too Unhealthy/ Overweight/Disabled to Exercise

Physical activity is necessary for everyone. It is not only encouraged, it is often prescribed as part of treatment for such conditions as diabetes, heart disease, arthritis, obesity, and osteopenia (low bone density). If you have knee or hip problems, lower-impact activities such as biking, swimming, water aerobics, and yoga may be more comfortable than walking or jogging. If you have physical limitations, some exercises can be done in a chair, in water, or even while lying in bed. Appropriate exercise often increases mobility, stamina, and emotional well-being. You may find it helpful to consult with your health care provider or a physical therapist to develop or adapt an exercise program.

I Get Bored Exercising

Boredom could mean that you haven't found the right activity yet. Or boredom could be a good sign: You've mastered this level and it's time to move on. Change some of the exercises, add new ones, or mix up your routine somehow. Find a friend to join you, or a new (and safe) place to walk. Try dancing to music or take a class you were too intimidated to take before. Once you get stronger, new activities are easier and more fun to do.

I Don't Have Enough Money to Exercise

It's not necessary to join a fancy health club or buy huge pieces of equipment. Although it helps to have good sneakers, walking is free. You can walk anywhere that is safe: on sidewalks, in parks, on high school tracks, or at shopping malls. It is often possible to buy inexpensive weights in discount stores or secondhand weights in the classified ads. You can make your own weights by filling small plastic soda bottles with sand or water. There are also many resistance exercises that can be done using the weight of your body alone. Short exercise routines at home don't take much space or equipment. To get your body moving, you can just turn on some music in your living room and dance.

SETTING GOALS

It's important to integrate into our lives a combination of aerobic exercise, which increases the capabilities of the heart and lungs, and strength training, which develops muscles and bone strength. Exercises designed to enhance flexibility are useful as a cooldown. Balance-training exercises may help prevent falls. Some activities, such as yoga and tai chi, develop flexibility and balance as well as strength, among their many other positive attributes. The aim is to reap the health benefits from regular, repeated exercise—exercise that has become a habit.

The best way to make exercise a habit is to start with an activity that's readily available and that you can enjoy or at least tolerate. Then set very specific goals for yourself. They should be reasonable goals, especially if you've never exercised in your life. An example: I will walk around the neighborhood for fifteen minutes after dinner three times a week for a month.

Keep track on paper how you're doing each week. Write down when you exercised, what you did, and how you felt. Note the times when you don't meet your weekly goal, but don't let yourself get frustrated by them. If you miss a session, don't let the negative voice inside your head tell you that you've blown it and might as well give up. Stay focused and confident about meeting your goal the next week. When the first month is over, evaluate if you need to continue on this first step or are ready to add more time or intensity.

Every single time you exercise, you are succeeding. Every success edges you closer to the goal of physical fitness. There is no such thing as a step backward as long as you keep trying to exercise.

I've been going to [a gym] three times a week for about a year and a half. I weigh about the same as when I began, but I am more muscular and I feel much stronger. My legs and arms aren't flapping in the wind.

THE PRESCRIPTION FOR FITNESS

Particularly for those of us who have little or no exercise in our lives, it is less overwhelming to break down our goals into manageable steps. It helps to integrate this new habit into our lives slowly, not adding more until we are comfortable with what we're doing, but not waiting too long either to push ourselves to do more.

In addition to planned exercise—aerobics and strength training—it is beneficial to also think in terms of becoming more physically active throughout the day. In this way, too, you will be raising your activity consciousness, burning more calories, and getting a sense of where you can insert more activity into your life. This means taking the stairs instead of the elevator, walking to talk to someone at work instead of calling him or her, or moving around the house more to put things away rather than letting them pile up. It could mean dancing

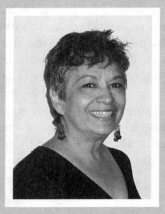

"I felt that I had to take better care of myself because of my children."

VIRGINIA VALENZUELA

While I was going through menopause, I was also going through a divorce. I was focused more on my children than myself. They were all teenagers at the time, or even younger, and it was a really tough time.

After menopause and my divorce, I increased my running and other exercise. I read about the best things to eat and focused more on eating right. I felt that I had to take better care of myself because of my children. If I didn't become healthier, what were they going to do without me?

As a matter of fact, if I came home stressed out, my children would say, "Mom, go run," because they knew it was something for me that made me feel good. If I was healthy and took care of myself, I could take better care of them.

I actually took a running and weight training class. Now I'm a runner and I do weight training regularly. I subscribe to health magazines, and I ask the doctor questions when I go.

My doctor recommended more calcium, so now I take calcium. I've also been on blood pressure medication the past couple of years, which I hope to get off. But that's it. I don't take anything else. I'm really trying to stay healthy.

---

while vacuuming or dusting, getting up to switch television channels rather than using the remote, or walking the dog. It could mean parking a little farther away to get in a brisk walk both to and from your workplace. Adding ten- or fifteen-minute segments of activity throughout the day has significant health benefits and can increase our awareness of and pleasure in our bodies.

When I am in the kitchen doing something at the counter, such as peeling or washing vegetables, I do little exercises. I lift my knees or kick my legs backwards. I run or walk in place while ironing. I do shoulder rolls while waiting in traffic in the car. I belong to a health club but don't go to it much, so I try to inject a few minutes of exercise into what I'm doing.

THE FIRST STEP

You've made the commitment. You're determined to become more active. You've been adding more physical movement to what you do at home, at work, or out shopping and doing errands. Now the first step is to plan to do any kind of moderate-intensity exercise three times a week for fifteen minutes. Brisk walking is a good way to start, as are programs at a local Y or fitness facility (including women-only facilities, which some women prefer). Or follow an exercise video in the privacy of your home.

Try to stick to your planned times by scheduling other responsibilities around them. If something comes up that you must do, reschedule another time that week to take its place—and stick to that. The important thing is consistency. It doesn't matter how little you do to start. Keep building on what you've accomplished, little by little.

STEP TWO

The next goal is to introduce a little strength training two days a week, if you haven't already, and to exercise a total of five days a week for at least thirty minutes each time.

Aerobic exercise (walking, biking, jogging, swimming): thirty minutes, three days a week.

Strength training: two days a week. Essential for heart and bone health, strength training also helps to reduce fat around the abdomen. Because muscles need time to recover, make sure to take at least one day off between strength-training sessions.

Starter Strength Exercises

Here are three exercises that require no equipment and will get you started.

Squat: strengthens hips, thighs, and buttocks. Squat ten times, rest one minute, then squat another ten times.

1. Stand directly in front of a sturdy chair. Your legs are hip-width apart and your arms are both directly out in front of you.

2. Bend your knees as you slowly lower your buttocks toward the chair, counting to four be-

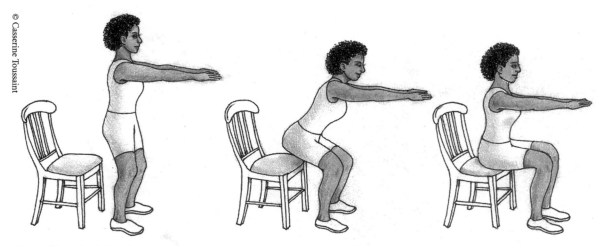

© Casserine Toussaint

Squat (described above)

fore you touch the chair. (If this is too difficult at first, put a pillow or two on the chair.)

3. Pause, sitting there, and then slowly rise back to a standing position. Keep your knees from coming in front of your ankles (not reaching too far in front, which puts pressure on your knee joints) and your back straight.

Wall push-up (or regular push-up, which is harder): strengthens arms, shoulders, and chest. Do ten, rest, then do ten more.

1. Stand facing a wall, a little farther than an arm's distance away. Lean forward with your arms straight out (shoulder height) and flatten your palms against the wall.

2. Bend your elbows as you lower your upper body toward the wall in a slow, controlled motion as you count to four. Keep your feet planted.

3. Pause. Then slowly push yourself back, counting to four. Don't lock your elbows or arch your back.

Toe stand: strengthens calves and ankles, and helps with balance. Do ten, rest a minute, do ten more.

1. Stand with your feet shoulder-width apart, facing a chair or counter. You may touch the chair or counter lightly for balance; don't lean on it.

2. Slowly push up onto the balls of your feet as you count to four. Hold this position for two to four seconds.

3. Slowly lower your heels back to the floor, counting to four.

(An advanced move is to do this exercise on a staircase, letting your heels hang over the edge of the stair; after the toe stand, you let your heels come down lower than the balls of your feet.)

STEP THREE

This is the optimal exercise program. It combines aerobic exercise three or more times a

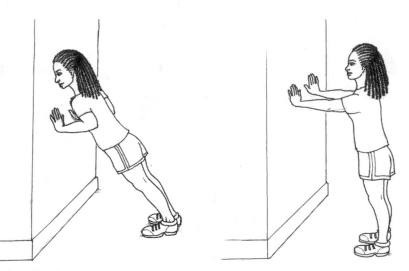

Wall push-up (described above)

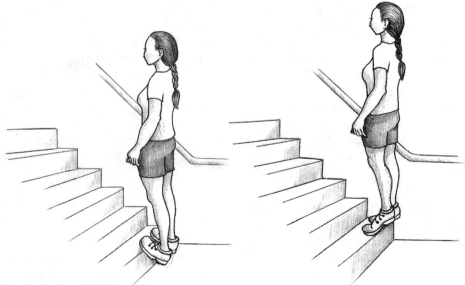

Toe stand (described on page 200)

week with two days of strength training exercises—for thirty minutes or more. Here are five more strength-training exercises you can add to the other three. This routine is designed[5] to have the greatest impact on the most muscles in the body in the least amount of time. It is also advisable to do some stretches after each exercise session, particularly if you have specific joints or muscles that are tight.

Knee extension: works the front thigh muscles (quadriceps). You will need ankle weights—strap-on cuffs with pockets that hold weighted bars. You can start with weights as light as one pound and keep adding more gradually as you become stronger.

1. Start by sitting in a chair with only your toes touching the ground. (Sit on a pillow if you need to be higher.)
2. Extend your left leg out as straight as possible as you count to three. Pause one second. Lower the leg slowly back to starting position, counting to four.

3. Do this 12 times with the left leg. Repeat with the right leg 12 times. Rest 30 seconds, and then do each leg 12 times again.

Knee curl: strengthens the hamstrings, the muscles in the back of the thigh. This is also done with ankle weights, which are gradually increased as you get stronger.

1. Stand tall behind a chair, legs hip-width apart, resting your hands on top of the chair's back for balance.
2. Maintaining good posture (do not let your back arch), slowly raise your left heel toward your buttocks as high as you can, or until your calf is parallel to the floor. Make sure that your thigh stays parallel to the other thigh and doesn't move forward. Pause one second. Lower to the count of four.
3. Do 12 repetitions with the left leg, and do 12 repetitions with the right leg. Rest 30 seconds, and then repeat 12 times on each side.

Overhead press: strengthens muscles in the arms and shoulders (tones "batwings" on the upper arms, for example) and improves flexibility. You will need dumbbells. Start with weights as light as 1 to 3 pounds and work your way up gradually to 10 pounds, or even 12 or 15 pounds, as you get stronger.

1. Stand straight with a dumbbell in each hand, feet shoulder-width apart, hands by your side. Bring the dumbbells up until they touch the front of your shoulders, your palms facing forward. (Note: this can also be done sitting in a chair.)

2. Push the dumbbells straight up to a count of three, until your arms are fully extended over your head. Pause for a breath, and lower, counting to three, to the starting position at shoulder height. (Do not arch your back; if you find yourself arching your back, the weights may be too heavy.)

3. Repeat 12 times. Rest a minute or two. Repeat 12 times.

Biceps curl: strengthens and tones muscles on the front of the upper arm, making it easier to lift groceries and other things.

1. Stand with good posture, your feet shoulder-width apart, arms at your sides, holding a dumbbell in each hand. Keeping your upper arms and elbows tight at your side, slowly lift the dumbbells up to your shoulders, counting to three. Your palms are facing your shoulders but not touching them.

2. Pause for a breath. Slowly lower your arms to the starting position, counting to four. Repeat 12 times. Rest a minute, and then repeat 12 more times.

Abdominal crunch: tightens your abdominal muscles.

1. Lie down face-up on the floor or a mat, bending your knees but keeping your feet flat on the floor. Interlock your fingers behind the back of your head (this helps support your head and neck).

2. Slowly lift your shoulders and head off the ground by gradually contracting your abdominal muscles. Your upper back need only come one to three inches off the ground. Think of the shoulders doing the lifting so you don't use

WHAT ABOUT THAT TUMMY?

I enjoy exercise and sports and have worked out in one form or another all of my life. I've never had a weight problem, although the past two years I have gotten a small layer of fat on my stomach that had previously always been very flat.

How do you get rid of that extra weight around the waist? I watch what I eat, but no matter what I do, I can't get rid of it.

There is no single exercise we can do to get rid of that "kangaroo pouch." The only way to reduce abdominal fat is to do a general well-rounded strength program as described in this chapter, to get enough aerobic exercise to burn calories and control body weight, and to eat sensibly. Research studies have shown reductions in abdominal fat with both strength and aerobic exercise.

your hands to push the head up. Also, your chin should be slightly tucked in but not touching your chest (for the correct position, imagine holding an apple between your chin and chest).

3. Pause for a breath, then, counting to four, slowly return to the floor. Repeat 12 times, rest for a minute, and then repeat 12 more times.

(An advanced follow-up exercise would be to lift off the ground as described above, twist your body to the right so your left shoulder is reaching toward the outside of your right knee, return to center, and slowly come back down to the ground. Repeat, twisting to the left.)

KEEP MOVING

Staying active or becoming more active is one of the best things we can do for ourselves at this time of life. Exercise helps us feel and look better as we go through menopause. In the long run, it helps us to remain healthy, independent, self-sufficient, and vibrant for many years to come.

NOTES

1. Ellen B. Gold, Barbara Sternfeld, Jennifer L. Kelsey, et al., "Relation of Demographic and Lifestyle Factors in a Multi-Racial/Ethnic Population of Women 40–55 Years of Age," *American Journal of Epidemiology* 152 (September 2000): 463–73; see also Ted Ivarson, Anna-Clara Spetz, and Mats Hammar, "Physical Exercise and Vasomotor Symptoms in Postmenopausal Women," *Maturitas* 29 (1998): 139–46; Mats Hammar, G. Berg, and R. Lindgren, "Does Physical Exercise Influence the Frequency of Postmenopausal Hot Flushes?" *Acta Obstetricia Gynecologica Scandinavica* 69 (1990): 409–12.

2. Centers for Disease Control and Prevention, 2003 data, accessed at apps.nccd.cdc.gov/PASurveillance/DemoCompareResultV.asp?State=1&Cat=3&Year=2003&Go=GO#result on May 23, 2005.

3. The President's Council on Physical Fitness and Sports, "Physical Activity Fact Sheet," accessed at www.fitness.gov/resources_factsheet.htm on May 23, 2005.

4. Michelle D. Holmes, Wendy Y. Chen, Diane Feskanich, Candyce H. Kroenke, and Graham A. Colditz, "Physical Activity and Survival after Breast Cancer Diagnosis," *JAMA* 293 (May 25, 2005): 2479–86; see also Kerry S. Courneya, "Exercise in Cancer Survivors: An Overview of Research," *Medicine and Science in Sports and Exercise* 35 (November 2003): 1846–52.

5. This strength-training program was designed by Miriam E. Nelson and adapted from her book *Strong Women Stay Slim* (New York: Bantam Books, 1998).

Health Concerns

CHAPTER 14

Uterine and Bladder Health

During the menopause transition, many women experience significant changes in our patterns of menstrual bleeding, and some of us may begin to experience urinary incontinence. It can be difficult to know when these changes related to our uterine and bladder health are a normal part of the menopause transition or of aging and when they may signify a health problem. This chapter discusses the uterine and bladder changes that can occur, common concerns, and how to maintain uterine and bladder health.

UTERINE HEALTH

UTERINE BLEEDING

A change in your bleeding pattern may be quite normal during the menopause transition. As the ovaries produce changing levels of estrogen and ovulatory periods become fewer, most women find that our menstrual periods change. For most women, the transition from having regular menstrual periods to having none occurs without problems.

What Is Considered Abnormal?

During the menopause transition, bleeding typically comes less often and is lighter in quantity over fewer days than premenopausal bleeding. However, more frequent menstrual periods can also occur, especially in the earlier stages of the menopause transition. Some women's cycles become shorter, with fewer days between the first day of one menstrual period and the next. It is not uncommon for women to miss one period or more, then resume bleeding. Missing a period may signal pregnancy, which remains possible until a woman has gone for a whole year without a period.

During the menopause transition, it is generally considered abnormal if periods come more often than every twenty days, bleeding becomes heavier or longer in duration, bleeding or spotting between periods occurs frequently, or menstrual cramping increases in severity.

Menopause is defined as one year without any bleeding or spotting. If you see any blood on your underwear or toilet paper after a full year without bleeding, consider other sites of possible bleeding such as the rectum or anus (you might have a hemorrhoid). To determine the source of bleeding, you can put your finger in your vagina and see if there is any blood. If the blood is coming from your vagina or you remain unsure of its source, contact your provider. The presence of any blood from your vagina, even a spot, after menopause may be important.

Reasons for Unusual Bleeding during the Menopause Transition

There are many reasons for unusual bleeding in the menopause transition. Among the more common reasons are hormone imbalance caused by your body secreting too much estrogen or not enough progesterone; the effects of hormone pills; fibroids; polyps; adenomyosis (see page 209); infection; abnormal growth of the uterine lining (endometrium); chronic endometritis (inflammation or infection of the lining of the uterus); and thyroid hormonal changes. An abnormal pregnancy is also a possibility. It is rare that the cause of bleeding is cancer.

A **hormone imbalance** may cause excessive bleeding. In general, the imbalance is caused by changes in natural levels of estrogen or progesterone or by hormone pills. In the menopause transition, most women do not ovulate regularly and therefore do not regularly produce progesterone. The lining of the uterus may be stimulated to grow by estrogen and not regularly exposed to progesterone, which counteracts the effect of the estrogen. The lining may become thickened by the overstimulation of the estrogen alone. The thickened lining sometimes produces irregular or heavy bleeding. The overgrowth of the endometrial lining may over time become abnormal or even precancerous or cancerous.

Polyps can also cause bleeding. A polyp is a small, usually benign (noncancerous) growth in the lining of the uterus. Polyps can generally be removed from the uterus by an endometrial aspiration, hysteroscopy (a minor surgery, see page 211), or dilation and curettage (D&C, see page 211). Not all polyps need to be removed. Some studies indicate that they go away on their own sometimes, particularly if they are small.

Another cause of unusual bleeding is **fibroids** (myomas or leiomyomas). Fibroids are generally benign (noncancerous), solid tumors, which can occur inside or outside the uterus. While as many as half of all women may have fibroids during our lifetimes, only about one-third of women with fibroids experience discomfort or pain associated with them.[1] The cause of fibroids is unknown, but there may be a genetic factor. Fibroids are more common in African-American women than in white women. Estrogen or progesterone may stimulate fibroids to grow. While fibroids may be very small and cause no symptoms, they may grow in rare instances to the size of a large melon or

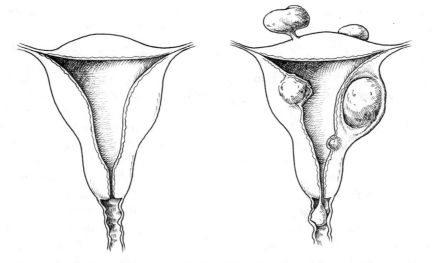

A uterus without fibroids (left), and a uterus with fibroids, or benign growths (right)

even larger. Fibroids are usually diagnosed during a routine gynecological exam. Frequently, an ultrasound is used for better evaluation.

Heavy and sometimes painful menstrual periods in women in our forties may be associated with a condition known as **adenomyosis.** Adenomyosis is the presence of endometrial tissue, the tissue that lines the inside of the uterus, in the uterine muscle, where it is not found normally. This condition is thought to cause heavy menstrual bleeding in about 70 percent of women who have it. Adenomyosis is like endometriosis in the uterus and sometimes responds to hormone treatments that suppress the menstrual period. Hysterectomy is the only way to diagnose adenomyosis definitively, and may be recommended to treat symptoms.

Infections of the vagina, cervix, or uterus can be the cause of minor bleeding or spotting. These may be sexually transmitted infections (STIs), such as gonorrhea or chlamydia. STIs are diagnosed by laboratory cultures. Antibiotics are used to cure the infection.

Cancer of the cervix or uterus is a rare cause of bleeding. The Pap smear, colposcopy, and cervical biopsy are used to diagnose cervical cancer. Uterine cancer is usually detected from an endometrial biopsy or aspiration, or dilation and curettage. (For more information, see Chapter 18, "Cancers.")

Reasons for Unusual Bleeding after Menopause

The most common reasons for bleeding or spotting after menopause are hormone treatments; vaginal atrophy (dryness); benign or cancerous tumors of any part of your reproductive system, including the lining of your uterus; or lesions of the labia, perineum, or vagina.

The reason for the bleeding will determine treatment options. A provider needs to take a complete history and do a gynecological exam to find the cause of the bleeding. Sometimes, the provider advises that other tests such as a pelvic ultrasound, endometrial sampling, or dilation and curettage (D&C) be done. Another possible diagnostic test is the saline hydrosonogram or sonohysterogram (also called SIS or HSN). This is a saline-enhanced ultrasound test that may be very effective at delineating polyps or fibroids or other growths within the cavity of the uterus. It can sometimes be done in a provider's office and may cause minor cramping.

Nonsurgical Treatments for Abnormal Bleeding

Nonsteroidal anti-inflammatory drugs called NSAIDS (such as ibuprofen, naproxen, or mefenamic acid) may be used to decrease menstrual bleeding during the perimenopause. These over-the-counter medications can occasionally cause stomach irritation. Eating food with the medications can decrease this effect. It is generally suggested that NSAIDS should be started a few days before you expect your period or at the start of the bleeding and continued through the menstrual period. NSAIDS are also used for menstrual cramps. In general, taking NSAIDS helps about 25 percent of women with heavy periods. You should not take NSAIDS if you have a stomach ulcer or are allergic to any anti-inflammatory medication.

Hormonal treatments, such as estrogen and progestin as pills, or progestin alone as pills, a shot, or an IUD may be recommended to control bleeding. For perimenopausal women who don't smoke or have high blood pressure, birth control pills can be used. Hormones may decrease the bleeding amount, correct irregular bleeding, and decrease menstrual cramps. A combination of estrogen and a progestin may be used to decrease irregular bleeding. Progestins are sometimes used for five to ten days before the period starts to help regulate and prevent heavy bleeding. Estrogen stimulates growth of the uterine lining; progestins mature these developing cells and promote regular sloughing of the lining. When the progestin is stopped, vaginal bleeding frequently starts. Progestin use may cause mood changes,

depression, fatigue, and blood cholesterol changes. For some women, progestins can cause a lot of spotting and continued bleeding and therefore can be a nuisance. An IUD that contains progestin (such as the Mirena IUS) releases a small amount of the hormone into the uterus. For perimenopausal women, using such an IUD ultimately reduces vaginal bleeding significantly and prevents pregnancy at the same time. An IUD can be inserted during a routine office appointment. IUDs are not currently approved for use in postmenopausal women.

Gonadotropin-releasing hormone agonists (GnRH agonists) may also be used in the treatment of fibroids *in perimenopausal women*. These are a class of medications that can temporarily shrink fibroids and stop bleeding by blocking the body's production of estrogen. Although these medications can relieve vaginal bleeding, they produce menopause-like effects such as hot flashes and vaginal dryness. They are rarely used for long-term treatment as they are expensive and can lead to bone density loss. If a woman is close to menopause, a brief treatment may be sufficient. GnRH agonists can also be used to shrink very large fibroids before surgery, in order to correct bleeding anemia and make removal of the uterus or fibroids easier.

Newer medications that block hormone production without decreasing bone density or causing other problems associated with menopause are being developed for treating fibroids.

Surgery for Evaluation or Treatment of Abnormal Bleeding

Surgery is considered when other treatments have been unsuccessful or if the problem can best be diagnosed or resolved by a more invasive procedure. If your provider suggests surgery, ask questions about the use of less invasive, nonsurgical treatments first, ask for pros and cons of each possible surgical treatment, and consider a second opinion. If a hysterectomy is suggested, ask if the procedure can be done vaginally or laparoscopically instead of abdominally. (See the section on hysterectomy below for more details.) If you agree to surgery, make sure the surgeon knows about any of your preferences, such as your feelings about receiving blood transfusions. (You may be able to store your own blood to use later in surgery.) The surgeon should also know whom to talk to about the outcome of the surgery while you are in recovery.

Hysteroscopy and Endometrial Biopsy

Two procedures to evaluate the lining of the uterus are generally done in a medical office. Hysteroscopy is done to look inside the uterus and sometimes take samples of tissue to evaluate the reason for abnormal bleeding. An endometrial biopsy or aspiration is usually done just to remove a sample of tissue from the uterus.

In both procedures, a woman is in the usual position for a gynecological exam with a speculum inserted in her vagina. The provider inserts a thin, long instrument about the size of a straw through the cervix into the uterus. In a hysteroscopy, the provider visually evaluates the lining of the uterus and sometimes removes a small amount of tissue from the uterus. In an endometrial aspiration or biopsy, the provider removes a small amount of tissue from the lining of the uterus.

During both procedures, most women feel discomfort like menstrual cramps for a minute or two. Sometimes the cervix needs to be dilated (opened slightly) so the instrument can be inserted into the uterus. Some women find that taking aspirin or an anti-inflammatory medication like ibuprofen or naproxen before the procedure lessens the discomfort. Local

anesthesia is generally used with a hysteroscopy but may also be used for a woman having a biopsy or aspiration. (Sometimes general anesthesia is used for hysteroscopy, if tissue removal is planned.)

The person performing an endometrial aspiration cannot see directly what she or he is trying to remove, so growths like polyps and very small fibroids can be missed. A hysteroscopy "sees" more than endometrial aspiration, but more dilation of the uterus is needed and not all practitioners perform this procedure in the office. A saline sonohysterogram, in which a vaginal ultrasound is enhanced by putting saline inside the uterus, can help define whether there are growths inside the uterus. It can sometimes be combined with an aspiration biopsy to get the same information that a hysteroscopy would provide.

Dilation and Curettage (D&C)

Dilation and curettage (D&C) is done under local, spinal, or general anesthesia. The procedure involves a more extensive removal of tissue from the endometrial or uterine lining than does an endometrial aspiration or biopsy. D&C may be done to aid in the diagnosis of a bleeding problem or as a treatment for abnormal bleeding. The tissue that is removed from the uterus is sent to a laboratory for evaluation. D&C is often performed in conjunction with hysteroscopy. Because D&C requires anesthesia and an operative setting and because endometrial biopsy techniques have improved, D&C is performed less frequently than in the past.

Endometrial Ablation

Endometrial ablation is a procedure done under hysteroscopy. During the procedure, an instrument is inserted into the uterus and used to destroy the lining (endometrium) with heat, an electric current, or cryosurgical (freezing) techniques. Only women who do not have a clotting problem, do not desire pregnancy after the procedure, do not have large fibroids, and do not have a diagnosis of cancerous or precancerous uterus should consider this procedure. During the procedure, most of the lining of the uterus is destroyed to limit regrowth of the lining.

Most women have little or no bleeding after the surgery. The hormones from the ovaries are not affected by the surgery. Endometrial ablation has become a well-established treatment for heavy menstrual bleeding and may be a good alternative to hysterectomy for some women. The procedure is frequently performed in the office or an outpatient surgery setting. Local, spinal, epidural, or general anesthetic is used. An endometrial ablation procedure leaves no surgical scar, can be done in an outpatient clinic, and is safer and costs less than a hysterectomy.[2] Menstrual periods do not disappear after ablation, and over time, bleeding may increase again. If you are considering having the procedure at age forty-eight or forty-nine and can expect to reach menopause within the next couple of years, this may not be a concern for you, but if you are younger, the possibility of recurrent bleeding may be more important to consider.

Myomectomy

Myomectomy is the surgical removal of uterine fibroids without removal of the entire uterus. This can be done through a small incision in the abdomen, through a laparoscope, or sometimes through a hysteroscope, depending on the location and size of the fibroids. Myomectomy is very effective, but fibroids can regrow. Women who are nearing menopause are less likely to have problems from fibroids again after myomectomy than younger women, because fibroids are less likely to develop after menopause.

Uterine Artery Embolization

Uterine artery embolization may be an alternative to surgery for symptomatic fibroids. Embolization reduces the blood flow to the uterus, particularly to the fibroids, so that the fibroids shrink. The procedure is usually done in a hospital, by a doctor called an interventional radiologist. While under mild sedation (sleepy but awake), a woman has a needle placed in an artery in her groin. A small catheter is placed into the artery and particles made of polyvinyl alcohol are injected to block the flow of blood to the uterus, which takes several minutes. When blood flow to the fibroid is reduced, the fibroid will have less oxygen and will begin to die. This process happens over days to weeks. During this time, the fibroid shrinks by approximately 40 to 50 percent and the uterus by approximately 30 to 40 percent. There can be some pain with the procedure and some women may stay overnight in the hospital for observation.

Hysterectomy and Oopherectomy

Removal of the uterus (hysterectomy) and sometimes the ovaries (oopherectomy) may be the solution for women whose symptoms do not respond to more conservative treatments. Less invasive medical and surgical procedures should be explored before hysterectomy is considered. Approximately one-third of all hysterectomies are performed to treat fibroids.

Hysterectomies are done vaginally, abdominally, or through a combination of these routes with a laparoscope. The selection of the approach is based on many factors, including the size of the uterus and the diagnosis. In general, if a vaginal hysterectomy is an option, most women prefer it because the recovery time is shorter and there is no visible scar.

There are several types of hysterectomy. The most common type is a complete or total hysterectomy, in which the cervix and uterus are

removed. In a subtotal or partial hysterectomy, the upper part of the uterus is removed and the cervix is left in place. In a radical hysterectomy, which may be done in some cases of cervical cancer, the cervix, uterus, upper part of the vagina, and supporting tissues are removed. At the time that any of the three types of hysterectomy is done, one or both ovaries and fallopian tubes may also be removed.[3] Women undergoing a hysterectomy should discuss with the surgeon the pros and cons of not removing the ovaries and cervix. Retaining the ovaries, particularly before menopause, will affect the body's hormone levels; retaining the cervix helps to maintain the natural sensation and integrity of the upper vagina. Some recent research has suggested that the ovaries should not be removed for most women undergoing hysterectomy before age sixty-five, unless ovarian cancer is a concern.[4]

UTERINE PROLAPSE

Uterine prolapse is the protrusion of the uterus (womb) or cervix into the vagina or even through the vagina to the outside of the body. Prolapse is caused by a weakening of the ligamentous and muscular support that surrounds the uterus. A major factor associated with prolapse is pregnancy, especially for women who had large babies, multiple pregnancies, and vaginal deliveries. Other factors that can lead to prolapse include a genetic predisposition, constipation with a habit of frequent straining to pass stool, chronic coughing, and smoking. White women experience uterine prolapse more often than women of other racial and ethnic backgrounds. As estrogen levels decrease with menopause, symptoms of prolapse may become worse.

The symptoms associated with uterine prolapse vary depending on the degree of prolapse. In many cases, there are no symptoms. But some of us may easily see or feel the uterus or cervix. We may feel a fullness or irritation in the vagina, or experience urinary hesitancy, frequency, or incontinence, especially the feeling of an urgent need to urinate. Sometimes we have bowel problems, including difficulty having a bowel movement, pain, and constipation. For some of us, prolapse may cause pain with vaginal intercourse.

If the prolapse does not cause problems, treatment is unnecessary. Kegel exercises (see page 214) may be helpful in decreasing symptoms. Preventing constipation by increasing fiber and water consumption, urinating frequently, and avoiding caffeine and alcohol also may be helpful. Treatment may involve use of a vaginal pessary, which is a device placed in the vagina for support. (For more information on pessaries, see page 219.)

If such measures do not give adequate relief, surgery may be needed to repair vaginal support. This may be done without hysterectomy (surgical removal of the uterus), but in many cases hysterectomy is recommended.

BLADDER HEALTH

As we age, as many as half of women experience unwanted urine loss, known as urinary incontinence.[5] It is unclear if this is related to menopause, but there is a marked increase in urinary incontinence between the ages of forty and fifty-nine.

Those of us who experience urinary incontinence may feel embarrassed or ashamed. We may avoid social events, because we fear others will notice our frequent bathroom trips or sense an unpleasant odor. We may try using panty liners, menstrual pads, or even toilet tissue to contain the leaking urine, although none of these products is designed for this use. We may stop exercising because we fear a leak may show.

A fifty-two-year-old woman from Texas says,

I wet myself every time I cough. I get so embarrassed. I can't be out very long because of this. If you have to wear a pad, you don't feel comfortable because it may shift and not protect you. You're always worried that if you wet yourself, others will notice the odor. You're afraid that you smell and you can't be around people. My husband comments that he didn't know he was traveling with a meona (person who pees a lot). This hurts my feelings because he doesn't understand.

We should not let embarrassment get in the way of finding help. Even if our health care providers don't ask about bladder problems, it is important to raise the issue.

Effective treatment is available for the three most common types of urinary incontinence women experience:

- Stress incontinence: occurs with coughing, laughing, lifting, or participating in any physical activity that increases pressure within the abdomen and pushes on the bladder
- Urge incontinence: includes an uncontrollable need to empty the bladder
- Mixed incontinence: combines urge and stress incontinence symptoms

For those of us who are not experiencing leaking now, specialized exercises and bladder training may help us stay dry long-term. Many health care providers recommend that women start this self-care to prevent incontinence later in life. Research in postmenopausal women shows that those who practiced pelvic floor muscle and bladder training for a year were twice as likely to remain continent as those who did not practice the exercises.[6]

SELF-CARE FOR TREATMENT OR PREVENTION

Not only is each of the three main types of urinary incontinence treatable, but initial treatment is based on simple behavior changes that can help us avoid medication and/or surgery. Urinary incontinence is not inevitable. Women can work with our own bodies to treat or prevent such problems.

PELVIC FLOOR MUSCLE TRAINING

Healthy pelvic floor muscles form a hammock that stretches across our pelvis, supports the bladder and urethra (see illustration below), and helps keep the urethra tightly closed, containing urine in the bladder. To understand how this works, picture the bladder as a balloon filled with water and turned upside down with its neck pinched closed. Coughing, sneezing, or sudden movements increase pressure on the

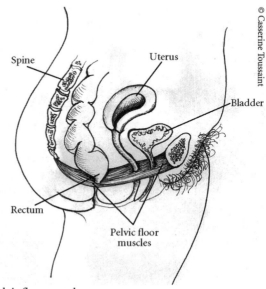

© Casserine Toussaint

Pelvic floor muscles

bladder, just as pressing on the top of the balloon increases pressure on it. Healthy pelvic floor muscles prevent urine from leaking by squeezing the urethra closed, in much the same way that squeezing the balloon neck prevents water from squirting out.

Pelvic floor muscle training is exercise to strengthen the muscles and make them more effective. Research has shown that many women had much less leaking—and sometimes eliminated incontinence entirely—when they practiced pelvic floor muscle exercises.[7] Obtaining this benefit took between two and six months, depending on the woman's age; older women needed to do the daily exercises for a longer time before seeing results.

Once you understand how to contract your pelvic floor muscles, you can consciously prepare for any event that might cause unwanted leakage. For example, if you feel a cough or a sneeze coming on or you are blowing your nose or lifting something heavy, you can tighten the pelvic floor muscles. Women have dramatically reduced the amount of urine leaked while coughing just by tightening and holding the pelvic floor muscles before and during a cough.[8]

I couldn't believe it! My underwear would get wet every time I coughed. The nurse showed me how to tighten up when I felt a cough coming and that was enough to keep me dry. Really, if I can remember to do it, I stay totally dry. For me, the hardest part is remembering to tighten down there when I feel like I'm getting ready to cough.

Pelvic floor exercises are sometimes called Kegel exercises (after Dr. Arnold Kegel, who popularized them in the early 1950s), strengthening exercises, or elevators. In addition to helping prevent urine leakage, they may lead to more pleasurable orgasms.

How to Exercise Your Pelvic Floor

The same muscles that help hold in urine and prevent intestinal gas release are used in pelvic floor muscle training. The muscles are tightened up and in, tightened around the rectum and vagina, and moved up toward the small of the back.

To better feel the muscles contracting when first learning to do a pelvic floor muscle contraction, it helps to lie flat with feet on the floor, knees bent and slightly apart. When contracting the pelvic floor, it's important to feel the muscles tighten inward and upward. Some women mistakenly think we are doing pelvic floor muscle training when we are actually bearing down, which won't strengthen the muscles. To avoid bearing down, try breathing in and out gently through the mouth while contracting the muscles. (It's difficult to both push down and breathe easily at the same time.) Try to relax your abdominal, thigh, and buttocks muscles. Tightening these muscles doesn't cause any injury, but it lessens the workout the pelvic muscles get.

A way to check if the right muscles are being contracted is to look at the vaginal area with a mirror. When your pelvic floor muscles are contracting correctly, the clitoris moves toward the vagina, and the rectal opening puckers inward. You may put your finger halfway inside your vagina and try to grip your finger with your vagina. Or if you have sex with a male partner, you can tighten the pelvic floor muscles around his penis during intercourse. Over time, he can tell if the contractions are getting stronger.

It takes time to build muscle endurance. Begin by holding each contraction for two seconds, and gradually increase the time to ten seconds. Over time, the number of seconds you will be able to hold each contraction will increase. Relax for at least ten seconds between contractions to give the muscles adequate rest.

Women who practice thirty to forty-five pelvic muscle contractions a day typically see results in six to eight weeks, but some women need to do the exercises longer before getting an effect. It takes about fifteen minutes to complete the recommended thirty to forty-five contractions a day. You can divide your exercises into two or three shorter sessions throughout the day with equal effectiveness.

Setting aside time for the exercises in your daily schedule or adding them to other daily workout routines may be helpful. Research shows that people who make the exercises a planned part of their day have been more successful at actually doing them over an extended period.[9] Reminders about pelvic floor muscle training also can be useful. You can post a note on the bathroom mirror or plan to do pelvic floor muscle exercises during a regularly watched TV program. Any daily event can serve as a reminder.

A sixty-two-year-old woman decided to do pelvic floor muscle training exercises five times a week:

I decided to do them at night when there were no distractions. It's become routine and I always complete the sequence. That is my time to relax.

Once comfortable with the technique, you can practice pelvic floor muscle exercises while standing or sitting. You can do these exercises anywhere and at any time, even while waiting for an elevator or at a red light.

BEHAVIOR CHANGES THAT BENEFIT BLADDER HEALTH

Behavior changes can directly benefit bladder health. If you are a smoker and have a smoker's cough, you may have experienced uncontrollable urine leakage accompanying bouts of coughing. Reducing the cough by quitting smoking will reduce the leakage. For the same reason, if you suffer from chronic bronchitis, asthma, or allergies, getting the condition treated and under control will mean a lot fewer sneezes and sessions of deep continuous coughing that can cause urine leakage. Drinking caffeine, artificial sweeteners, or alcohol can irritate the bladder and make us more likely to leak urine. Cutting back intake of these irritants can make a big difference in the frequency of urination, bothersome urges to empty, and actual leakage.

Some women are too rushed to allow time to relax and let their bladder empty normally. Trying to squeeze out all the urine quickly by contracting abdominal muscles and bearing down intensely interferes with the normal bladder function and keeps the bladder from emptying completely. When we are relaxed, the involuntary muscle of the bladder can do its job by smoothly contracting and efficiently emptying its contents. We can intentionally allow ourselves to relax by taking a few slow, deep breaths in through the nose and slowly exhaling through the mouth. Some women can empty better by double-voiding (urinate once, wait a short while without getting up from the toilet, then urinate again). It can be pretty surprising how much urine comes out the second time. Still other women benefit from pressing firmly on their bladder with their hands just over the pubic bone. This can help the bladder empty more completely.

BLADDER TRAINING

How often we need to urinate is a mark of bladder health. A number of research studies have shown that women are less likely to have incontinence problems when the average time between our trips to the bathroom is three hours or longer over a twenty-four-hour day.[10] Put another way, six to eight visits to the bathroom in a given day is considered normal and healthy.

Extending the time between one visit to the bathroom and the next (the voiding interval) is a recommended first treatment for urinary urge incontinence, as well as for women who are going to the bathroom on average more often than every two hours.[11] This is called bladder training. Bladder training simply means that instead of emptying the bladder every time the urge arises, you gradually train your bladder to hold urine for longer periods of time. The end goal is 3.5 to 4 hours between trips to the bathroom during waking hours.

It takes from one to six months to see results; older women need a longer time before seeing an effect. Women who do bladder training need to urinate less often and report significant decreases in leaking. Approximately 60 percent of women in a three-month bladder training program became completely dry or experienced only mild incontinence following the training.[12]

Bladder training recognizes that the bladder first sends a signal to urinate when it's about half full. You can quiet this urge and wait for the bladder to fill. The trick to doing this is to use a combination of pelvic floor muscle contractions, relaxation techniques, and mental distraction.

Many women don't know how long we can go between trips to the bathroom. Some of us were taught when we were growing up to empty our bladder at every possible opportunity. This teaching may have been based on the mistaken belief that more frequent urination would prevent bladder infections. Some of us who have experienced incontinence try to use the bathroom more frequently because we think having less urine in our bladder will decrease the potential for accidental leakage. But

this belief, too, is inaccurate. A bladder that is emptied more frequently becomes trained to signal an urge to empty when it's less full.

The first step in bladder training is to track your current habits on a daily bladder diary (see illustration on page 218). A bladder diary should be kept for at least three consecutive days during a period of typical daily life. During this period, record every visit to the bathroom to urinate and any episodes of urine leakage. Calculate the average voiding interval by tallying the total number of urinations, dividing it by however many days the diary was kept, and then dividing 24 by that number. For example, if you urinated 12 times on Monday, 14 times on Tuesday, and 13 times on Wednesday, you would have a total of 39 voids for the three days or, upon dividing the total by the three days of diary keeping, an average of 13 voids per day. Twenty-four hours divided by 13 yields an average voiding interval of 1 hour and 45 minutes. This is considerably less than the healthy three-hour or more intervals that are recommended and suggests that you could benefit from bladder training.

If you find that you currently average at least three hours between trips to the bathroom, there's no need for further action. But many women find we have a much shorter interval.

If you decide to begin bladder training, start by trying to increase the time between trips to the bathroom by ten to fifteen minutes each week. When an earlier urge to urinate arises, you can:

• do a pelvic floor muscle contraction. Two or three rapid contractions are often enough to quiet the bladder's signal to urinate.
• relax by breathing slowly and deeply, inhaling through the nose and exhaling through the mouth. Focus on breathing and relaxation, not on needing to empty the bladder. This strategy often decreases or erases the urge to empty.

Your Daily Bladder Diary

This diary will help you and your health care team. Bladder diaries help show the causes of bladder control trouble. The "sample" line (below) will show you how to use the diary.

Your name: _____

Date: _____

Time ☼	Drinks — What kind? How much?		Urine — How many times?	How much? (circle one)			ACCIDENTS — Accidental leaks — How much? (circle one)			Did you feel a strong urge to go? Circle one		What were you doing at the time? Sneezing, exercising, having sex, lifting, etc.
Sample	Coffee	2 cups	✓✓	⊙ sm	○ med	○ lg	⊙ sm	◉ med	○ lg	Yes	(No)	Running
6–7 a.m.				○	○	●	○	○	●	Yes	No	
7–8 a.m.				○	○	●	○	○	●	Yes	No	
8–9 a.m.				○	○	●	○	○	●	Yes	No	
9–10 a.m.				○	○	●	○	○	●	Yes	No	
10–11 a.m.				○	○	●	○	○	●	Yes	No	
11–12 noon				○	○	●	○	○	●	Yes	No	
12–1 p.m.				○	○	●	○	○	●	Yes	No	
1–2 p.m.				○	○	●	○	○	●	Yes	No	
2–3 p.m.				○	○	●	○	○	●	Yes	No	
3–4 p.m.				○	○	●	○	○	●	Yes	No	
4–5 p.m				○	○	●	○	○	●	Yes	No	
5–6 p.m.				○	○	●	○	○	●	Yes	No	
6–7 p.m.				○	○	●	○	○	●	Yes	No	

Courtesy of the National Kidney and Urologic Diseases Information Clearinghouse

• shift attention from the urge to urinate by focusing on something else, for instance, making a telephone call or reading an article.

As the extended time period becomes more comfortable (usually after a week, but it may take several weeks), extend the time between trips to the bathroom a little more.

Practice bladder training only when you are awake. If you need to urinate during the night, get up and go. Also, bladder training doesn't require slavish adherence to the schedule; ten minutes' leeway on either side of the scheduled time is fine.

Every woman is different, and special considerations should be taken into account when beginning bladder training. When drinking caffeine or taking a diuretic or other medication, you may not be able to delay urination in those hours right after caffeine or medication is consumed. It doesn't hurt to try to delay, but if the schedule can't be maintained, just resume once caffeine or medication effects ease off.

MEDICATION AND SURGERY

Sometimes urinary incontinence is so severe that medication, a device called a pessary, or surgery is the only option to get it under control.

Some medications can lessen an intense urge to urinate and decrease urine leakage related to urgency. These medications also can cause other effects, such as dry mouth or mental confusion, so some women use bladder training and pelvic floor muscle training along with the medication, aiming to reduce medication use as soon as it's feasible. Some newer medications do not cause problems with mental confusion, but most women prefer to manage without medication if they can.

Pessaries are flexible, soft plastic devices inserted into the vagina to support the pelvic organs. They can markedly lower the amount of leakage. Pessaries have to be taken out, washed, and reinserted regularly. They must be fitted by a health care provider but can be inserted and removed by the user daily or weekly. A well-fitted pessary should provide relief but otherwise be unnoticed by the wearer. They generally have no adverse effects and are both easy to use and easy to stop using.

For women with stress incontinence (leaking with coughing, sneezing, or exercise), common surgical treatments are bladder neck suspensions and vaginal tape insertions. Surgery isn't always successful and sometimes it fails after a few years. However, new minimally invasive procedures have success rates of 80 to 90 percent in the treatment of stress incontinence when done by qualified surgeons. As a general practice, all possible nonsurgical options should be tried before surgery is decided on. If you choose surgery, be sure to find a surgeon experienced in continence surgery on women. A new specialty called urogynecology provides training in pelvic floor surgery.

Consulting with your health care provider and doing some independent research can help you decide whether medication, pessary, or surgery is an option you should consider. Whichever option you select, pelvic floor muscle training and bladder training can enhance the treatment effects. To learn more about urinary incontinence treatment, consult the National Association for Continence website (NAFC.org) and the American Urogynecologic Society website (www.augs.org).

NOTES

1. Gordon P. Flake, Janet Anderson, and Darlene Dixon, "Etiology and Pathogenesis of Uterine Leiomyomas: A Review," *Environmental Health Perspectives* 111, no. 8 (June 2003): 1037–55.

2. Diane D. League, "Endometrial Ablation as an Alternative to Hysterectomy," *AORN Journal* 77, no. 2 (February 2003): 322–24, 327–38.

3. Office on Women's Health in the Department of Health and Human Services, "Hysterectomy," November 2002, accessed at www.4woman.gov/faq/hysterectomy.htm on August 8, 2005.

4. William H. Parker, Michael S. Broder, Zhimei Liu, Donna Shoupe, Cindy Farquhar, and Jonathan S. Berek, "Ovarian Conservation at the Time of Hysterectomy for Benign Disease," *American Journal of Obstetrics and Gynecology* 106 (August 2005): 219–26.

5. Carolyn M. Sampselle, Sioban D. Harlow, Joan Skurnick, Linda Burbaker, Irina Bondarondo, "Urinary Incontinence Predictors and Life Impact in Ethnically Diverse Perimenopausal Women," *Obstetrics and Gynecology* 100 (December 2002): 1230–38.

6. Ananias C. Diokno, Carolyn M. Sampselle, A. Regula Herzog, Trivellore E. Raghunathan, Sandra J. Hines, Kassandra L. Messer, et al., "Prevention of Urinary Incontinence by Behavioral Modification Program: A Randomized Controlled Trial among Older Women

in the Community," *Journal of Urology* 171 (March 2004): 1165–71.

7. Jean Hay-Smith, Peter Herbison, and Siv Mokved, "Physical Therapies for Prevention of Urinary and Fæcal Incontinence in Adults (Cochrane Review)," in *The Cochrane Library,* no. 2 (Oxford, UK: Update Software, 2002).

8. Janis M. Miller, James A. Ashton-Miller, and John De-Lancey, "A Pelvic Muscle Precontraction Can Reduce Cough-Related Urine Loss in Selected Women with Mild SUI," *Journal of the American Geriatric Society* 46 (1998): 870–74.

9. Sandra J. Hines, Julia S. Seng, Kassandra L. Messer, Trivellore E. Raghunathan, Ananais C. Diokno, and Carolyn M. Sampselle, "Factors Contributing to Adherence to a Pelvic Floor Muscle Exercise Regimen to Prevent Urinary Incontinence: A Mixed-Method Analysis" (in progress).

10. Carolyn M. Sampselle, "Behavioral Interventions in Young and Middle-Aged Women: Simple Interventions to Combat a Complex Problem," *American Journal of Nursing, Supplement, State of the Science on Urinary Incontinence* 3 (March 2003): 9–19.

11. Phillip D. Wilson, Kari Bo, Jean Hay-Smith, Ingrid Nygaard, David Staskin, Jean F. Wyman, et al., "Conservative Treatment in Women," in Paul Abrams, Linda Cardozo, Saad Khoury, and Alan Wein, eds., *Incontinence,* 2nd ed. (Plymouth, UK: Plymbridge Distributors, 2002), 571–624.

12. Andrew Fantl, Jean F. Wyman, Donna K. McClish, Stephanie W. Harkins, R. K. Elswick Jr., et al., "Efficacy of Bladder Training in Older Women with Urinary Incontinence," *JAMA* 265, no. 5 (1991): 609–13.

CHAPTER 15

Memory and Mood

When I started having hot flashes, I also started having these waves of emotional distress . . . I was in a meeting a few weeks ago, and suddenly, for no apparent reason, I just felt like bursting into tears. And I didn't, but I really struggled with whether I needed to leave the room. These waves seem to come out of nowhere. They remind me of the days right before I would get my period, when I was in my early twenties and had awful premenstrual tension.

I was so surprised when I walked into the store and for the life of me could not remember why I had gone there. I decided to just walk around looking at the products, hoping that [the reason] I was there would come to me. Luckily, it popped into my brain. Sometimes I have the experience of going into another room or a store to do or buy a few things. If I don't write down what I need to do, I often end up with only half [the things] done. The things I find myself forgetting are small and not so important, but it is nonetheless a great shock when these things simply "slip my mind." It seems that this started around the change of life.

As we go through the menopause transition, some of us experience mood swings, irritability, depression, and memory problems. This chapter examines the changes some of us experience, the factors that influence them, and how to get help.

Many women who have memory and mood problems at this life stage attribute them to shifting hormones, but the connection is not clear. For example, there is no proof that natural menopause is linked to changes in memory beyond those associated with aging. But women who experience sleep problems associated with menopause sometimes have memory difficulties that are linked to sleep loss and fatigue. Evidence for a correlation between natural menopause and clinical depression is mixed. Perimenopausal women do report significantly more psychological distress than pre- or postmenopausal women.[1] In addition, two recent studies suggest that the menopause transition is a time of increased risk for depression for women without a history of depression.[2] But other studies have not found an increase in depression among women at this life stage. Surgical menopause and medically induced menopause are sometimes associated with memory or mood problems that are specific to a woman's circumstances, age, and medical treatments.

MEMORY AND MENOPAUSE

OUR BRAIN, THINKING, AND MEMORY

Most of us take our brain for granted. We assume that our thinking, memory, and ability to manipulate knowledge will always be there for us. It is thus a great shock to most when we have the first experience of not being able to find a word that we use frequently, or not being able to remember a phone number, or simply forgetting why we went into the kitchen. This can happen throughout life because of stress, too much multitasking, or simply fatigue. When it happens after a surgically induced menopause or during a natural menopausal transition, the challenge is to determine if it is just the same old problem experienced before or something new associated with the change in hormones.

Medical science refers to two main categories of brain function. One is *cognition* and the other is *memory*.

Cognitive Functioning

Cognition includes many of the ways we use our brain as a tool of our intellect, or *intellectual (thinking) functioning*. These functions include perception and the ability to learn new material, to remember what we have learned, to acquire language, to reason and to work with abstract ideas and thoughts, and to make judgments.

Memory

Memory is multidimensional. We have conscious recollection of recently encountered information. This is referred to as *new learning*. The immediate memory for events that have just happened is called *short-term memory*.

An easy and common way to test short-term memory is to have a friend give you a list of words, generally three, and then ask you to say all the words five minutes later. This kind of test is called a delayed recall task. It is a rough measure of recall; more sophisticated ways to test memory include testing after twenty minutes and distracting the person whose memory is being tested.

I laughed when my friend said to remember apple, tree, and the Brooklyn Bridge. I repeated them to myself. Five minutes later, she said to me to repeat them back, and by golly, I got them all. Then she gave me some numbers to remember; I was able to do that, too. It seems that when I am doing only one thing and concentrating, I can remember just fine.

Quick or short-term memory is in contrast to what is called *long-term memory*. Our brain seems to have different banks for memory, the immediate bank and the long-term bank. Memories move from the immediate bank to the long-term bank by a series of neurochemical processes in our brain.

I was worried about my loss of ability to remember numbers and names. I went to my clinician to discuss this. She spoke to me about all the ways age and day-to-day life can impact this. She asked me to remember what my own mother was like at the end of her life when she had a dementia associated with her small strokes and high blood pressure. I remembered that Mom could tell wonderful stories about us as children, herself as a child, and had the clearest mind when it came to the past. When I would ask her about my daughter's visit to her yesterday, she would give me a blank look. My clinician explained to me that my mother had lost her ability to make these new memories and park them in new long-term storage, but that she was able to remember the things she had successfully parked in long-term storage years ago. My mother's memory problems were related to her [progressive] dementia, and my memory problems were common at midlife but did not mean I was "demented." That was a great relief to hear.

Age and Memory

Intellectual functioning involving all aspects of the brain's ability to work with information steadily declines with age. Not all aspects change equally, and there is much variation from person to person. How we continue to use our brain and how much practice our brain has doing different aspects of "brain work" will also affect how our brain changes with age. The longer we live, unfortunately, the less quickly our brain is able to function. The most common type of change is trouble recalling someone's name or numbers. This is not a sign of a "dementia." It may be simply a sign of age; it also can be a sign of stress, mood problems, or poor sleep. As we age, older information is more easily remembered than new information.

MIDLIFE AND MEMORY

Many of us who are going through the menopause transition complain of problems with concentration and memory. Researchers have been attempting to quantify and describe these changes. Few scientific studies to date have been able to show a change in mental function during the menopause transition. Subtle changes in memory and word finding concentration are most likely attributable to other aspects of our lives, such as aging, physical health problems, sleep problems, stress, or depression.

Some researchers believe that if there are changes in memory and cognitive ability during the natural menopause transition, these changes may be too subtle to measure in clinical studies.[3] Medical researchers have shown that women who have had our ovaries removed surgically (through complete hysterectomy or oophorectomy) and experience problems in memory will generally experience improved memory by taking estrogen.[4] Some researchers theorize that the suddenness of the loss of estrogen with loss of the ovaries may make it easier to identify memory problems and resolve them with treatment than in natural menopause, a process that may take many years. For the woman going through natural menopause, there is no consistent proof yet of associated loss of cognitive function or memory.

The Role of Estrogen in Brain Wellness

Estrogen has many beneficial effects on the brain. Scientists have been looking at whether decreasing estrogen levels may cause problems with our brain's ability to function at its best. Estrogen has been found to affect the brain in several ways, by:

- protecting neurons from the stress of aging (loss of blood, oxidative changes).
- stimulating nerve cell growth (branching).
- stimulating blood flow and increase in the uptake of glucose (the body's sugar) into the brain.

- affecting patterns of brain activation during intellectual tasks.
- reducing formation of a protein associated with Alzheimer's disease known as beta-amyloid.
- influencing neurotransmitters that among other things affect memory and mood (acetylcholine, norepinephrine, serotonin).
- blunting the stress response (hypothalamic-pituitary-adrenal axis reactivity).[5]

The fact that estrogen serves these particular physiological roles doesn't mean that women's brains can't work as well after menopause, when circulating estrogen levels go down. There is no strong clinical evidence that women have a change in mental function or cognitive ability outside the normal range after menopause.

Despite all of the research on estrogen's beneficial effects on the brain, estrogen treatment has not been shown to improve memory or brain function when a woman takes it during or after the menopause transition. Rather, research shows that other problems associated with menopause lead to problems with memory and thinking. Sleep problems due to hot flashes and night sweats have been shown to influence cognitive performance and memory. If the sleep problems are resolved, then the cognitive performance returns to normal. If the sleep problems are not resolved, there is no evidence for a long-term impact on the woman's memory.

Stress also affects memory, as does depression and anxiety. Midlife is a phase of life full of challenges. If these challenges lead to increased stress, sleep problems, or mood problems, then memory and cognitive performance may be affected.

I have been beside myself. Starting at age forty-nine, I would wake up a few times a night soaked in sweat. I didn't pay much attention to this at first, as I had grown up in the heat in Texas. We were hot at night there in the summer and it was just normal. This felt different. After a while, I noticed that I was feeling more irritable during the day and drinking more coffee. I started to feel fatigued all the time. I also found it was hard to concentrate and do my job. Things would slip my mind. Thankfully, this all went away when my hot flashes got better. I was lucky, as they only lasted about a year. Had they lasted any longer, I think I would have needed to ask for some help. For that year, I woke up each morning as though I had not gotten enough sleep, and the whole day seemed to be worse for this. After the hot flashes went away, my rested and energetic old self returned. And, with it, my brain!

WHO HAS MEMORY PROBLEMS AT MIDLIFE?

Few studies look at the percentage of women who may have cognitive problems during the menopause transition. One study of one hundred women attending a menopause clinic found that 75 percent complained of memory loss.[6] But the women attending the clinic were likely to be experiencing many problems associated with menopause that might be causing the problems in memory. Most studies find that women's memories in menopause are fine and that women with many menopause-related problems, including night sweats, may experience memory problems. However, it is unclear if the night sweats or other menopause-related concerns are the cause of the perceived memory problems.

We may perceive ourselves as having memory loss but still perform well on testing. These memory problems can be very annoying.

I can't remember the phone numbers told to me by directory assistance. I am at the point where I simply push number 1 when the recording prompts me and pay the fifty cents for the service (the charge in California). I feel this is a waste of money, but at least I know that I will be connected correctly. When I try to remember the numbers, half the time I get them wrong. I asked my clinician to test me. After testing, she said that my memory was fine. She told me that I am tired, working a lot, with much responsibility for my family. She says that these stressors distract my ability to remember things like numbers and names. When she tested me, I was rested and I concentrated so as to do well. And I did well. I asked her what I could do to help my memory outside her office. She said more rest, exercise, and slowing down. I said that would be hard to do. She then said to do the best I can and be patient with myself . . . just laugh when it happens rather than get frustrated.

Treatments

The best way to treat perceived changes in memory and cognitive function is to tackle the underlying causes. The most common in midlife are:

- depression
- stress
- severe hot flashes and night sweats (that disrupt sleep)
- change in life circumstances.

The least common would be early symptoms of dementia.

If you have persistent symptoms of memory problems that go beyond the normal amount, check with your health care provider about getting a formal neuropsychological assessment and medical workup. It may also be helpful to do more brain and physical exercises and to adopt healthy lifestyle habits such as eating a good diet and living smoke-free.

I started to worry when I could not keep the orders at work straight. At first I thought I was just tired. Then I noticed that it was more than names or forgetting what I went into the room for, I was confusing instructions and having trouble performing normal tasks at work. I had had some anxiety and mood problems in life, but they had never been bad enough to require me to make an appointment with my clinician. I started to think maybe it was my menopause. I went to get a checkup and the clinician was also worried. She thought that my steady loss of ability to perform at work was more than the normal amount seen with the anxiety and mood problems I described to her. She sent me to a neurologist and to a neuropsychologist for evaluation. It was a great shock to my husband and me when the tests came back showing significant problems with memory and mental functioning. After many tests, they told us that I had some kind of early dementing process but they didn't know what the cause was or how it would progress. They put me on a neurologic drug for early dementia to help my memory. My husband and I are taking life day by day and embracing the time we have, however long that may be. We are also attending a support group for patients such as myself.

Developing a progressive dementia at menopause is *very uncommon*. It is more common to develop progressive dementia at much older ages. However, if you are deeply troubled by a steep decline in your memory and mental abilities, you can talk with your health care provider.

Hormone Treatment

Hormone treatment is not recommended to improve thinking or prevent dementia, although research on its effects is ongoing. The Women's Health Initiative found an increased risk of dementia for women older than sixty-five who took hormones—both the estrogen-progestin combination and estrogen only—and no improvement in overall cognitive function.[7]

(For more information about the WHI results, see Chapter 7, "Hormone Treatment.")

There is some controversy about whether the WHI results provide the definitive answer to the question of estrogen's effect on cognitive decline. Observational studies have shown a 30 percent reduction in risk of developing dementia due to Alzheimer's disease by taking hormone treatment.[8] But observational studies are not as trustworthy as randomized, double-blind studies such as the WHI. More studies have been proposed to investigate the theory that there is a critical "window of opportunity" for hormone treatment to be beneficial; such studies will examine the timing of hormone treatment (during or after the menopause transition) and its effect on long-term cognitive function and the risk of developing Alzheimer's.[9] So far, no large, randomized, double-blind studies have shown improvement in memory and cognition with hormone treatment, whether taken early or at any time after menopause.

Alternatives to Hormones and Medications

Memory and attention, concentration, and ability to perform daily tasks of the brain are highly dependent on how our mood is, whether or not we are anxious, how much multitasking we are doing, how distractible we are, and whether we are rested. Long-term maintenance of our ability to use our brain is greatly helped by continuing to use our brain. Helpful natural brainpower treatments include:

- doing one thing at a time.
- protecting your sleep, so your brain can restore itself. (See "Squeaky Clean Sleep," page 84.)
- relaxing at least once per day and, if possible, practicing some type of relaxation exercise, such as yoga, stretching, meditation, tai chi, or chi gong.
- taking time to exercise.
- taking time to eat healthily and properly.
- looking at the stresses in your life and taking steps to reduce them.
- creating or maintaining positive interpersonal relationships and social support.
- if your mood or anxiety does not improve, seeking help from a knowledgeable provider.

(For more information on relaxation and stress reduction, see Chapter 11; for information on eating well and staying active, see Chapters 12 and 13.)

MOOD AND MENOPAUSE

MOOD PROBLEMS AND DEPRESSION

Many of us experience low mood or just feel sad and blue when we are disappointed, stressed, have losses, or simply have a "down day." Some women experience these low moods consistently, and a smaller percentage of women have the symptoms of clinical depression. Clinical depression is defined as a depressed mood or loss of interest or pleasure, along with at least four of the following:[10]

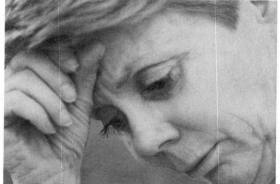

© Leah Hogsten

- weight loss or weight gain
- changes in sleep
- agitation or a feeling of being slowed down
- fatigue
- feeling of worthlessness or guilt
- trouble thinking or concentrating
- thoughts of death or suicide.

If some of the above symptoms cause significant distress or affect your ability to work or socialize, and if they last for more than two weeks, consider seeking help from a knowledgeable health care provider. If you feel like you are in immediate danger, call a suicide hotline or go to an emergency room.

I had had a hard year. I have an upbeat temperament and am known as an optimist. This year was rough on me. First, my husband got a demotion at work; this impacted our finances. Then my daughter started to have trouble with her eating. She was starving herself and getting thinner. I could not get my mind off my husband's stresses and my daughter's eating problems. Even though things were improving in both arenas, I found myself not rebounding as I usually do. I started feeling low all the time, even if it was a basically good day. Then I started to have trouble sleeping and was not enjoying the hobbies I had always enjoyed. My husband noticed that I was unusually down. When this lasted for three months, I decided to seek out professional help.

The majority of women do not experience depression during the menopause transition. It is not clear if we are at any greater risk for developing clinical depression than at any other time of life. However, women with a past history of depression, particularly depression related to menstruation, pregnancy, or childbirth, may be more prone to depression in the perimenopause.[11] This is especially true if the woman's menopausal transition is marked by many hot flashes lasting over many months or years, or if she is experiencing severe life stresses, such as divorce, the death of a loved one, or a new illness. Women have a higher rate of developing depression than men from puberty to old age. The reasons for this difference are unclear but may be related to discrimination, victimization, psychosocial expectations, cognitive style, physiology, and research bias. A woman who experiences depression during the menopausal transition may simply be experiencing depression unrelated to menopause.

Although treatments for depression do not always work, and some health care providers have problematic biases with respect to women, it may be well worth it to seek help.

I had had a depression when I was in college. It was a rough year. My mother had died in a car accident and I had broken up with my high school boyfriend. I felt kind of lost in college to begin with, as I didn't really fit into any group of friends well. I started to slip into a depression. I had never been depressed like this before. I was always a sensitive girl but not particularly moody. I went to the college counseling service and was helped greatly by the psychologist who saw me weekly that year. It really was not until my menopause that I got that sticky depressed feeling again. The circumstances were similar. My marriage had been on the rocks for a number of years. It was no surprise when my husband came in and said he wanted a divorce. I am not sure if I was relieved, sad, or both. Our marriage had not been good for a long time, but I was ambivalent about what to do about it. The kids had gone off to college, and we seemed not to have enough to keep us together anymore. My father was diagnosed with terminal cancer this same year. I started to sink into the same depressed feeling I had had in college. I thought at first it was my menopause, as my girlfriends were talking about menopause and how they read it can cause mood problems. I was not having any menopausal symptoms, but I sure felt depressed. I went to see a psychiatrist, who said that I was having a hard time and this had led to the depression, similarly to what had happened in college. I started talk therapy and slowly pulled out of it.

CAUSES FOR MOOD PROBLEMS AND DEPRESSION DURING THE MENOPAUSE TRANSITION

Many studies suggest that women have more feelings of being "sad and blue" as well as more changes in mood during the menopause transi-

ANTIDEPRESSANT MEDICATIONS

The two most common treatments for depression are psychotherapy and antidepressant medications. The most widely prescribed antidepressants belong to a class of drugs called selective serotonin reuptake inhibitors, or SSRIs, and include the medications Prozac, Zoloft, Paxil, Luvox, Celexa, and Lexapro. Wellbutrin, Remeron, and Effexor are also widely prescribed; while these drugs are not SSRIs, they act in similar ways on the brain, affecting neurotransmitters. All of these drugs are considered "second generation" antidepressants because they have, since their creation in the 1980s and 1990s, largely replaced older tricyclic antidepressants such as Elavil and Sinequan.

Over the past fifteen years there has been a dramatic increase in the number of people taking these drugs, with women far outnumbering men. Most people think—and pharmaceutical companies would have us believe—that these medications are a cure-all for depression. However, research trials have shown them to be only slightly to moderately more effective than placebos.[12]

In addition, the negative effects of the second generation antidepressants, including agitation, digestive problems, and sexual problems, as well as a possible increased risk of suicide, tend to be downplayed or even concealed by the companies that sell them.[13] Many of the clinical trials conducted to evaluate the safety of these drugs lasted only six weeks, with relatively few lasting up to six months or a year. Because women often take antidepressants for extended periods of time—often for years—this lack of data on long-term effects is particularly troublesome.

For women with mild to moderate depression, alternatives to medications such as talk therapy and exercise may be as or more effective than drug therapy, and have few, if any, harmful effects.

Women who experience severe clinical depression may find it helpful to combine drug and nondrug treatments. Because it is important to be monitored while taking these medications, and because finding the best drug or combination of drugs and the appropriate dosage can be difficult, it is best to work with an experienced physician, psychiatrist, or psychopharmacologist (a psychiatrist who specializes in psychoactive drugs).

Discontinuing these medications can cause withdrawal symptoms such as a worsening of depression, appetite changes, insomnia, and agitation. Women who decide to stop taking the medication should do so slowly and under the supervision of a knowledgeable health care provider.

tion, but only a few studies show more depression that requires treatment.[14] Depression is more likely if the transition is prolonged (greater than twenty-seven months) with more symptoms or stressors.[15]

It seems like I am more easily upset these days. Ever since my periods have become infrequent and my monthly bleed has lightened, I have been a bit more irritable, but then at times I am fine. It is like my personality is not as consistent as it used to be. My friends have asked if I am depressed, but I really don't feel depressed. I just don't feel as steady in my emotions as I used to be.

There are many theories as to why some women may find ourselves more moody during the menopause transition:

- Estrogen affects neuronal function, so it is possible that falling levels of estrogen during the perimenopause affect mood.
- Hormones have been shown to increase endorphins; thus a change in a woman's hormones may increase or decrease her feelings of well-being.
- Serotonin receptors, part of the mood mechanism in the brain, have been shown to increase in women who received estrogen patch therapy after menopause, suggesting that estrogen levels may affect mood.
- The menopause transition may magnify the effect of stress on depressed mood.
- Sleep disturbance and nighttime sweating associated with menopause may lead to increasing levels of fatigue and irritability, which may cause depressed mood.

Various research studies (double-blind trials, longitudinal population-based studies, and longitudinal analysis) support the conclusion that bothersome signs of menopause adversely affect mood.[16]

WOMEN AND STRESS

There is building evidence that women experience acute stress more intensely after menopause than before. Midlife is often a time for many stressors, including demanding family responsibilities, lack of time for oneself, lack of sleep, and financial concerns. Recent research is also showing that women exposed to more stressful events may be more likely to experience subsequent low mood as well as hot flashes and night sweats during the menopause transition. Reducing stress at any time in a woman's life may help protect her from mood problems; this is especially true in the menopause transition and after menopause.

WHO EXPERIENCES MOOD PROBLEMS AT MENOPAUSE?

Women develop mood problems and depression more if we are experiencing hot flashes and night sweats than if we are not. Women who have a very long menopause transition have been shown to be at a higher risk of developing mood problems. Mood problems may coincide with the time when menstrual periods are skipped. The exact percentage of women who have mild to moderate mood problems versus those with more serious mood problems is hard to say, as the medical studies have used different ways of measuring mood.

Certain risk factors increase a woman's chance of developing mood problems or depression with menopause, although some women may have these risk factors and not develop mood problems. The risk factors are:

- a history of having depressed mood or depression
- having had a postpartum depression or premenstrual syndrome
- stressful life events

- living or working in a high-stress environment
- an unhealthy lifestyle—smoking, getting little exercise
- difficulty paying for the basics
- lower educational level
- health problems
- lack of a partner or single parenthood
- negative attitudes toward aging and menopause
- hot flashes or night sweats along with other bodily symptoms of menopause
- an early natural menopause (before age forty).

My doctor didn't seem surprised that I was having a tough time with my change of life. I had had this gynecologist since my first child in my early twenties. We have gone through thick and thin together. I always had PMS but not so bad that exercise, vitamins, and patience could not cure. Then, after my second child was born, a sadness came over me for no reason at all. I sank into it and felt more and more low. Eventually a postpartum depression was diagnosed, and when psychotherapy did not work, I ended up taking an antidepressant. It worked, and after nine months of treatment, I went off them and was well. I had not thought about any of this until lately. I had been on my own for these last ten years. My partner had died suddenly of a heart attack. I had thought I had gotten over it, but with the kids entering college, my having these bothersome hot flashes and bodily aches and pains, I just felt like I was sinking into a low mood. I finally went in to see my gynecologist, who felt that it was no surprise that a time of hormonal change might knock me into a depression again. Also, she felt that I had a lot of stressors in my life. We restarted the antidepressant that had worked so well after I had my sweet Sara. It worked again, and I was thankful to return to my old self.

TREATMENTS

The critical aspect of treating problems at menopause is to determine what is most bothersome to you. Are you primarily bothered by sleep problems, temperature problems, memory, or mood? Once the bothersome issue(s) have been identified, you may be able to figure out if changing hormones are the culprit or if your problems are a function of stress, depression, anxiety, or some combination.

If stress, low mood, and anxiety are causing the problems and the problems are mild, many approaches may help alleviate them. Exercise, a support group, relaxation training, and any form of meditation, whether it be a moving one like tai chi, chi gong, or yoga or a nonmoving one such as sitting meditation or focused breathing, often help. (For more information, see Chapter 11, "Emotional Well-Being and Managing Stress.") More serious mood and anxiety problems may require more intensive approaches such as psychotherapy and possibly medication.

If you and your clinician determine that hormonal change might be the primary cause of the problems, a number of solutions can be explored. Stress reduction, exercise, a support group, relaxation training, and meditation may be helpful. (For more information, see Chapter 11.) If night sweats are contributing to mood problems, simply sleeping in a cool room and layering one's clothing can often ameliorate them. (For more information, see Chapter 5, "Hot Flashes, Night Sweats, and Sleep Disturbances.")

If those approaches do not bring some relief, you may have other options. If you have had a hysterectomy with your ovaries removed and you are on hormone treatment, the problems you are experiencing may be reduced if your hormone formula is adjusted.

If you are experiencing a natural menopause transition and have severe hot flashes that are affecting sleep (and therefore memory and mood), you may benefit from hormone treatment. Hormone treatment is recommended only if you have significant problems associated with menopause and then at the lowest dose for the shortest time that is effective. (For more information, see Chapter 7, "Hormone Treatment.")

NOTES

1. J. T. Bromberger, P. M. Meyer, K. M. Kravitz, et al., "Psychologic Distress and Natural Menopause: A Multiethnic Community Study," *American Journal of Public Health* 91 (2001): 1435–42.

2. L. S. Cohen, C. N. Soares, A. F. Vitonis, M. W. Otto, and B. L. Harlow, "Risk for New Onset of Depression During the Menopausal Transition," *Archives of General Psychiatry* 63 (April 2006): 385–90; see also E. W. Freeman, M. D. Sammel, H. Lin, and D. Nelson, "Associations of Hormones and Menopausal Status with Depressed Mood in Women with No History of Depression," *Archives of General Psychiatry* 63 (April 2006): 375–82.

3. E. Anderson, S. Hamburger, J. H. Liu, and R. W. Rebar, "Characteristics of Menopausal Women Seeking Assistance," *American Journal of Obstetrics and Gynecology* 156, no. 2 (1987): 428–33; see also V. W. Henderson, J. R. Guthrie, E. C. Dudley, H. G. Burger, and L. Dennerstein, "Estrogen Exposures and Memory at Midlife: A Population-Based Study of Women," *Neurology* 60, no. 8 (2003): 1369–71; and P. M. Meyer, L. H. Powell, R. S. Wilson, et al., "A Population-Based Longitudinal Study of Cognitive Functioning in the Menopausal Transition," *Neurology* 61, no. 6 (2003): 801–6.

4. S. M. Phillips and B. B. Sherwin, "Effects of Estrogen on Memory Function in Surgically Menopausal Women," *Psychoneuroendocrinology* 17, no. 5 (1992): 485–95.

5. V. W. Henderson, *Hormone Therapy and the Brain* (New York: Parthenon Publishing Group, 2000); M. R. Foy, V. W. Henderson, T. W. Berger, and R. F. Thompson, "Estrogen and Neural Plasticity," *Current Directions in Psychological Science* 9, no. 5 (2000): 148–52; M. R. Foy, J. Xu, X. Xie, R. D. Brinton, R. F. Thompson, T. W. Berger, "17 Beta-Estradiol Enhances NMDA Receptor-Mediated EPSPs and Long-Term Potentiation," *Journal of Neurophysiology* 81, no. 2 (1999): 925–29; R. D. Brinton, "Investigative Models for Determining Hormone Therapy-Induced Outcomes in Brain: Evidence in Support of a Healthy Cell Bias of Estrogen Action," *Annals of the New York Academy of Science* 1052 (2005): 57–74; G. J. Brewer, J. D. Reichensperger, and R. D. Brinton, "Prevention of Age-Related Dysregulation of Calcium Dynamics by Estrogen in Neurons," *Neurobiology of Aging* 2005, accessed at pharmweb.usc.edu/brintonlab/_new_papers/Neurob%20Aging%202005.pdf on September 15, 2005.

6. Anderson et al.

7. M. A. Espeland, S. R. Rapp, S. A. Shumaker, et al., "Conjugated Equine Estrogens and Incidence of Probable Dementia and Mild Cognitive Impairment in Postmenopausal Women: Women's Health Initiative Memory Study," *JAMA* 291, no. 24 (2004): 2959–68; see also S. A. Shumaker, C. Legault, S. R. Rapp, et al., "Estrogen Plus Progestin and the Incidence of Dementia and Mild Cognitive Impairment in Postmenopausal Women: The Women's Health Initiative Memory Study: A Randomized Controlled Trial," *JAMA* 289, no. 20 (2003): 2651–62; S. R. Rapp, M. A. Espeland, S. A. Shumaker, et al. "Effect of Estrogen Plus Progestin on Global Cognitive Function in Postmenopausal Women: The Women's Health Initiative Memory Study: A Randomized Controlled Trial," *JAMA* 289, no. 20 (2003): 2663–72; Writing Group for the Women's Health Initiative Investigators, "Risk and Benefits of Estrogen Plus Progestin in Healthy Postmenopausal Women," *JAMA* 288, no. 3 (2002): 321–33.

8. E. S. LeBlanc, J. Janowsky, B. K. Chan, and H. D. Nelson, "Hormone Replacement Therapy and Cognition: Systematic Review and Meta-Analysis," *JAMA*

285, no. 11 (2001): 1489–99; see also K. Yaffe, G. Sawaya, I. Lieberburg, and D. Grady, "Estrogen Therapy in Postmenopausal Women: Effects on Cognitive Function and Dementia," *JAMA* 279, no. 9 (1998): 688–95.

9. B. B. Sherwin, "Estrogen and Cognitive Aging in Women," *Neuroscience* 138 (2006): 1021–6; see also P. M. Maki, "Hormone Therapy and Cognitive Function: Is There a Critical Period for Benefit?" *Neuroscience* 138 (2006): 1027–30; V. W. Henderson, "Estrogen-Containing Hormone Therapy and Alzheimer's Disease Risk: Understanding Discrepant Inferences from Observational and Experimental Research," *Neuroscience* 138 (2006): 1031–9; V. W. Henderson, K. S. Benke, R. C. Green, L. A. Cupples, L. A. Farrer, "Postmenopausal Hormone Therapy and Alzheimer's Disease Risk: Interaction with Age," *Journal of Neurology, Neurosurgery and Psychiatry* 76, no. 1 (2005): 103–5; and Y. Z. Bagger, L. B. Tanko, P. Alexandersen, G. Qin, and C. Christiansen, "Early Postmenopausal Hormone Therapy May Prevent Cognitive Impairment Later in Life," *Menopause* 12, no. 1 (2005): 12–17.

10. American Psychiatric Association, *Diagnostic and Statistical Manual for Mental Disorders*, 4th ed. (Washington, DC: 1994).

11. N. F. Woods, A. Mariella, E. S. Mitchell, "Patterns of Depressed Mood across the Menopausal Transition: Approaches to Studying Patterns in Longitudinal Data," *Acta Obstetricia et Gynecologica Scandinavica*, 81, no. 7 (2002): 623–32.

12. I. Kirsch, T. J. Moore, A. Scoboria, and S. S. Nicholls, "The Emperor's New Drugs: An Analysis of Antidepressant Medication Data Submitted to the U.S. Food and Drug Administration," *Prevention & Treatment* 5, no. 1 (July 2002); see also J. Moncrieff, S. Wessely, and R. Hardy, "Active Placebos Versus Antidepressants for Depression," *The Cochrane Database of Systematic Reviews* 2004, Issue 1, Art. No. CD003012, DOI 10.1002/14651858.CD003012; J. R. Geddes, N. Freemantle, J. Mason, M. P. Eccles, and J. Boynton, "Selective Serotonin Reuptake Inhibitors (SSRIs) Versus Other Antidepressants for Depression," *The Cochrane Database of Systematic Reviews* 1999, Issue 4, Art. No. CD001851, DOI 10.1002/14651858.CD001851.

13. See D. Healy, *Let Them Eat Prozac: The Unhealthy Relationship Between the Pharmaceutical Industry and Depression* (New York: New York University Press, 2004).

14. N. Rasgon, S. Shelton, and U. Halbreich, "Perimenopausal Mental Disorders: Epidemiology and Phenomenology," *CNS Spectrums* 10, no. 6 (2005): 471–78; P. J. Schmidt, N. Haq, and D. R. Rubinow, "A Longitudinal Evaluation of the Relationship between Reproductive Status and Mood in Perimenopausal Women," *American Journal of Psychiatry* 161, no. 12 (2004) 2238–44.

15. J. T. Bromberger and K. A. Matthews, "A Longitudinal Study of the Effects of Pessimism, Trait Anxiety, and Life Stress on Depressive Symptoms in Middle-Aged Women," *Psychology of Aging* 11, no. 2 (1996): 207–13; M. Hunter, "The South-East England Longitudinal Study of the Climacteric and Postmenopause," *Maturitas* 14, no. 2 (1992): 117–26; A. Baker, S. Simpson, and D. Dawson, "Sleep Disruption and Mood Changes Associated with Menopause," *Journal of Psychosomatic Research* 43, no. 4 (1997): 359–69; L. Dennerstein, P. Lehert, H. Burger, and E. Dudley, "Mood and the Menopausal Transition," *Journal of Nervous and Mental Disease* 187, no. 11 (1999): 685–91.

16. Ibid.

CHAPTER 16

Bone Health

Imagine that you look in your local newspaper and find a special section on women's health. In it you see an article by a prominent physician about bone health and osteoporosis prevention that asks you:

Do you know if you are one of the 30 million American women who have osteoporosis or low bone mass? (Fifty-five percent of women over fifty do!) If so, you are at higher risk for pain and disability from fractures of your wrists, spine, and hips. Annual expenditures for direct medical care of osteoporotic fractures in the U.S. total over $15 billion. The number of Americans with osteoporosis is expected to rise to 14 million, with another 48 million having low bone mass by 2020.

On the same page you see advertisements for free bone density testing at a drugstore in your neighborhood and for a medication that you are told can prevent these fractures.

If this information causes you to feel concerned and think about getting a bone density test, you will have been successfully affected by pharmaceutical company propaganda. These companies want even more women to take medication, not to treat a disease, but to modify one risk factor (low bone density) for fractures.

The mother of a close friend is seventy-three years old, weighs ninety-two pounds, and has advanced Parkinson's. She falls every day. So far, in her falls she has broken

a toilet tank and made holes in the walls, but she has not broken any bones.

With enough impact, anyone's bones will break. The bones of a person with osteoporosis tend to break more easily, but osteoporosis may or may not contribute to a particular fracture, and many women with osteoporosis never break a bone.

Scaring women about our bone strength has become a profitable industry. Consumer ads show women slumped in wheelchairs and urge us to "talk to our doctors about osteoporosis before it's too late." Bone density tests, which are easily available and either free or covered by Medicare and other health plans, can tell us "how much we have lost."

Before we let fear drive us toward more tests and medication, it is important to understand osteoporosis, the likelihood of broken bones and problems associated with them, and other options we have to increase our bone strength and decrease our chance of fractures.

REDEFINING OSTEOPOROSIS

Osteoporosis is *not* a disease but a risk factor. It does not by itself predict whether a woman will have a bone fracture. Preventing, detecting, and treating osteoporosis are significant in fracture prevention, but other risk factors are more important.

A woman with osteoporosis has fragile bones that break more easily. Osteoporotic bones have less mass—that is, they weigh less—than normal bones. In addition to weighing less, osteoporotic bones have lost some of the microscopic architecture that gives bones more strength (see illustration below).

The definition of osteoporosis is based on bone mineral density (BMD). In 1994, the World Health Organization announced these categories for women:

Normal: BMD within 1.0 standard deviation of the average for young adult women

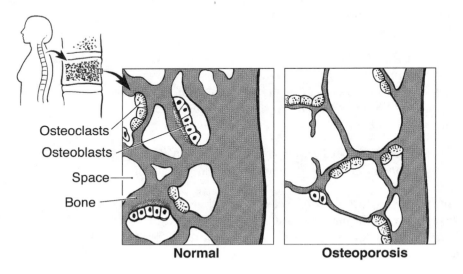

Normal **Osteoporosis**

Normal bone (left) weighs more than osteoporotic bone (right). Osteoporotic bones have lost some of the microscopic architecture that gives bones strength. Osteoclasts destroy bone, while osteoblasts help form new bone. When more bone is destroyed than created, bones can become brittle and more likely to break.

Osteopenia: BMD 1.0 to 2.5 standard deviations below the average for young adult women

Osteoporosis: BMD more than 2.5 standard deviations below the average for young adult women

Severe osteoporosis: BMD more than 2.5 standard deviations below the average for young adult women and one fracture related to osteoporosis.[1]

SYMPTOMS

Osteoporosis has no symptoms until a bone breaks.

Last July, my mother, a woman in her early eighties, went with me to the grocery store. She was in excellent health, walked two miles daily, and took no prescription medications. When she leaned forward to get out of the car, she suddenly felt a severe pain in her low back. An X-ray showed a compression fracture of her third lumbar vertebra. On X-ray, her entire spine appeared osteoporotic, but there was no sign of a previous fracture.

HOW COMMON IS OSTEOPOROSIS?

Using the WHO definition of osteoporosis, the most conservative estimate is that about 20 percent of postmenopausal women have osteoporosis.[2] Some researchers estimate the number as closer to 50 percent.[3]

WHO IS AT RISK OF BONE FRACTURE?

Fractures are a major problem for older women in the United States and Northern Europe. For older women in other areas of the world, including Japan, fractures are a lesser problem.

What explains these differences? Although the exact reasons are unknown, it is clear that race, ethnicity, body build, diet, smoking, and physical activity have tremendous impact on a woman's risk of fracture as she ages.

White women are more likely to have osteoporotic fractures than are women of any other racial or ethnic group.[4] Lifetime risk of hip fracture (a break in the upper thigh bone) is about 16 percent for white women at age fifty, but only 6 percent for fifty-year-old African-American women.[5] Within each racial and ethnic group, women who weigh less are more likely to have fractures than heavier women. Women who are physically active have denser bones and fewer fractures in old age.

Some medications—for example, prednisone, an oral steroid used to treat severe asthma or rheumatoid arthritis—can cause loss of bone density. Some medical conditions also may increase the risk of fracture. These include kidney disease, liver disease, and diseases of the adrenal, thyroid, and parathyroid glands. Women using Depo-Provera may lose significant bone mineral density.[6] This appears to be reversible after Depo-Provera use is stopped, but the impact on later fracture risk is not known.[7]

Fractures differ in their health implications. For example, a hip fracture (a fracture in the upper thigh bone or femur), especially in a frail, elderly woman, may lead to extended time in bed, which increases the risk of pneumonia, pulmonary embolism, and death. Not all vertebral fractures are painful and most often they are not life-threatening. Osteoporosis and vertebral fractures can lead to a loss of height and curvature of the spine so that the person appears bent over. A wrist fracture is painful but does not compromise a woman's ability to walk, unless she needs to use a cane or walker.

WHAT CAN I DO?

I added more walking to my schedule, hand weights, 1,500 mg of calcium a day, and calcium-rich foods. I also continued Pilates and yoga. . . . [I] felt so much better, it was like a new life.

Preventing osteoporosis depends on two things: making the strongest, densest bones possible during the first thirty years of life and limiting the amount of bone loss in adulthood. While we can't go back to our first thirty years, the following wellness strategies can help minimize bone loss as we age.

EXERCISE TO STRENGTHEN MUSCLES AND BONES

Any exercise that is weight-bearing (done standing up) can help prevent or slow bone loss and may even modestly increase bone density. This includes walking, jogging, stair climbing, dancing, and tennis. Swimming is not weight-bearing and riding a bike is only partially weight-bearing. Exercise also decreases fracture risk by improving strength and balance.

Many women exercise more consistently when we include other people, whether family, friends, or strangers. Showing up for an aerobics class three times a week can be much easier than deciding alone every day when, where, and what your exercise will be.[8]

Six years ago, two friends and I began walking together before work. There are many days when I know I would stay in bed if I were going by myself. But knowing that my friends will be coming by in the next ten minutes and that we will start our day by walking and talking together airlifts me into my sweats and out the door.

GET ENOUGH CALCIUM

Adequate calcium for people of all ages, from children to the elderly, is necessary for optimal skeletal health. Getting an adequate amount of calcium can help reduce the risk of osteoporosis. (People over sixty-five who take calcium and vitamin D are also less likely to lose teeth.[9])

However, contrary to popular belief, the healthiest or safest amount of dietary calcium hasn't yet been established.[10] The National Academy of Science recommends that women over the age of fifty consume 1,200 mg per day; a similar British committee recommends 700 mg a day.[11] Foods high in calcium include milk, cheese, and other dairy products; dark leafy greens; beans; and foods such as orange juice that are calcium fortified.

GET ENOUGH VITAMIN D

We have all heard of vitamin D, but we may not appreciate its important role in bone health for adults. Vitamin D also may help prevent common cancers, hypertension, and even type 1 diabetes.[12]

Unlike other fat-soluble vitamins that are plentiful in a healthy diet, vitamin D is in very few foods naturally. Foods with high vitamin D content include oily fish such as salmon and mackerel and cod liver oil. To obtain adequate vitamin D from natural food sources alone, you would need to eat these fish three to four times a week or take cod liver oil daily. Some foods, including milk, some breads, and calcium-supplemented soy milk and orange juice, are fortified with vitamin D. However, the majority of our vitamin D requirement (80 to 95 percent) comes not from foods but from exposure to sunlight.

Surprisingly, vitamin D deficiency is common in adults in the United States. More than half of elderly women, whether living at home or in a nursing home, are vitamin D deficient. We don't absorb oral vitamin D as well as we get older. However, young and middle-aged adults are also at risk for vitamin D deficiency. Many of us work and spend our free time indoors and have little sun exposure. Also, because we now are aware of the connection between sun expo-

FACTORS THAT INCREASE RISK OF FRACTURE[13]

advancing age (especially over eighty)
female sex
being white
low bone density
prior fracture after age fifty
hypogonadism
smoking
inactivity
history of falls
anticonvulsant therapy
glucocorticoids (a type of steroids)
hyperthyroidism
alcoholism
excess dietary protein
family history
being below ideal body weight

CALCIUM SUPPLEMENTS

The Women's Health Initiative, a study of more than 36,000 postmenopausal women ages 50 to 79, found that taking calcium and vitamin D supplements did not affect bone density but did reduce fractures. After an average of seven years, there was no overall difference in hip bone density between women who were given a placebo and women assigned to take 1,000 mg of calcium and 400 IUs of vitamin D a day. However, hip fractures were significantly reduced in several groups who took calcium and vitamin D for the study: women over sixty, women who were not previously taking calcium and vitamin D supplements, and women who took the calcium and vitamin D supplements regularly.

Women who took the full doses of both supplements had a 29 percent decrease in their risk of hip fractures. Women over sixty had a 21 percent reduction in hip fracture risk. About a third of all participants in the study had been taking calcium and vitamin D supplements previously. In women who were not taking supplements before the study began, calcium and vitamin D supplementation reduced hip fracture risk by 30 percent.

The supplements increased the risk of kidney stones by 17 percent. However, other research has indicated that calcium supplements increase kidney stone risk if taken between meals, but may decrease risk if taken with meals. Therefore, taking calcium with meals is recommended.

Vitamin D may be even more important for bone health than calcium, and older people are often deficient in this vitamin. There is a high rate of vitamin D deficiency among people with hip fracture; for example, a study in London of 103 people with hip fractures found low levels of vitamin D in almost every one.[14]

sure and the risk of skin cancer, many women use sunscreen consistently. A sunscreen with an SPF of 8 will reduce vitamin D synthesis by 97.5 percent.[15]

A recent CDC report indicated that 41 percent of African-American women between the ages of fifteen and forty-nine were vitamin D deficient at the end of winter.[16] In one study, 32 percent of medical students and residents at a medical center in Boston were found to be vitamin D deficient also.[17]

Chronic vitamin D deficiency has many consequences for bone health and for overall health. Vitamin D deficiency results in decreased intestinal absorption of calcium. This causes increased production of a hormone that leaches calcium from bone. Vitamin D deficiency can both cause and increase osteoporosis. Also, vitamin D deficiency can cause osteomalacia, a condition that causes muscle aches, muscle weakness, and bone pain.

Blood tests can measure vitamin D levels. An effective immediate treatment for vitamin D deficiency is to take 50,000 IU of vitamin D weekly for eight weeks.[18]

However, some women cannot absorb vitamin D owing to chronic problems with intestinal malabsorption (related to conditions such as sprue, chronic liver disease, cystic fibrosis, Crohn's disease, and Whipple's disease). Exposure to natural sunlight or tanning bed radiation that has a component of ultraviolet-B radiation is recommended in these cases.

The National Academy of Sciences recently

CALCIUM CONTENT OF SELECTED FOODS[19]

Dairy Food	Content Calcium (mg)	Nondairy Food	Content Calcium (mg)
Skim milk, 1 cup	300	Calcium-fortified orange juice, 1 cup	300
Low-fat milk, 1 cup	295	Salmon, canned, with bones, 3 oz	167
Whole milk, 1 cup	290	Oysters, raw, 13–19 medium	226
Yogurt (plain, low-fat), 1 cup	415	Sardines, canned with bones, 3 oz	372
Frozen yogurt (fruit), 1 cup	240	Shrimp, canned, 3 oz	98
Swiss cheese, 1 oz	270	Collard greens, cooked, 1 cup	357
Cheddar, mozzarella, or Muenster cheese, 1 oz	205	Turnip greens, cooked, 1 cup	252
Cottage cheese (low-fat), 4 oz	78	Broccoli, cooked, 1 cup	100
Part-skim ricotta cheese, 4 oz	335	Soybeans, cooked, 1 cup	131
Vanilla ice cream, 1 cup	176	Tofu, 4 oz	108 *
Soft-serve vanilla ice cream, 1 cup	236	Almonds, 1 oz	75

* Calcium content of tofu varies depending on processing method; check nutritional label on package for precise calcium content.

recommended that middle-aged and elderly adults increase daily vitamin D intake. New recommendations for daily doses are for 200 IU for ages 1–50, 400 IU for ages 51–70, and 600 IU for those over 70 years. However, other researchers have estimated that in an absence of exposure to sunlight, the requirement should be closer to 1,000 IU of vitamin D daily.

GET ENOUGH VITAMIN A, BUT NOT TOO MUCH

In addition to helping maintain good vision, Vitamin A helps our bodies process calcium. Vitamin A comes in two forms: Preformed vitamin A, found in animal foods such as milk and eggs, can be used by our bodies immediately, while betacarotenes in dark yellow and green vegetables and fruits are converted into vitamin A after we eat them. Because excessive intake of preformed vitamin A may increase the risk of hip fractures, it's best to avoid vitamin supplements that contain the full RDA (5,000 IU) of vitamin A as preformed vitamin A.

AVOID EXCESSIVE CAFFEINE

Caffeine increases calcium losses in the urine, but only some studies have found a higher risk of fracture in people who consume large amounts (the equivalent of at least three cups of coffee per day). The effect of caffeine on calcium balance is only pertinent or potentially harmful in those with very low calcium intake.

DECREASE RISK FOR FALLS

Nine out of ten hip fractures in older Americans are the result of a fall.[20] To reduce your risk of falling:

- Avoid or decrease medications that can cause dizziness or drowsiness. These include muscle relaxants, tranquilizers, and some heart disease and high blood pressure drugs.
- Get your eyes checked regularly. Poor vision increases the risk of falls.

SAFETY TIPS FOR FALL PREVENTION[21]

- Remove throw rugs and make certain that carpet edges are securely fastened to the floor.
- Reduce clutter, especially in traffic areas.
- Install or maintain sturdy handrails at stairs.
- Increase wattage of lighting in hallways, bathrooms, kitchens, stairwells, and entrances to home.
- Install safety handrails in shower, tub, and around toilet; bathtubs and shower stalls should have nonskid surfaces.
- When you must reach for something high, use a safety step stool (one with wide steps and a friction surface to stand on); a type equipped with a high handrail is preferred.
- If a cane or walker has been recommended, use it to help increase your stability.
- Wear supportive, cushioned, low-heeled shoes; avoid scuffs (backless bedroom slippers) and high heels.
- Avoid rushing to answer the phone or doorbell; a portable phone that you can take from room to room with you is a good idea for security and safety.
- Have sand or salt available to spread on porches, stairs, and sidewalks during snowy, icy weather.

- Practice muscle strengthening and balance exercises.
- Evaluate your environment for "fall hazards," such as scatter rugs, clutter, and poor lighting.

MEDICAL TREATMENT

The treatment of osteoporosis consists of diet, exercise, and sometimes medication. In the recent past, estrogen treatment was considered a

THE MERCK LAUNCH OF FOSAMAX

In 1995, the pharmaceutical company Merck submitted Fosamax (alendronate) to the FDA for approval. Ads to physicians followed immediately. However, Merck realized that many consumers were not yet worried about osteoporosis. Therefore, Merck gave a large grant to a leading consumer group for older women with the explicit instructions to use the money to "educate" women about osteoporosis. To reinforce this campaign, Merck began direct-to-consumer ads that contrasted frail older women in pain with vivacious seniors in control of their lives. The text with the ads implied that Fosamax made the difference.

Next Merck began to market bone density testing, first by making it more available and then by making it more affordable.[22] Even before Fosamax received FDA approval, Merck had purchased a company that manufactured bone density testing equipment and expanded its production capacity. Merck also sponsored the National Osteoporosis Risk Assessment (NORA) study, which found that almost half the postmenopausal women participating unknowingly had low bone density.[23] According to a Merck chairman, this study showed that such women were at risk of fracture and "underscore(d) the significant medical need that *Fosamax* can help fulfill."[24]

Merck is also a major contributor to the National Osteoporosis Foundation, which promotes a toll-free number for consumers, now having been "educated," to find the location of a nearby bone density screening center. Because bone density screening is expensive, Merck added a final piece to its campaign: a public policy initiative to persuade the federal government to pay for bone density screening tests through Medicare. Merck also targeted private insurers at the state level with slick educational materials and drew up model legislation for distribution to state legislators, who could then argue for state funding so women could get free or inexpensive bone scans.

Having successfully persuaded women to worry about the strength of our bones and to have our bone density measured, Merck had created the perfect environment to sell its product. Every component of its campaign contributed to the sales of Fosamax, the only nonhormonal drug approved at the time for osteoporosis prevention.[25]

In 2005, the Merck-funded National Osteoporosis Foundation launched a campaign using ivory-colored lace ribbons (to match the red ribbons for HIV and pink ones for breast cancer) to increase "awareness" (or fear?) of osteoporosis and to promote bone density testing.[26] Perhaps Merck was also thinking of the likely consequence of this campaign—increased prescription of Fosamax.

primary therapy for postmenopausal osteo-porosis. At the time, health providers thought that estrogen also had the advantages of treating other problems associated with menopause and preventing or delaying cardiovascular disease. However, data from the Women's Health Initiative have shown that estrogen-progestin therapy does not reduce the risk of coronary heart disease and increases the risk of breast cancer, stroke, and blood clots.

As a result of the Women's Health Initiative findings, other medications are now preferred and are prescribed more frequently for treatment of postmenopausal osteoporosis. The medications most frequently used now are the bisphosphonates alendronate (brand name Fosamax) or risedronate (Actonel) and a selective estrogen receptor modulator (SERM) called raloxifene (Evista).

Bisphosphonates increase bone mass and reduce the incidence of both vertebral and nonvertebral fractures, even in women who already have had fractures.[27] But be aware that statistics can create an exaggerated impression of the effectiveness of these drugs: At its best, alendronate (Fosamax) is reported to reduce the risk of hip fracture by 56 percent (in women with osteoporosis at an average age of sixty-eight).[28] This sounds like a huge benefit, but the 56 percent reduction is known as the *relative risk reduction*. This means that the women who took alendronate developed 56 percent fewer hip fractures than the women given placebos. The important number is not the relative reduction in risk, but how many hip fractures are actually prevented by women who fit this description taking alendronate (known as the *absolute risk reduction*). Women in this drug company–sponsored study who took the placebo had a 99.5 percent chance of getting through each year without a broken hip. The women who took alendronate, on the other hand, had a 99.8 percent chance of getting

through each year without a fracture.[29] So the dramatic relative risk reduction of 56 percent translates into an absolute risk reduction of 0.3 percent each year. This means that if 1,000 women with osteoporosis take alendronate for a year, about three hip fractures will be prevented.

Raloxifene currently is the only SERM approved by the U.S. Food and Drug Administration for the treatment of osteoporosis. It increases bone mineral density without stimulating the growth of endometrial tissue or increasing risk for vaginal bleeding. However, it has been proven to reduce only vertebral fractures, not hip fractures.[30]

ESTROGEN-PROGESTIN TREATMENT

Estrogen-progestin therapy is no longer a first-line approach for osteoporosis treatment because it increases the risk of breast cancer, stroke, blood clots, and probably coronary artery disease. It may be recommended for some postmenopausal women who have persistent severe problems associated with menopause and women who cannot tolerate a bisphosphonate or a SERM.

Within two months, I suffered a vertebral compression fracture and I fell, fracturing both my hip and wrist. I had already been on high doses of calcium and vitamin D. My nurse practitioner and I decided that I needed medication to decrease my high risk of another fracture. I have been on medication for two years and follow the directions closely, and my most recent test showed improved BMD in both my hip and spine.

AGE FOR BONE DENSITY TESTING

The U.S. Preventive Services Task Force (USPSTF) recommends that women who are

BONE DENSITY TESTS

Measurement of bone mineral density (BMD) can establish a diagnosis of osteoporosis, before or after a fracture occurs. (Remember: Osteoporosis is a risk factor, not a disease.) There are no randomized controlled clinical trials that show that bone density tests lead to better health outcomes.

Several methods measure BMD:

- Dual energy X-ray absorptiometry (DEXA) is the most popular method because it provides precise readings at important bone sites, such as the hip, spine, and forearm, with minimal radiation. During a DEXA scan, an X-ray detector scans a bone region and the varying amounts of X-rays that pass through the bone are measured, allowing the calculation of bone density values.
- Single energy X-ray absorptiometry may be used to measure BMD of the forearm and the heel. However, DEXA scans are better predictors of fracture risk.
- Quantitative computerized tomography (CT) provides accurate measurements of spine BMD. It is seldom used because it involves more radiation exposure and is more expensive than other methods.
- Ultrasonography (ultrasound) can be used to measure the density of the calcaneus (the bone in the heel). Sound transmission through bone is related to bone density and skeletal strength. This method is not as accurate as DEXA.

sixty-five years old and older be screened routinely for osteoporosis, although there have been no gold standard studies—randomized controlled clinical trials—showing that testing of bone mineral density (BMD) leads to better health outcomes. The USPSTF recommends that routine screening begin at age sixty for women who are at "increased risk" for osteoporotic fractures. The exact risk factors that should trigger screening in women between sixty and sixty-five are debated. Lower body weight (under 155 pounds) is the single best predictor of low BMD. At any given age, African-American women on average have higher BMD than white women and are less likely to benefit from screening.[31] This difference may be accounted for by differences in body size. African-American women with risk factors (such as low body weight or previous fractures) should be evaluated for bone health in the same way that white women are. The prevalence of osteoporosis in Mexican-American women is similar to that in white women.[32]

No studies have evaluated the optimal intervals for repeated screening. Because of the limited precision of BMD testing, a minimum of two years or longer is needed to measure a change in BMD reliably. There are no data to determine when osteoporosis screening should stop and little data on osteoporosis treatment in women older than eighty-five.[33]

NOTES

1. "Report of a WHO Study Group. Assessment of Fracture Risk and its Application to Screening for Postmenopausal Osteoporosis," *WHO Technical Report*

Series 843, (Geneva: World Health Organization Press, 1994).

2. A. Looker, et al., "Prevalence of Low Femoral Bone Density in Older U.S. Women NHANES3 [third annual National Health and Nutrition Examination Survey]," *Journal of Bone Mineral Research* 10, no. 5 (1995): 796–802.

3. L. J. Melton, et al., "How Many Women Have Osteoporosis?" *Journal of Bone Mineral Research* 7, no. 9 (1992): 1005–10.

4. National Women's Health Network, *The Truth about Hormone Replacement Therapy: Breaking Free of the Medical Myths of Menopause* (New York: Prima Publishing/Random House, 2002), 147.

5. Ibid.

6. "Physician Information," accessed at www.fda.gov/medwatch/SAFETY/2004/DepoProvera_Label.pdf on October 13, 2005.

7. National Women's Health Network, "Fact Sheet: Depo Provera and Bone Mineral Density," February 2005, accessed at www.nwhn.org/publications/factdetails.php?fid=21 on October 13, 2005.

8. Charles Massion and Adriane Fugh-Berman, "Exercise Counseling for Women," *Alternative Therapies in Women's Health* 2, no. 1 (January 2000): 3–5.

9. E. A. Krall, et al., "Calcium and Vitamin D Supplements Reduce Tooth Loss in the Elderly," *American Journal of Medicine* 111 (2001): 452.

10. For more information, see www.hsph.harvard.edu/nutritionsource/calcium.html.

11. The Food Standards Agency (UK). Expert Group on Vitamins and Minerals, 2003, accessed at www.food.gov.uk/multimedia/pdfs/evm_calcium.pdf on June 14, 2005.

12. M. Holick, "Importance of Vitamin D for Adult Health," *Alternative Therapies in Women's Health* 5, no. 1 (January 2003): 1–3.

13. Christine K. Cassel, Rosanne M. Leipzig, Harvey Jay Cohen, Eric B. Larson, and Diane E. Meier, eds., *Geriatric Medicine: An Evidence Based Approach,* 4th ed. (New York: Springer-Verlag, 2003).

14. C. Moniz, T. Dew, and T. Dixon, "Prevalence of Vitamin D Inadequacy in Osteoporotic Hip Fracture Patients in London," *Current Medical Research and Opinions* 21, no. 12 (2005): 1891–94.

15. L. Y. Matsuoka et al., "Sunscreen Suppressed Cutaneous Vitamin D3 Synthesis," *Journal of Clinical Endocrinology and Metabolism* 64 (1987): 1165–68.

16. S. Nesby-O'Dell et al., "Hypovitaminosis D Prevalence and Determinants among African American and White Women of Reproductive Age," Third National Health and Nutritional Examination Survey, 1988–1994, *American Journal of Clinical Nutrition* 76 (2002): 187–92.

17. V. Tanpricha et al., "Vitamin D Insufficiency among Free-Living, Healthy Young Adults," *American Journal of Medicine* 112 (2000): 659–62.

18. Holick.

19. Mindy Smith and Leslie Shimp, *20 Common Problems in Women's Healthcare* (New York: McGraw-Hill Companies, 2000), 650.

20. National Resource Center, The National Institutes of Health, "Preventing Falls and Related Fractures." Accessed at www.niams.nih.gov/bone/hi/preventfalls.htm on March 28, 2006.

21. Smith and Shimp, 646.

22. E. Tanouye, "Merck's Osteoporosis Warnings Pave the Way for Its New Drug," *Wall Street Journal,* June 28, 1995.

23. Ethel S. Siris, Paul D. Miller, Elizabeth Barrett-Connor, Kenneth G. Faulkner, Lois E. Wehren, Thomas A. Abbott, Marc L. Berger, Arthur C. Santora, and Louis M. Sherwood, "Identification and Fracture Outcomes of Undiagnosed Low Bone Mineral Density in Postmenopausal Women: Results from the National Osteoporosis Risk Assessment," *JAMA* 286, no. 22 (December 2001): 2815–22.

24. Raymond V. Gilmartin, "Chairman's Report," Merck & Co., Inc. Annual Meeting of Stockholders, April 23, 2002, accessed at http://www.merck.com/newsroom/executive_speeches/042302.html on February 3, 2006.

25. National Women's Health Network, "*The Truth about Hormone Replacement Therapy,*" 168–69.

26. National Osteoporosis Foundation, "A Symbol of the

Fight for Bone Strength & Independence." Accessed at http://www.nof.org/new_ribbon.htm on February 3, 2006.

27. U.S. Preventive Services Task Force, "Screening for Osteoporosis," September 2002, accessed at www.preventiveservices.ahrq.gov on May 5, 2005.

28. S. R. Cummings, D. M. Black, E. Thompson, et al., "Effect of Alendronate on Risk of Fracture in Women with Low Bone Density but without Vertebral Fractures: Results from the Fracture Intervention Trial," *JAMA* 280, no. 24 (1998): 2077–82.

29. Ibid.

30. U.S. Preventive Services Task Force.

31. U.S. Preventive Services Task Force.

32. Ibid.

33. Ibid.

CHAPTER 17

Heart Health

Problems with our hearts and blood vessels are a leading cause of death among older women.[1] These problems are known as cardiovascular disease. (*Cardio* refers to the heart and *vascular* refers to blood vessels, including those supplying the brain, legs, and other parts of the body.) Our likelihood of developing cardiovascular disease increases steadily with age. Luckily, there are steps each of us can take to improve our cardiovascular health. These include quitting smoking, eating a healthy diet, and participating in regular physical activity.

Although women of all ages benefit from heart-healthy lifestyle choices, the need for effective prevention of heart disease is particularly important as we grow older. A sixty-three-year-old woman shares her strategies for avoiding the health problems that run in her family:

My dad had bypass surgery and so did his sister. I was looking into the family tree and seeing a pattern of heart attacks and many relatives with diabetes. So I started to change my diet. . . . I don't eat what I grew up on. My family cooked with lard and ate a lot of fatty foods. I eat a lot of fish and tofu. I really watch sodium and saturated fat. I mostly cook at home, but when I eat at restaurants, I'm careful what I order. I walk every day for thirty minutes and twice a week I run two miles. Since I'm retired now, I have more time for exercise. I expect to be doing that into my seventies.

TAKING CARE OF OURSELVES

RISK FACTORS

Some factors associated with increased risk of heart disease, such as age, we cannot change. But others, such as smoking, we can modify (see chart below). Our own choices make a difference.

CHOLESTEROL LEVELS WITH MENOPAUSE

Menopause provokes a number of changes in our blood levels of cholesterol and other blood fats. Total cholesterol generally rises by about 6 percent, low-density lipoprotein (LDL) cholesterol (so-called bad cholesterol) by 10 percent, and triglycerides, another type of blood fat, by 11 percent. HDL ("good" cholesterol) begins to fall two years before the last menstrual cycle and declines gradually after menopause. There is considerable controversy about the effects of these changes on heart disease. (For more information, see "Questioning the Role of Cholesterol," page 248.)

I used to take no medications. My blood pressure was normal; my cholesterol was only slightly elevated. Now, a few years after menopause, I find myself having to take two blood pressure drugs, another pill for cholesterol, and thyroid medication as well. I do aerobic exercise most days, haven't gained any weight, and find this all very frustrating. But since my mother died of a heart attack at sixty-six, and her mother died of a stroke even younger, I have been very motivated to take care of myself.

BLOOD PRESSURE WITH MENOPAUSE

Blood pressure increases with age in both men and women. Menopause is associated with a steeper increase in blood pressure than that due to age alone.[2] Even modest increases in blood pressure affect heart disease risk. Optimal blood pressure is below 120/80. Women with a

RISK FACTORS FOR HEART DISEASE AND STROKE		
RISK FACTOR	FOR HEART DISEASE	FOR STROKE
Nonmodifiable		
AGE	+	+
FAMILY HISTORY (HEART ATTACK OR SUDDEN DEATH IN CLOSE MALE RELATIVE—PARENT, SIBLING, OR CHILD—YOUNGER THAN 55, OR CLOSE FEMALE RELATIVE YOUNGER THAN 65)	+	
Modifiable		
HIGH BLOOD PRESSURE	+	++
DIABETES	++	+
CIGARETTE SMOKING	++	+
HIGH CHOLESTEROL OR TRIGLYCERIDES OR LOW LEVEL OF HIGH-DENSITY LIPOPROTEIN (HDL) CHOLESTEROL	+*	+
PHYSICAL INACTIVITY	+	+
OBESITY	+	+
DEPRESSION, SOCIAL ISOLATION, AND LACK OF SOCIAL SUPPORT	+	
+ Indicates risk factor.		
++ Indicates especially strong risk factors.		
* There is considerable controversy about whether cholesterol levels affect heart disease risk for women. (For more information, see "Questioning the Role of Cholesterol," page 252.)		

top number (for systolic blood pressure) between 120 and 140, or a second number (diastolic blood pressure) between 80 and 90 had heart disease and stroke almost six times more often than women with blood pressure of 120/80.[3]

To measure blood pressure, a cuff is inflated to block blood flow to the arm. Air is released from the cuff gradually; as the pressure in the cuff falls, the level on the dial or mercury tube at which pulsing is first heard is the systolic pressure. As the air continues to be let out, the pulsing sounds will disappear. The point at which the sound disappears is the diastolic pressure (the lowest amount of pressure in the arteries as the heart rests).

I knew my body well for fifty years. Suddenly I didn't recognize my body anymore. There was tremendous change. I always had low blood pressure. Now my blood pressure is higher than it used to be . . . and my cholesterol shot up.

STRESS AND THE HEART

Stress is widely believed to contribute to heart disease, but the connection is not clear. Some studies have concluded that stress increases heart disease, while others have said it does not.

A recent meta-analysis of the research on stress and heart disease came to two conclusions. First, it said that people who experience chronic life- and work-related stresses, "Type A" personality characteristics (such as impatience, competitiveness, and intolerance), or anxiety and panic disorders have no greater risk of heart disease than people who do not. However, it also concluded that depression, social isolation, and lack of quality social support are associated with higher rates of heart disease.[4]

These results point to the importance of addressing the depression and isolation that some of us experience while going through the menopause transition. Building a close network of friends and family, exercising, eating well, getting support, and working to change conditions that contribute to women's isolation can help. (For more information, see Chapter 11, "Emotional Well-Being and Managing Stress;" Chapter 15, "Memory and Mood;" and Chapter 21, "Finding Our Power, Organizing for Change.")

Stress management and other forms of psychological intervention are frequently recommended for people with heart disease. Such interventions do not appear to reduce the risk of heart attack or death.[5] Their effects on other forms of heart disease remain unclear. However, these and other self-care techniques may help us reduce stress and anxiety and increase our sense of well-being. (For more information, see "The Fine Art of Effective Coping," page 168.)

Better research could help us understand stress and heart disease more fully. The scientific research on this topic is often constrained by the lack of a uniform definition of stress. (For example, does it mean being stuck in traffic or living in chronic poverty?) Interpreting the results of research is also difficult because people who report high levels of stress in their lives are more likely to smoke and less likely to exercise, two factors that are known to increase heart disease. In addition, it is hard to separate correlation (two factors being associated) from cause and effect (one factor causing the other).

OPTIMAL LEVELS OF CORONARY RISK FACTORS

Body mass index (BMI) = your weight (in kilograms) divided by your height (in meters) squared. A BMI calculator can be found at www.nhlbisupport.com/bmi.

Normal: 18.5-24.9; lower ranges have been suggested for people of Asian descent.
To be in the normal range, a woman of average height (5 feet 3.7 inches) would weigh between 105 and 140 pounds.

Overweight: 25-29.9
The overweight range for a woman of average height is 141 to 169 pounds.

Obese: above 30
To have a body mass index over 30, a woman of average height would weigh more than 170 pounds.

(The average height for an American woman between the ages of 20 and 74 is 5 feet 3.7 inches; the average weight is 164.3 pounds.)[6]

Another useful measure that can help predict heart disease risk is the waist-to-hip ratio. Evidence shows that extra fat around the abdomen places a person at higher risk of heart disease. This extra fat often gives a person an "apple shape," with a waist larger than the hips. Having a waist that is smaller than one's hips, called a "pear shape," is an indicator of lower heart disease risk.

Blood pressure (upper number is the systolic pressure; lower number is the diastolic pressure; in millimeters of mercury)

Optimal: below 120/80

Prehypertension: systolic pressure 120-139 *or* diastolic pressure 80-89

Hypertension: systolic pressure above 140 *or* diastolic pressure above 90

Treatment indicated when above 140/90 or, in people with diabetes or chronic kidney disease, above 130/80

Fasting blood sugar, mg/dL

Normal: less than 100

Impaired: 100-125

Possible diabetes (requires additional confirmation): 126 or higher

WEIGHT CHANGE
WITH MENOPAUSE

Being overweight increases heart disease risk in women.[7] Most American women over age forty weigh more than recommended for our height, and we tend to gain weight during our middle years, although this increase is not clearly linked to menopause.[8] Significant weight gain in our middle years, especially in the waist area, increases the risk of diabetes and cardiovascular disease.

CARDIOVASCULAR
DISEASE PREVENTION

Women of all ages can reduce the risk of developing heart disease by avoiding the initial development of risk factors such as high blood pressure and diabetes. We can do this through healthy lifestyle practices such as avoiding cigarette smoking, engaging in physical activity, eating a healthy diet, and managing stress.

PREVENTION

In a fourteen-year study, heart disease was 80 percent lower among women who did not smoke cigarettes, were not overweight, maintained a prudent diet, engaged in moderate to vigorous physical activity for thirty minutes each day, and consumed alcohol in moderation, when compared with all other women.[9]

Healthy Lifestyle

A heart-healthy diet includes a variety of fruits, vegetables, grains, low-fat or nonfat dairy products, fish, legumes, sources of protein low in saturated fat, and unsaturated fats such as those found in fish, most plants, oils, nuts, and seeds. Vegetarian and vegan diets can also be heart-healthy. (For more information, see Chapter 12, "Eating Well.") The Mediteranean diet is recommended for women who have heart disease. (For more information, see page 259.)

Becoming physically active is recommended to promote health, psychological well-being, and a healthy weight.[10] To reduce the risk of chronic disease, engage in at least thirty minutes of moderate-intensity physical activity (see list on page 251) on most days of the week. People who don't exercise regularly are 4.3 times more likely to have a stroke than people who engage in frequent vigorous exercise.[11] Some people may need to consult with a health care provider before participating in this level of activity. Flexibility and resistance exercises such as stretches and weights are recommended. (For suggestions to get you moving, see Chapter 13, "Staying Active.")

If you smoke, quitting is probably the most important behavioral change you can make. Avoiding secondhand smoke is recommended for everyone. (For more information on smoking, and quitting, see page 279.)

Drug Treatment to Prevent
Diabetes, High Blood Pressure,
or High Cholesterol

Maintaining a healthy weight and exercising regularly have been shown to prevent diabetes. No

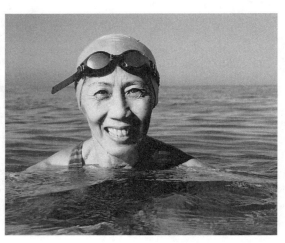

drugs are approved by the Food and Drug Administration for diabetes prevention. More than 90 percent of diabetes cases in one study were attributed to unhealthy habits such as lack of exercise, poor diet, and smoking.[12] A randomized clinical trial showed that people at high risk of developing diabetes who participated in a program to improve health habits reduced their risk by 58 percent; in the same study, metformin (a diabetes drug) was less effective, reducing the likelihood of developing diabetes by 31 percent.[13] Drug therapy has not been shown to prevent high blood pressure or high cholesterol.

TREATING RISK FACTORS TO PREVENT HEART DISEASE AND STROKE

Despite our best efforts, as we move into the postmenopausal years, we may develop risk factors for heart disease and stroke such as high blood pressure. We may then turn to strategies directed at delaying or preventing the onset of disease.

Low-dose aspirin has been shown to reduce heart attack risk in men, but the findings differ for women. Routine use of aspirin by low-risk women is not recommended. In a study of 39,876 healthy women, who were fifty-five years old on average, the women who were assigned to take aspirin every other day had the same number of heart attacks as those who took inactive (placebo) pills.[14] Stroke was reduced 17 percent by aspirin, but gastrointestinal bleeding, ulcers, blood in the urine, and nosebleeds were all more common among the women who took aspirin.

TREATMENT OF HYPERTENSION

High blood pressure, or hypertension, affects about one in four adults in the United States and is especially common among African-Americans. Effective treatment has been shown to prevent heart disease and stroke.[15] Weight loss, physical activity, and dietary changes can reduce blood pressure. The DASH (Dietary Approaches to Stop Hypertension) eating plan,[16] which is low in sodium and fat while rich in fruits, vegetables, and low-fat dairy products, reduces blood pressure as much as a single blood pressure–lowering antihypertensive drug, without drugs' negative effects.

In general, individual blood pressure–lowering drugs reduce blood pressure by only small amounts, averaging reductions of about 9 mm of mercury in systolic and 5 in diastolic blood pressure.[17] Because of these limited effects, women may be prescribed more than one drug. The best medication for most people with high blood pressure is usually a diuretic.[18] Other drugs used to lower blood pressure include thiazides, beta-blockers, angiotensin-converting enzyme inhibitors, angiotensin receptor blockers, and calcium channel antagonists.

Some women find that eating well and staying active are enough to maintain healthy blood pressure and cholesterol levels, but for other women, they may not be sufficient. A slim nurse practitioner who eats a low-fat diet with lots of fruits and vegetables and walks to and from work experienced a rise in her blood pressure:

I was reluctant to believe that my blood pressure was elevated, so I had it checked repeatedly. I increased my exercise even more and lowered my salt intake, which was already low, but [these changes] didn't have a noticeable effect. So after about a year, we started some medication. It was frustrating because the dosage had to be increased twice. Now I'm on two medications.

TREATMENT OF HIGH CHOLESTEROL

More than 16 million women in the United States have what is considered to be high cholesterol.[19] Standard recommendations suggest that it is optimal to keep LDL cholesterol below 100 mg/dL, HDL cholesterol above 50, and triglycerides below 150. Dietary changes may help prevent or manage high cholesterol. (For more information, see page 182.) Drug treatment to lower cholesterol levels has not been proven to reduce risk of developing heart disease for women who do not have heart disease or diabetes. (For more information, see "Questioning the Role of Cholesterol," below.)

For women who have heart disease or diabetes, the group of cholesterol-lowering drugs known as *statins* can prevent heart attack and stroke.[20] Statins available in the United States include atorvastatin (Lipitor), fluvastatin (Lescol), lovastatin (Mevacor), pravastatin (Pravachol), rosuvastatin (Crestor), and simvastatin

QUESTIONING THE ROLE OF CHOLESTEROL

Many of us have been advised to monitor our cholesterol levels and take cholesterol-lowering drugs to prevent heart disease. But cholesterol may not be as important as we are often told.

Cholesterol-lowering statin drugs have been on the market since 1987 and are the best-selling class of drugs in the United States. But still there is not a single "gold standard" randomized controlled trial that shows that these drugs are beneficial to women who do not yet have heart disease. Furthermore, a study that followed the health of 7,300 Chicago women for thirty-one years found that elevated cholesterol levels played a small but statistically insignificant role in their risk of death due to heart disease and had no effect at all on their overall rate of death.[21]

Another study showed that statins not only fail to reduce the risk of heart attack and stroke in people between seventy and eighty-two years old who don't already have heart disease, but they significantly increase the risk of cancer in this population (by 25 percent).[22]

Other studies have not found a higher cancer risk with statin use, but the people in those studies were much younger.

Another study found that for women who have reached the age of sixty-five, not only is high cholesterol not a health risk, but—going directly against our common wisdom—the *higher* older women's bad (LDL) cholesterol levels, the *longer* they live.[23] The catch is that the women in this study lived in small Italian towns, almost certainly eating healthier diets and getting more exercise than most Americans.

So why are millions of women without heart disease taking cholesterol-lowering drugs?

The answer is found in the recommendations of the supposedly "evidence-based" guidelines issued by the National Cholesterol Education Program. This program is coordinated by a division of the National Institutes of Health, but many of the authors of the guidelines have financial ties to companies that manufacture cholesterol-lowering drugs. Section II of these guidelines states definitively that clinical trials show statins reduce the risk of coronary heart disease in women without heart disease (so-called "primary prevention").[24] Readers are referred to a table that convincingly cites seven studies that supposedly support this claim. But in fact, not a single one of these studies actually provides such evidence. Only one of the seven included any women who didn't already have heart disease, and in this study there were only a total of twenty heart events that developed in the women, not nearly enough to provide a statistically significant finding.[25]

Section VIII of the same 284-page document says that there are no clinical studies that support the claim that statins are beneficial for women who are at increased risk but have not yet developed heart disease: "Clinical trials of LDL lowering generally are lacking for this risk category. . . ."[26] In other words, the statement made in Section II, which appears to justify millions of women taking these drugs, is simply not true.

Women and health care providers are being misled by such guidelines, which often are developed by experts with financial ties to drug makers. (For more information, see "Can We Trust the Evidence in Evidence-Based Medicine?" page 24, and the book *Overdosed America,* by John Abramson.)

If you are considering taking a statin to lower cholesterol and you do not already have heart disease, you may want to weigh the potential risks against the lack of proven benefit. Learn what you can and discuss your individual situation with a knowledgeable health care provider. If lowering cholesterol plays a role in improving your health, it is far less important than each of these healthy ways of living:

- Exercise routinely
- Eat a Mediterranean-style diet
- Don't smoke
- Reduce chronic stress
- Avoid eating foods containing trans fats (partially hydrogenated fats)

Adopting and maintaining these healthy habits is the most effective, safest, and least expensive way to prevent heart disease and improve your chances of living a long and healthy life.

(Zocor). Statins reduce LDL up to 60 percent. They also raise HDL ("good" cholesterol) a few percent and lower triglycerides. Adverse effects of statins may include muscle aches or weakness, liver problems, constipation, gas, indigestion, and stomach pain.

HDL is also raised by exercise, red wine, and niacin (vitamin B3). The doses of niacin needed to raise HDL are high enough to require medical supervision and monitoring blood tests for safety. Large doses of niacin can also lower triglycerides. Triglycerides are type of blood fat that confers heart disease risk. Triglycerides can be lowered by weight loss and eating a diet low in simple sugars. The best drugs for lowering triglycerides are fibrates, two of which are available in the United States, gemfibrozil (Lopid) and fenofibrate (Tricor). But while these drugs reduce triglycerides, they do not reduce death rates.[27]

TREATMENT OF DIABETES

Diabetes, epidemic in the United States, is strongly related to the increasing number of people who are overweight. In type 2 diabetes, formerly known as adult-onset diabetes, insulin is still produced, but our ability to use the insulin is impaired, leading to high blood sugar and blood insulin levels.[28] Poor control of

blood sugar damages small blood vessels in the eyes, kidneys, and feet.

Managing high blood pressure and cholesterol in those of us who have type 2 diabetes reduces coronary heart disease, which is by far the leading cause of death in people with diabetes.[29] While medication may be helpful, becoming physically active can reduce the mortality rate four times more for diabetics than does taking a statin.[30] The data are so strong that the target blood pressure for individuals with type 2 diabetes is lower than for the general population (see "Optimal Levels of Coronary Risk Factors" on page 249).

Costs of medication to treat blood pressure, cholesterol, and diabetes are a concern to many of us. Health care providers can help by prescribing generic medications, pills combining two medications in a single tablet, or prescribing one-half of a 20 mg tablet rather than a single 10 mg pill. Also, pharmaceutical companies have programs on their websites to help make their products available to all.

POSTMENOPAUSAL HORMONE TREATMENT

For decades, estrogen was thought to lower heart disease risk, based on observational studies in which women who took estrogen developed heart disease less often than women who

---

MYTH OR REALITY?

• *Estrogen prevents heart disease and stroke.*

Myth. Estrogen with progestin actually appears to increase the risk of heart attack and stroke. Estrogen alone, which is generally taken by women who have had a hysterectomy or oophorectomy, neither increases nor decreases the risk of heart attack, but does increase the risk of stroke.

did not take estrogen. However, the women who chose to take estrogen had other healthy behaviors, such as exercising more, eating a healthier diet, and being leaner, so it was not clear if the lower rate of heart disease was due to estrogen or the other behaviors.

The Women's Health Initiative, funded by the National Institutes of Health, set out to answer that question, among others. It included two randomized trials to find out if post-menopausal estrogen really did prevent heart disease. In one study, women with a uterus were assigned to either estrogen with progestin or to a placebo. The progestin was given to prevent cancer of the uterus, which estrogen can induce. Estrogen with progestin increased heart attack, breast cancer, stroke, dementia, and blood clots in the legs. Fractures and colon cancer were reduced by estrogen with progestin, but these benefits were not enough to offset the hormones' risk.[31]

In a separate study, women who had previously had a hysterectomy were assigned to estrogen alone or a placebo. The number of heart attacks was similar in the two treatment groups, but stroke was increased by estrogen.[32] Therefore, postmenopausal hormone treatment is considered not useful or effective, and possibly harmful, in terms of cardiovascular disease. (For more information, see Chapter 7, "Hormone Treatment.")

HOW HEART DISEASE DEVELOPS

The heart is a muscle; its job is to pump blood to the brain, kidneys, and the rest of the body. The coronary arteries deliver needed oxygen and nutrients to the heart muscle. If a coronary artery becomes partially or completely blocked, the heart muscle won't get enough oxygen. These blockages usually develop over time, as deposits of fat, cholesterol, and inflam-

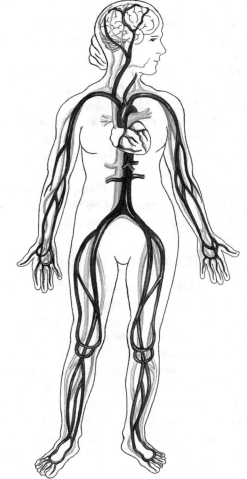

The cardiovascular system circulates blood through the entire body. Damage to just one area can negatively affect the whole system.

matory cells (like those involved in fighting infection) build up in the artery wall. The deposits are called *plaques,* and the process of plaque buildup is known as *atherosclerosis.*

Occasionally a plaque may rupture, triggering a blood clot to form in the coronary artery. This can lead to chest pain (called *angina*) or to a heart attack. Less commonly, heart attacks can also be caused by spasm of a coronary artery. If we have a heart attack, the area of heart muscle supplied by the blocked coronary artery is damaged and doesn't pump as well as it should (a process called *ischemic cardiomyopathy*).

Heart damage can also be caused by high blood pressure, diabetes, viral illnesses, pregnancy, and other factors. Heart damage can lead to heart rhythm problems and heart failure, when the heart can't pump as much blood as we need, leading to fatigue and shortness of breath.

Effective treatments are available for most types of heart disease, so we shouldn't hesitate to get any symptoms evaluated.

CEREBROVASCULAR DISEASE

Problems with arteries supplying blood to the brain are called *cerebrovascular disease.* If a plaque ruptures in one of the large arteries in our necks (carotid arteries), it can cause a stroke. Strokes can also be caused by blood clots or other bits of circulating debris, which may circulate to the brain, where they eventually block a small artery, obstructing blood flow and causing either a stroke or a *transient ischemic attack* (TIA). TIAs are strokelike symptoms that last less than twenty-four hours. They can serve as a warning sign of stroke risk.

PERIPHERAL ARTERIAL DISEASE

Problems in arteries other than those supplying the heart and brain are known as *peripheral arterial disease.* A blockage in the arteries supplying the legs can cause buttock, thigh, or calf pain, changes in skin color, sores or ulcers, and difficulty walking. Total loss of circulation to the legs and feet can cause gangrene and loss of a limb.

WHEN TO SUSPECT CARDIOVASCULAR DISEASE

SIGNS OF HEART DISEASE

Plaques in the coronary arteries (which supply blood to the heart muscle) usually expand gradually with no symptoms until the artery is narrowed at least 70 percent. At that point, the heart muscle's need for oxygen and nutrients may exceed the artery's ability to deliver it. In high-demand situations, such as during exercise or in cold weather, we may develop chest heaviness, which is relieved by rest. This symptom, called angina, can also feel like pressure, squeezing, fullness, or pain and may be accompanied by shortness of breath. Not everyone has typical angina; some of us might have discomfort in the arm, jaw, or stomach, or shortness of breath without discomfort, or fatigue.

Plaques may become fragile and rupture, causing complete obstruction of the artery—a heart attack. So, if chest discomfort or shortness of breath lasts for more than a few minutes or waxes and wanes, particularly if you also experience nausea, cold sweat, or lightheadedness, seek immediate medical attention. Time is of the essence in treating heart attack, so dial 911 and let the emergency medical system perform its role.

A woman who collapsed on a cross-country plane trip at age seventy-three because of severely blocked arteries did not recognize the warning signs:

I knew that I was at risk for a heart attack. I was taking medications for hypertension and had a strong family history of cardiac disease, including an older sister who had had bypass surgery fifteen years earlier. I thought that I knew the symptoms of an impending heart attack, yet I did not recognize those signs the evening before the flight, when I felt a strange tingling and mild inflam-

mation and discomfort around the neck and shoulders as well as flu-like symptoms. Since there were no chest pains, nor any obvious heart-related symptoms, I did not think it was a heart attack. Instead, I thought that I might be experiencing a reaction to my crab dinner or perhaps the beginning of a viral infection.

Only in the hospital did I learn that women exhibit different symptoms for a heart attack than do men, and that mine were typical. I believe that it is important for others to know that women's symptoms are not the same as men's and that medical advice should be sought immediately when they occur.

SIGNS OF STROKE

Strokes are caused by complete obstruction of an artery supplying blood to the brain. This can either result from a ruptured plaque or from a blood clot migrating from elsewhere in the body. Signs of a stroke include sudden numbness or weakness of the face, arm, or leg, especially on one side of the body, sudden confusion, trouble speaking or understanding, sudden trouble seeing in one or both eyes, sudden loss of coordination or a sudden, severe headache with no known cause. Suspected stroke is a medical emergency; if you are in this situation, do not hesitate to dial 911.

SIGNS OF PERIPHERAL ARTERIAL DISEASE

Peripheral arterial disease is plaque blocking arteries supplying blood to other areas of the body, often the legs, arms, or kidneys. If a leg artery is narrowed, it may be unable to increase blood flow to meet oxygen and nutrient requirements of the leg, causing leg cramping with exercise, relieved by rest. Narrowing of arteries supplying the kidneys can aggravate high blood pressure or impair kidney function.

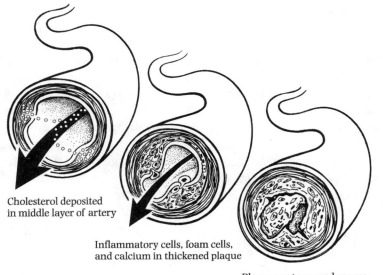

© Marcia Williams

Cholesterol deposited in middle layer of artery

Inflammatory cells, foam cells, and calcium in thickened plaque

Plaque ruptures and causes clot that clogs artery

Plaque formation can slow or even stop the movement of blood through the arteries. When plaque ruptures or erodes, blood clots can develop and result in a heart attack or stroke.

TESTING FOR HEART DISEASE

A variety of medical tests can help sort through symptoms to find out which indicate arterial blockages and which may be due to other causes such as acid reflux, stomach problems, respiratory problems, or thyroid disease. In some cases, women who have no symptoms should be evaluated for possible heart disease, for example, individuals with risk factors such as diabetes, or sedentary women planning to start exercise programs.

A fifty-three-year-old woman recovering from bypass surgery shares her story:

I'd never had any heart symptoms that I was aware of, although in retrospect, I think I had a lot of fatigue. In addition to being diabetic, I had well-controlled hypertension for many years and was on cholesterol medication as well. So it seemed to make sense to have the [stress] test. . . . During the test, I noticed jaw pain, but it went away when the test was over. On my way back to work, I got a call on my cell phone to come back and see the doctor the next day. I was scared. On Thursday, I had an angiogram, which turned out worse than we anticipated. Friday morning, I had quadruple bypass, with four vessels 80 percent blocked. It had all happened so quickly. For almost two months after the surgery, I had weakness and pain. Now things are improving. I'm in cardiac rehab and back to work two days a week. The rehab program is slowly giving me my energy back, and there is support and camaraderie from the other men and women.

TESTS TO EVALUATE CHEST DISCOMFORT

A *resting electrocardiogram* (ECG) records the electrical activity of the heart and has the advantages of being inexpensive, widely available, and risk-free. On the other hand, it does not catch all problems. An ECG may identify problems with the heart's electrical system but will usually not detect partial arterial blockages; that's the role of stress testing.

Stress tests can identify flow-limiting narrowing of the coronary arteries, usually those obstructing at least 70 percent of the blood vessel, but are unlikely to detect less severe narrowings. The simplest type of stress test is an exercise ECG, during which the ECG is recorded while you walk on a treadmill. The workload is gradually increased until you develop chest discomfort, shortness of breath, or fatigue, usually in about ten minutes. Stress testing is susceptible to both false negative test results (in which people with significant narrowings have a normal test) and false positive test results (in which people with no significant narrowings have abnormal test results). For reasons that aren't clear, exercise ECG is less accurate in women than men.[33]

The accuracy of stress testing is improved by adding imaging to the ECG monitoring. In a *stress echocardiogram,* ultrasound pictures of the heart are taken at rest and immediately after exercise. Areas of the heart with inadequate blood flow may not pump normally during stress. In nuclear imaging, a small amount of a radioactive tracer is injected in a vein, and a picture of the heart is acquired before and after exercise using a nuclear camera. By comparing the rest and stress pictures, areas of the heart getting enough blood flow at rest but not during stress can be detected. For those who may be unable to walk on a treadmill, intravenous medications can substitute. Although imaging studies are more accurate than plain exercise ECG, they can still provide false negative or false positive results.

The gold standard for detecting coronary blockages is *coronary angiography.* If suspicion of coronary disease is high, a health care provider may recommend skipping the stress test and proceeding directly to coronary angiogram, also called *cardiac catheterization.* This is a procedure performed by a cardiologist in which a thin plastic tube is inserted in an artery, usually in the groin, via needlestick, and advanced up to the heart. X-ray dye is injected through the tube into the coronary arteries and pictures are taken of the coronary arteries. A coronary angiogram will detect both severe and nonsevere coronary artery blockages.

A fifty-seven-year-old woman with high cholesterol in her family reflects on her double bypass surgery:

When I was forty-six, I started experiencing chest pains, angina. They sent me off for a stress test but I couldn't complete it. Then I had an angiogram. One artery was shut down and the other 90 percent blocked. A week later I had double bypass.

Although most tests don't result in such dramatic treatments, they can alert us to the need for effective intervention.

OTHER TESTING

Another test that may be useful in those of us without symptoms is an X-ray or scan to detect calcium deposits in coronary arteries. The amount of calcium may predict heart attack risk.[34]

An echocardiogram is a resting ultrasound picture of the heart, a painless and risk-free test useful for evaluating heart structure. Pictures of the heart valves and pumping chambers are recorded. Echocardiography can help detect problems with valves and determine if the heart is not able to pump strongly enough, but it does not provide information about coronary blockages.

Ultrasound is also useful for evaluating arteries supplying our extremities, kidneys, or brain. Plaque in the carotid arteries, which supply blood to the brain, can lead to stroke. In addition to ultrasound pictures, another useful noninvasive test for evaluating these arteries is magnetic resonance angiography, a painless, non-X-ray test using a magnet and radiowaves to make a picture. A contrast agent called gadolinium is often injected so the blood vessels can be seen better. The machine makes loud banging, buzzing, and clicking noises during the exam.

TREATMENTS FOR HEART DISEASE

Once we have heart disease, our goal is to stay as healthy and functional as possible for as long as possible.

LIFESTYLE

Regular participation in physical activity can help us manage heart disease. In addition, one diet that appears to reduce the risk of subsequent heart attack among those of us with heart disease is the Mediterranean diet:[35]

- daily consumption of whole-grain products, fruits (4–6 servings/day), vegetables (2–3 servings/day), olive oil, non- or low-fat dairy products (1–2 servings/day), wine (1–2 glasses/day)
- weekly consumption of fish, poultry, potatoes, olives, beans, and nuts (4–6 servings/ week), eggs and sweets (1–3 servings/week)
- monthly consumption of red meat (4–5 servings/month)
- moderate consumption of fat and a high ratio of monounsaturated to saturated fat.

A fifty-year-old woman originally from Peru had heart disease diagnosed in her thirties, shortly after moving to the United States. She has been following a low-fat diet since then and teaching it to her children:

We tried to cook meals that were low in fat, since we knew it was a hereditary disease and we didn't know who had it and who didn't. We started eating more chicken and fish, using olive oil, and avoiding red meats. We all went to the supermarket and everybody would look for the things that were low in fat. We became label readers. Now my kids have grown and only the youngest, who is now fifteen, is at home. We like Peruvian food, but it is too elaborate to prepare on a daily basis, so I stick to simple recipes I can make after work. All of my kids have kept the healthy habits they learned at home.

HERBS AND VITAMINS

No herbal treatments have been shown to prevent heart disease. Antioxidant vitamins such as vitamins A, C, and E were prescribed for cardiovascular prevention for decades, but a number of large, randomized trials have found no benefit and, in some cases, found harm from antioxidant vitamins.[36]

PROTECTIVE AND NONPROTECTIVE DRUGS

Aspirin is of clear-cut benefit for preventing subsequent heart attacks in those of us with coronary disease. In a pooled analysis of 287 research trials, aspirin reduced the heart attack, stroke, and cardiovascular death rate by 23 percent.[37] The American Heart Association recommends aspirin (75 to 162 mg daily) for women considered at high risk, including those with known coronary disease.

Clopidogrel (Plavix) is a prescription drug that impedes blood clotting and that has been shown to reduce heart attack, stroke, or cardio-

vascular death by 9 percent in people who already have heart disease.[38]

Beta-blockers are a family of drugs that block the effect of adrenaline, slowing heart rate and lowering blood pressure. They've been around for a long time and are effective for treating high blood pressure, angina, and heart failure. In pooled data analyses, beta-blockers reduced death by 21 percent and heart attack by 24 percent in people who already had heart disease.[39] Examples of beta-blockers include propranolol (Inderal), atenolol, metoprolol (Lopressor, Toprol), and carvedilol (Coreg).

Angiotensin-converting enzyme (ACE) inhibitors and *angiotensin receptor blockers* expand blood vessels, allowing blood to flow more easily and making the heart's work easier or more efficient. These drugs treat heart failure symptoms and lower blood pressure. Both ACE inhibitors and angiotensin receptor blockers improve survival and prevent hospitalization for heart failure;[40] their role for preventing heart attack remains controversial. Commonly prescribed ACE inhibitors include enalapril, fosinopril, lisinopril, ramipril (Altace), and trandolapril (Mavik). Angiotensin receptor blockers may be easier to tolerate than ACE inhibitors because they are less likely to make you cough. Examples include candesartan (Atacand), irbesartan (Avapro), losartan (Cozaar), and valsartan (Diovan).

The benefits of cholesterol-lowering with *statins* to prevent subsequent heart attack in women with coronary disease are well established, with risk reductions ranging from 15 percent to 43 percent.[41] But statins have not been shown to decrease the death rate in women with coronary artery disease.[42] Commonly prescribed statins include lovastatin, simvastatin (Zocor), atorvastatin (Lipitor), rosuvastatin (Crestor) and pravastatin (Pravachol).

Postmenopausal hormone treatment does

not protect women with existing coronary disease from subsequent heart attacks. Like antioxidant vitamins, estrogen is categorized by the American Heart Association as not useful/effective and possibly harmful.

NOTES

1. Heart and Stroke Facts, American Heart Association, accessed at www.americanheart.org/downloadable/heart/1056719919740HSFacts2003text.pdf on May 2, 2005.

2. Jan A. Staessen, Christopher J. Bulpitt, Robert Fagard, et al., "The Influence of Menopause on Blood Pressure," *Journal of Human Hypertension* 3, no. 6 (1989): 427–33.

3. Ramachandrans S. Vasen, Martin G. Larson, Eric P. Leip, et al., "Impact of High-Normal Blood Pressure on the Risk of Cardiovascular Disease," *New England Journal of Medicine* 345, no. 18 (2001): 1291–97.

4. Stephen J. Bunker et al., " 'Stress' and Coronary Heart Disease: Psychosocial Risk Factors," *Medical Journal of Australia* 178, no. 6 (2003): 272–76.

5. K. Rees, P. Bennett, R. West, G. Davey Smith, and S. Ebrahim, "Psychological Interventions for Coronary Heart Disease." The Cochrane Database of Systematic Reviews Issue 2. Article No.: CD002902. (2004) DOI: 10.1002/14651858.CD002902.pub2.

6. Centers for Disease Control and Prevention, "Americans Slightly Taller, Much Heavier than 40 Years Ago," accessed at www.cdc.gov/od/oc/media/pressrel/r041027.htm on October 25, 2005.

7. Kathryn M. Rexrode, Vincent J. Carey, Charles H. Hennekens, et al., "Abdominal Adiposity and Coronary Heart Disease in Women," *JAMA* 280, no. 21 (1998): 1843–48.

8. Barbara Sternfeld, Hua Wang, Charles P. Quesenberry Jr., et al., "Physical Activity and Changes in Weight and Waist Circumference in Midlife Women: Findings from the Study of Women's Health Across the Nation," *American Journal of Epidemiology* 160, no. 9 (2004): 912–22.

9. Meir J. Stampfer, Frank B. Hu, JoAnn E. Manson, et al., "Primary Prevention of Coronary Heart Disease in Women through Diet and Lifestyle," *New England Journal of Medicine* 343, no. 1 (2000): 16–22.

10. Dietary Guidelines for Americans 2005, accessed at www.health.gov/dietaryguidelines/dga2005/document/html/executivesummary.htm on May 2, 2005.

11. Ralph L. Sacco, Robert Gan, Bernadette Boden-Albala, I-Feng Lin, Douglas E. Kargman, W. Allen Hauser, Steven Shea, and Myunghee C. Paik, "Leisure-Time Physical Activity and Ischemic Stroke Risk: The Northern Manhattan Stroke Study," *Stroke* 29, no. 2 (February 1998): 380–87.

12. F. B. Hu, J. E. Manson, M. J. Stampfer, G. Colditz, S. Liu, C. G. Solomon, and W.C. Willett, "Diet, Lifestyle, and the Risk of Type 2 Diabetes Mellitus in Women," *New England Journal of Medicine* 345 (September 13, 2001): 790–97.

13. William C. Knowler, Elizabeth Barrett-Connor, Sarah E. Fowler, et al., "Reduction in the Incidence of Type 2 Diabetes with Lifestyle Intervention or Metformin," *New England Journal of Medicine* 346, no. 6 (2002): 393–403.

14. Paul M. Ridker, Nancy R. Cook, I-Min Lee, et al., "A Randomized Trial of Low-Dose Aspirin in the Primary Prevention of Cardiovascular Disease in Women," *New England Journal of Medicine* 352, no. 13 (2005), 1293–304.

15. Blood Pressure Lowering Treatment Trialists' Collaboration, "Effects of Different Blood-Pressure-Lowering Regimens on Major Cardiovascular Events: Results of Prospectively-Designed Overviews of Randomized Trials," *Lancet* 362, no. 9395 (2003): 1527–35.

16. The DASH eating plan, accessed at www.nhlbi.nih.gov/health/public/heart/hbp/dash/ on May 2, 2005.

17. M. R. Law, N. J. Wald, J. K. Morris, and R. E. Jordan, "Value of Low Dose Combination Treatment with Blood Pressure Lowering Drugs: Analysis of 354 Randomised Trials," *British Medical Journal* 326, no. 7404 (2003): 1427–31.

18. ALLHAT (Antihypertensive and Lipid-Lowering Treatment to Prevent Heart Attack Trial) Officers and

Coordinators for the ALLHAT Collaborative Research Group, "Major Outcomes in High-Risk Hypertensive Patients Randomized to Angiotensin-Converting Enzyme Inhibitor or Calcium Channel Blocker vs. Diuretic: The Antihypertensive and Lipid-Lowering Treatment to Prevent Heart Attack Trial (ALLHAT)," *JAMA* 288, no. 23 (December 18, 2002): 2981–97.

19. Donald O. Fedder, Carol E. Koro, and Gilbert J. L'Italien, "New National Cholesterol Education Program III Guidelines for Primary Prevention Lipid-Lowering Drug Therapy. Projected Impact on the Size, Sex, and Age Distribution of the Treatment-Eligible Population," *Circulation* 105, no. 2 (2002): 152–56; see also "Implications of Recent Clinical Trials for the National Cholesterol Education Program Adult Treatment Panel III Guidelines," accessed at www.nhlbi.nih.gov/guidelines/cholesterol/atp3upd04 .htm on May 2, 2005.

20. John C. LaRosa, "New and Emerging Data from Clinical Trials of Statins," *Current Atherosclerosis Reports* 6, no. 1 (2004): 12–19.

21. Martha L. Daviglus, Jeremiah Stamler, Amber Pirzada, Lijing L. Yan, Daniel B. Garside, Kiang Liu, Renwei Wang, Alan R. Dyer, Donald M. Lloyd-Jones, and Philip Greenland, "Favorable Cardiovascular Risk Profile in Young Women and Long-Term Risk of Cardiovascular and All-Cause Mortality," *JAMA* 292 (2004): 1588–92.

22. J. Shepherd, G. J. Blauw, M. B. Murphy, et al., on behalf of the PROSPER study group, "Pravastatin in Elderly Individuals at Risk of Vascular Disease (PROSPER): A Randomized Controlled Trial," *Lancet* 360, no. 1 (2002): 1623–30.

23. Valerie Tikhonoff, Eduardo Casiglia, Alberto Mazza, et al., "Low-Density Lipoprotein Cholesterol and Mortality in Older People," *Journal of the American Geriatrics Society* 53, no. 2 (2005): 159–64.

24. National Cholesterol Education Program, "Third Report of the Expert Panel on Detection, Evaluation, and Treatment of High Blood Cholesterol in Adults (Adult Treatment Panel III)," accessed at www.

nhlbi.nih.gov/guidelines/cholesterol/atp3_rpt.htm on March 17, 2006.

25. J. R. Downs, M. Clearfield, S. Weis, et al., "Primary Prevention of Acute Coronary Events with Lovastatin in Men and Women with Average Cholesterol Levels: Results of AFCAPS/TexCAPS," *JAMA* 279, no. 1 (1998): 615–22.

26. National Cholesterol Education Program, "Third Report of the Expert Panel on Detection, Evaluation, and Treatment of High Blood Cholesterol in Adults (Adult Treatment Panel III)," page VIII-3, accessed at www.nhlbi.nih.gov/guidelines/cholesterol/atp3_rpt. htm on March 17, 2006.

27. RxList, "Gemfibrozil: Clinical Pharmacology," accessed at www.rxlist.com/cgi/generic/gemfib_cp.htm on October 28, 2005; RxList, "Fenofibrate: Warnings, Precautions," accessed at www.rxlist.com/cgi/gen eric3/fenofibrate_wcp.htm on October 28, 2005.

28. Type 2 Diabetes, accessed at www.diabetes.org/type-2-diabetes.jsp on May 2, 2005.

29. Peter Gaede and Oluf Pedersen, "Intensive Integrated Therapy of Type 2 Diabetes: Implications for Long-Term Prognosis," *Diabetes* 53, supplement 3 (2004): S39–47.

30. E. W. Gregg, R. B. Gerzoff, C. J. Caspersen, et al., "Relationship of Walking to Mortality Among U.S. Adults with Diabetes," *Archives of Internal Medicine* 163 (2003): 1440–47.

31. Women's Health Initiative Participant website, accessed at www.whi.org on May 2, 2005.

32. Women's Health Initiative Steering Committee, "Effects of Conjugated Equine Estrogen on Post-menopausal Women with Hysterectomy: The Women's Health Initiative Randomized Controlled Trial," *JAMA* 291, no. 14 (2004): 1701–12.

33. Poul Flemming Høilund-Carlsen, Allan Johansen, Henrik Wulff Christensen, et al., "Usefulness of the Exercise Electrocardiogram in Diagnosing Ischemic or Coronary Heart Disease in Patients with Chest Pain," *American Journal of Cardiology* 95, no. 1 (2005): 96–99.

34. Mark J. Fletcher, Jeffrey A. Tice, Michael Pignone,

Warren S. Browner, "Using the Coronary Artery Calcium Score to Predict Coronary Heart Disease Events: A Systematic Review and Meta-analysis," *Archives of Internal Medicine* 164, no. 12 (2004): 1285–92.

35. Christina Chrysohoou, Demosthenes B. Panagiotakos, Christos Pitsavos, et al., "Adherence to the Mediterranean Diet Attenuates Inflammation and Coagulation Process in Healthy Adults," *Journal of the American College of Cardiology* 44, no. 1 (2004): 152–58.

36. Heart Protection Study Collaborative Group, "MRC/BHF Heart Protection Study of Antioxidant Vitamin Supplementation in 20,536 High-Risk Individuals: A Randomised Placebo-Controlled Trial," *Lancet* 360, no. 9326 (2002): 23–33.

37. Antithrombotic Trialists' Collaboration, "Collaborative Meta-Analysis of Randomised Trials of Anti-platelet Therapy for Prevention of Death, Myocardial Infarction and Stroke in High Risk Patients," *British Medical Journal* 324, no. 7329 (2002): 71–86.

38. CAPRIE Steering Committee, "A Randomised, Blinded, Trial of Clopidogrel versus Aspirin in Patients at Risk of Ischaemic Events (CAPRIE)," *Lancet* 348, no. 7329 (1996): 1329–39.

39. Åke Hjalmarson, "International Beta-Blocker Review in Acute and Postmyocardial Infarction," *American Journal of Cardiology* 61, no. 3 (1988): 26–29.

40. Victor C. Lee, David C. Rhew, Michelle Dylan, et al., "Meta-Analysis: Angiotensin-Receptor Blockers in Chronic Heart Failure and High-Risk Acute Myocardial Infarction," *Annals of Internal Medicine* 141, no. 9 (2004): 693–704.

41. LaRosa.

42. Judith M. E. Walsh, "Drug Treatment of Hyperlipidemia in Women," *JAMA* 291 (2004): 2243–53.

CHAPTER 18

Cancers

Cancer is a disease in which cells grow out of control. It is often described as a disease of aging, because the risk of developing most cancers increases as people age. The incidence of most common cancers gradually increases until it peaks in people who are just past their middle years, which for most women means the years following menopause. One reason is that cancer often starts to develop when we are young, but tumors or symptoms may take a long time to be detected.

Apart from the more common types of skin cancer, which are generally not life-threatening, the cancers most frequently diagnosed among women in the United States are breast, lung, colorectal (colon plus rectum), and endometrial cancer.[1] This chapter describes the cancers that particularly affect women in our middle and older years, including the "female" cancers, or those that affect our breasts and reproductive organs (less than 1 percent of all breast cancer occurs in men). Research has shown that in some cases these cancers may be hormone-sensitive or hormone-related, thus the hormone changes of menopause can be considerations in evaluating risk, prevention, and treatment. This chapter discusses how widespread these cancers are, whom they affect, their symptoms, the screening practices used to find them, the options available to treat them, and issues to consider if you are diagnosed with one of them.

There is a great deal of apparently conflicting information about some risk factors for particular cancers. It is helpful to understand what is known—and what isn't—about the risks for cancers that develop as women age.

When I was diagnosed with cancer, I was terrified. It really was happening to me and I didn't want to believe it. I found I longed to go to sleep at night so I could escape the nightmare of being awake. Those first phone calls from my friends and family across the country meant the world to me. I have saved every e-mail, every card. Knowing that people cared really helped me get through it. Everything shifted when I got my diagnosis, but now I can say some good things came of it. I gained a deeper understanding about life and relationships, and what was meaningful and what I had to let go of. I am very lucky seven years later to be alive and feel so grateful to be able to help others who are going through the same thing.

SCREENING FOR EARLY DETECTION

Cancer screening is often recommended for people who don't have symptoms or a diagnosis of cancer. Most screens are used for individuals who are at higher than average risk of cancer, which means that screens increasingly become part of our care as we get older. The purpose of screening is to detect cancer at an early stage, when it theoretically can be more effectively treated. A screening test can involve collecting blood, urine, or other body substances to look for abnormal amounts of proteins or other molecules. Alternatively, screening can use an imaging method, such as mammography, which looks for breast cancer, or a technical procedure, such as a colonoscopy to look for colon cancer.

A good screen must detect all or most cancers for which it is designed and not identify benign or normal conditions as cancer. Unfortunately, many screening tests too often fail to detect cancer (false negatives) or detect too many abnormalities that are not cancer (false positives) or both.

Raising a false alarm about something that is not cancer can have negative consequences. In order to verify the presence of cancer, you may have to undergo invasive tests that can be expensive and time-consuming and have their own negative effects. Many of us may experience anxiety just worrying about whether we have cancer, when, in the end, the initial finding of possible cancer may turn out to be wrong.

An ideal cancer screen would detect all cancers and nothing else. Unfortunately, no screen is perfect, and only a few are good enough to be routinely recommended. For postmenopausal women, the commonly recommended screens are for breast, cervical, and colon cancers. Most clinicians recommend annual mammography beginning at age forty or fifty, but routine mammograms remain a controversial topic. Pap smears are used to detect changes in the cervix that might lead to cervical cancer; for many women, they are recommended annually. Screening of some kind is usually recommended after the age of fifty for colorectal cancer, with screening thereafter at regular intervals, depending upon the test and the results of your first screen.

TREATMENTS AND EFFECTS

Cancer treatments vary, but most include one or a combination of the following: surgery, radiation, chemotherapy, and hormonal treatment. All of these treatments have proven benefits, but also, to varying degrees, can have negative effects. These are usually temporary but sometimes permanent. For some women, certain treatments may also trigger early menopause. (For more information, see Chapter 4, "Sudden and Early Menopause.")

Complications from surgery may include pain, bleeding, and infection. Some women go through radiation with virtually no negative effects, although in many cases there are incidences of "sunburn" of the skin, fatigue, and, depending on the type of cancer being irradiated, nausea, vomiting, and diarrhea. Different types of chemotherapies are used in different situations for different cancers, but common effects include temporary hair loss, anemia, infection, nausea, fatigue, numbness, and tingling in the fingers and toes. Hormonal treatments are generally prescribed for years at a time with a wide variation in reported adverse effects. The commonly used drug tamoxifen often causes hot flashes, vaginal discharge, menstrual irregularities, temporary nausea and vomiting, weight gain, mood disturbances, fatigue, and, rarely, endometrial cancer and blood clots in the leg veins and lungs. Newer hormone treatments such as anastrozole, letrozole, and exemestane, which belong to a class of drugs called aromatase inhibitors, are beginning to be used instead of and in addition to tamoxifen in postmenopausal women with breast cancer. These drugs have fewer adverse effects than tamoxifen, though they have not been used long enough for their long-term effects to be known. The major problem with these drugs so far is that they can decrease bone density and increase bone fractures.[2] They also can cause hot flashes, nausea and vomiting, fatigue, and mood changes.[3]

BREAST CANCER

DEMOGRAPHICS, RISK FACTORS, AND SCREENING

Breast cancer describes a number of different kinds of cancer that start in breast tissue. Breast cancer is not deadly if it is confined to the breast, but it can be if it spreads to life-sustaining organs or bone.

Breast cancer is by far the most common cancer in women, apart from nonmelanoma skin cancer. Until the late 1990s, the incidence of breast cancer was rising in the United States, and it appears to continue to increase slightly among women fifty and older.[4] The number of deaths due to breast cancer in the United States has been decreasing overall. But African-American women, who are less likely than white women to get breast cancer, are more likely to die of the disease once diagnosed with it.[5] This disparity may be the result of more aggressive tumors in African-American women, differences in socioeconomic status (such as employment, income, and education), and differences in access to diagnosis and treatment programs.[6]

All women are at risk of developing breast cancer, and this risk increases as we grow older. On average, a woman has a one in seven chance of being diagnosed with breast cancer over her lifetime, if she lives to age eighty-five.[7] The risk of getting breast cancer increases at the greatest rate as a woman reaches and passes through menopause; then, after her late seventies, the risk begins to decrease but never goes away completely.[8] The reason for increasing risk at the time of menopause is not well understood. The rate of increase slows down after menopause, possibly due to lower levels of estrogen in the body.[9]

Many researchers believe that most breast cancers that occur before menopause are different from postmenopausal breast cancers. The premenopausal breast cancers tend to have different protein markers in their cells and generally are more aggressive than those in postmenopausal women. A woman's hormonal status very likely contributes, directly or indirectly, to the type of breast cancer she may develop.

Some of us are at higher than average risk for getting breast cancer, perhaps because we are exposed to more estrogen.[10] The growth of breast cancer and some of the other "female" cancers, such as endometrial cancer, is strongly stimulated by reproductive hormones, especially estrogen. While all women produce estrogen, some women's bodies produce estrogen for longer periods during our lifetimes. This increase in exposure happens in those of us who have more menstrual cycles (such as women who start menstruating earlier or stop menstruating later or do not have menstrual cycles interrupted by pregnancy), or have our first child after age thirty. Our risk is also elevated if we happen naturally to have higher levels of estrogen in our blood.[11] Exposure to estrogenlike compounds such as certain pesticides may also have an effect, and questions have been raised about additional estrogen exposure through fertility drugs and hormones in meat and milk.

Increased estrogen may also come from postmenopausal hormone treatment, which either contains estrogen alone or estrogen plus another hormone, progesterone. Several studies, including the Women's Health Initiative, a recent very large trial, have shown that using combined hormone treatment (estrogen plus progesterone) for a long time increases the risk of breast cancer.[12] Hormone use is recommended only for severe hot flashes or vaginal dryness that does not respond to other treatments, and then at as low a dose and for as short a time as possible. (For more information, see Chapter 7, "Hormone Treatment.") It is not clear whether taking oral contraceptives, which also contain estrogen, affects breast cancer risk. If you are taking oral contraceptives currently or have used them in the previous ten years, you may be at slightly increased risk.

Those of us who have one or more close relatives who have been diagnosed with breast cancer are also at increased risk. The more such relatives, particularly those who are diagnosed before menopause, and the closer they are to you, the greater the risk. For example, if your mother or your sister has breast cancer, your risk will be higher than if your grandmother or your aunt has breast cancer.

Some women have inherited a mutation, or change in the DNA, of certain "breast cancer genes," called BRCA1 and BRCA2, from a parent.[13] If you have one or both of these mutations, you have a much higher risk of getting breast cancer, as well as ovarian cancer. The type of breast cancer is one that tends to occur at an earlier age than most breast cancers and sometimes occurs in both breasts at the same or different times. Even though the risk of getting breast cancer if you have one of these mutations is very high, the mutation itself is uncommon, occurring in only 5 to 10 percent of all women who develop breast cancer.[14] In contrast, other factors, like being exposed to estrogen, are far more common, but they increase breast cancer risk only by a small amount.

In postmenopausal women, breast cancer risk seems to increase as weight increases, although the relationship is complex. Some studies have shown that gaining weight as an adult actually has a stronger association with risk than the weight itself.[15] Taller women also appear to be at greater risk.[16] Other risk factors include having dense breasts, because more dense breasts are more difficult to screen via mammography.[17]

Drinking two or more alcoholic drinks a day appears to increase risk of developing breast cancer.[18]

Finally, if you were treated with chest radiation for another disease, especially when you were young, your risk of breast cancer is very high.

For average-risk women, screening for breast cancer takes two forms: a breast X-ray, called a mammogram, and a physical exam either by a health care provider (clinical breast exam) or by the woman herself (breast self-exam).[19] Although doctors often recommend all of these approaches, the only screening test

• *At the time you experience menopause, your risk of getting breast cancer is 1 in 7.*

Myth. The risk of developing breast cancer increases with age until ages 75 to 79; then it decreases. In an average woman, the risk that you will have developed breast cancer by the time you are between 40 and 59 years old is about 1 in 24; by the time you are 60 to 79 years old, 1 in 13, and only by the time you reach 80 or 85 is there as high as a 1 in 7 chance that you will have developed breast cancer at some point.[20]

for which scientific evidence shows a benefit for women after menopause is an annual mammogram. If you see or feel a change in your breast, see a health care provider, but remember that not every lump is cancer. In fact, most are not. One type of breast cancer, called Paget's disease, can cause a change in the nipple's appearance so that it looks scaly, like eczema. Even without a lump and with a normal mammogram, this sort of tissue change should be biopsied if it does not disappear in a few weeks. Paget's disease occurs in about 1 percent of all breast cancer cases;[21] most people who are diagnosed with it are over fifty. Some studies suggest that breast cancers associated with Paget's disease tend to have a higher mortality rate than other types, because they are often not diagnosed early and providers are more apt to miss them.

Those of us who are at high risk because of a family history of breast cancer or a known genetic mutation may benefit from discussions with a specially trained genetic counselor.[22] We may be counseled to have more frequent screening mammography and to consider other methods of breast cancer risk reduction. Some women at high risk choose to undergo prophylactic mastectomy, in which both breasts are surgically removed (the most effective risk reduction method).[23] Sometimes women diagnosed with cancer in one breast, knowing that

they remain at high risk, will opt to have both removed during surgery.

Another way to decrease breast cancer risk is to take the drug tamoxifen, though it poses considerable risks of negative effects and is not as well studied in women with genetic mutations as in women with other risk factors.[24] In women at high risk of breast cancer, tamoxifen reduces risk by about 50 percent.[25] Although this may seem like a large decrease in risk, it's important to consider the reduction in absolute risk for high-risk women. For example, a woman who has a 5 percent risk of developing breast cancer in the next five years is considered to be at high risk, and tamoxifen will reduce this 5 percent risk by half, to about 2.5 percent.

Another drug that appears to decrease breast cancer risk is raloxifene, which was originally developed to treat osteoporosis. Preliminary results from a large study suggest that raloxifene is as effective as tamoxifen in preventing breast cancer in postmenopausal women considered at high risk of developing the disease.[26] The same preliminary results suggest that raloxifene causes fewer serious problems such as blood clots and cancer of the uterus than tamoxifen. As of April 2006, raloxifene (which is sold under the brand name Evista) had not been federally approved for use in preventing breast cancer.

There are no measures that reduce the risk of developing breast cancer to zero.

DIAGNOSIS AND TREATMENT

If a mammogram shows a suspicious area, or if a lump is felt during a breast exam, the next step is usually a biopsy. The simplest type of biopsy is a fine-needle aspiration or core biopsy, in which a biopsy needle is used to obtain the sample. The breast tissue obtained in this way is examined under a microscope by a pathologist, who determines whether it contains cancer and if so, what kind and with what features. These details are needed in order to decide how best to treat the cancer. Because decisions about treatment are so important, you may wish to seek a second opinion rather than immediately accepting a treatment recommended by your initial doctor. If possible, a good place to seek a second opinion is a research-oriented academic center or a hospital in a large city, where treatments are usually decided by a team of cancer experts, called oncologists.

Breast cancers that are diagnosed in postmenopausal women often have a good outcome, or prognosis. When found by a mammogram, they are generally small and often are confined to the breast. Such early-stage cancers usually can be treated by a surgical procedure called a lumpectomy, which removes only the cancerous tissue, rather than the entire breast. At the same time, one or more lymph nodes that are in the adjacent armpit are often removed and examined for the presence of cancer cells. Until recently, the standard practice for this was a procedure called axillary node dissection (AND), which generally removed a dozen or more lymph nodes in the armpit, often resulting in permanent arm difficulties including stiffness and lymphedema, or swelling. Nowadays, the preferred surgery is sentinel node biopsy (SNB), wherein the surgeon removes only a few primary lymph nodes to examine for cancer. If cancer is found, a complete axillary node dissection may be necessary. If you are

This self-portrait of journalist and photographer Marlies Bosch on the eve of her second mastectomy appears in her book *Life of My Breasts,* which documents her experience with breast cancer. "I would like to break the taboos surrounding breast cancer that seek to render it invisible," writes Bosch in the introduction to her book. "I would like an open discussion about the tendency of doctors and women alike to hide the effects of a mastectomy with implants, prostheses, and invasive reconstructive surgery methods. . . . Although it is delightful to have two intact breasts, a woman can live a full and beautiful life without them."

being evaluated for breast cancer surgery, it is important to ask if your surgeon is experienced with SNB, and if not, get a second opinion from someone who is. Determining whether cancer has spread to the lymph nodes helps the oncologist determine what further tests, such as CT scans, or treatments, such as radiation or chemotherapy, may be necessary. Cancer that has spread beyond the lymph nodes is referred to as metastatic or stage 4.

Breast cancers diagnosed when they are small can be surgically removed by a lumpectomy, in which only the cancer itself is removed. However, large cancers often require a mastectomy, or removal of the breast. If you have a mastectomy, you have the option of breast reconstruction. This can be done either by placing implants in the area of the mastectomy or by creating a breast mound, called a TRAM flap, from your own muscle tissue to replace the breast that was removed. An ongoing controversy at the FDA involves questions about the safety of some products used for breast implants. (For more information about breast implants, see page 129.)

I had a mastectomy. I avoided breast reconstruction because I really didn't want surgery again. So I only have one breast, and I sometimes feel deformed. I have had many conversations about it. People—some of them are my friends—have been troubled by the idea of my being asymmetrical. Even years later, some friends continue to encourage me to have reconstruction. But in a situation like this, what you want is to be the way you were, and even with reconstruction, you can never be that. So I still don't like it, but I think it's the best choice for me, and I feel comfortable with the choice. For me, though not for everyone, this is a more honest way of being.

The treatments for breast cancer for postmenopausal women sometimes differ from those for premenopausal women, partly because of hormonal differences in these two groups. There are two main types of breast cancer, distinguished by whether the cancer cells contain a protein, the estrogen receptor, that responds to estrogen by making the cell divide, causing the cancer to grow. Until recently, most postmenopausal women with an estrogen receptor–positive breast cancer (a cancer that has the estrogen receptor) have been prescribed the oral drug tamoxifen for five years after the initial surgery or radiation, to help prevent recurrence. Tamoxifen combines with the estrogen receptor and prevents the cell from dividing. In the last few years, however, a new group of drugs called aromatase inhibitors, which prevent estrogen from being made, are beginning to be used either after a few years of tamoxifen or instead of tamoxifen immediately after surgery or radiation. Premenopausal women with estrogen receptor–positive cancers did not receive tamoxifen in the past but now do. However, premenopausal women are not prescribed aromatase inhibitors, because these drugs have not yet been properly tested in this group.

Initial treatment may take several months. When it is complete, your health care provider will schedule regular follow-up appointments to check for symptoms resulting from your treatment and for possible recurrence.

OVARIAN CANCER

DEMOGRAPHICS, RISK FACTORS, AND SCREENING

Ovarian cancer is a serious cancer that is often diagnosed in its late stages,[27] because it pro-

---

MYTH OR REALITY?

• *Using oral contraceptives puts me at risk for gynecologic cancers.*

Myth. Although there is some debate about whether oral birth control pills may slightly raise a woman's risk of developing breast cancer, the use of the "pill" can actually reduce a woman's risk of ovarian cancer by up to 50 percent. Use of oral contraceptives is also protective against endometrial cancer.

duces very nonspecific symptoms and to date there is no truly effective screening method available. Approximately 75 percent of women diagnosed with ovarian cancer have a tumor that has spread beyond the ovary. Over your lifetime, you have approximately a one in seventy risk of developing ovarian cancer, and the highest incidence occurs between ages fifty-four and sixty-four.[28]

Many of the risk factors for ovarian cancer are the same as for breast cancer. For example, a strong family history of ovarian cancer or breast cancer or inheritance of the BRCA1 or BRCA2 gene mutation significantly raises a woman's chance of developing an ovarian cancer. In addition, if you have had a personal history of breast cancer or if you were ever exposed to talc, your risk is elevated. (One theory is that talcum powder entering the uterus and ovarian area may be associated with inflammation that promotes the cancer.) Increasing age, not bearing children, and a history of infertility also increase a woman's likelihood of developing ovarian cancer. Though it is not clear if exposure to estrogen and progesterone hormone supplementation increases the risk of ovarian cancer, the use of birth control pills has been shown to reduce a woman's chance of developing an ovarian cancer by up to 50 percent.[29]

DIAGNOSIS AND TREATMENT

Ovarian cancer symptoms are vague and varied and are often mistaken for a gastrointestinal problem.[30] One woman with ovarian cancer describes how she missed the signs of the disease:

There is a difference between an intense exhaustion and a bone-deep fatigue. I know that now. My intuitive voice was probably trying to tell me, but I was too busy to listen.

The most common symptoms of ovarian cancer include abdominal discomfort, bloating, gastrointestinal distress, nausea, vomiting, diarrhea, constipation, change in waist size, indigestion, getting full after eating only small amounts of food, frequent need to empty the bladder, intense urges to empty the bladder, weight loss, fatigue, pelvic pressure, vaginal bleeding, and pain with intercourse or other vaginal penetration. As one woman with ovarian cancer says,

I had been exercising regularly, eating a healthy diet, and doing daily sit-ups for three months, and my stomach just kept getting bigger.

All of these symptoms also occur in women who do not have ovarian cancer. However, if you experience these symptoms for more than a few days and, certainly, weeks, consult with a knowledgeable health care provider. If your provider or gynecologist suspects you have an underlying ovarian tumor, the most appropriate approach is for you to be referred to a gynecologic oncologist, a doctor who specializes in cancers of the female organs. Unfortunately, in the United States, only 40 to 60 percent of women found to have ovarian cancer are treated initially by a gynecologic oncologist. If you think you may need to see a specialist, it is important to speak with your care providers about your concerns or to seek the advice of a local or national cancer center or other health care support organization.

The diagnosis of ovarian cancer is typically made when a pelvic mass or thickening is discovered during a detailed physical exam that includes both a pelvic and rectal exam, or by pelvic or vaginal ultrasound. This is usually followed by X-rays, including a CT scan of the abdomen and pelvis and blood tests for tumor markers that are associated with ovarian tumors, especially CA-125.

Ovarian cancer is generally confirmed with surgery, which involves making a long vertical cut on your abdomen that extends from just above your pubic bone to above the belly button. During such surgery, the ovaries and uterus can be removed, along with any visible cancer. However, if the cancer is felt to be at an early stage or the diagnosis is not certain, it may be reasonable to complete the initial evaluation using laparoscopic techniques, which are minimally invasive and less traumatic than open surgery. Laparoscopic surgery usually involves placing a small camera in the belly button to enable the surgeon to see all around the abdominal and pelvic cavities and use instruments introduced through separate small incisions. Though this is not the standard surgery for ovarian cancer, the laparoscopic approach offers special cases a reasonable alternative that commonly results in less postoperative pain, less blood loss, shorter hospital stays, and a faster recovery time.[31] When considering surgical options, ask if your surgeon recommends a minimally invasive approach and, more important, if he or she is comfortable offering this option to you.

Except for a small number of women whose ovarian cancers are slow-growing and limited to only one ovary, most women will have chemotherapy after surgery. This treatment leads to better chances for overall survival.

When I was diagnosed with third-stage ovarian cancer over eight years ago, I thought it was a death sentence. But being driven by having two young children (who are now teenagers!), I learned everything I could about my disease including treatment options, diet, exercise, vitamins, and spiritual and psychological effects. I've had over a dozen chemotherapies, three major surgeries, and radiation. I am part of a team of doctors, nurses, nutritionist, family, and friends who support my health. I do have days when I am sad, angry, or depressed. But . . . I am determined to live my life to the fullest and for the longest time possible.

Ovarian cancer initially responds to surgery and chemotherapy in women with advanced disease in 60 to 80 percent of cases. But it comes back, or *relapses,* in as many as 70 to 80 percent of women with this diagnosis. Relapse may take place months or even years after the initial treatment.

If you have no more symptoms or clinical findings after treatment, you will have achieved a *clinical remission.* Whether your cancer responds to treatment or not, follow-up will involve seeing your gynecologic oncologist at recommended intervals.

ENDOMETRIAL/ UTERINE CANCER

DEMOGRAPHICS, RISK FACTORS, AND SCREENING

Ninety-four percent of uterine cancers begin in the lining of the uterus, also called the endometrium. Therefore, the terms *endometrial cancer* and *uterine cancer* are often used interchangeably. In the United States, endometrial cancer is the most common cancer of the gynecologic organs; worldwide, it is second to cervical cancer.[32]

Estrogen stimulates growth of cells in the uterine lining. When there is an increased amount of this hormone in a woman's body, an endometrial cancer may develop. The number one risk factor for this cancer is obesity: Fat tissue synthesizes estrogens, so greater amounts of fat tissue lead to higher levels of estrogens in the blood. Other risk factors include diabetes, hypertension, estrogen therapy (without progesterone), tamoxifen therapy (for breast cancer treatment or prevention), late menopause, and lack of childbearing. In some families, a high risk of endometrial cancer is inherited. Some of these risk factors can be controlled by exercising regularly, eating a healthy diet, and keeping blood sugar and blood pressure under control.

If you are postmenopausal, potential warning signs of endometrial cancer include *any* bleeding in the vaginal area. Before menopause, periods that get progressively heavier or bleeding between periods could be an indication. Other symptoms include abnormal vaginal discharge, pelvic pressure, and uterine enlargement. Currently, there are no routine screening tests for endometrial cancer.[33]

DIAGNOSIS AND TREATMENT

If you are experiencing abnormal bleeding or other symptoms, your health care provider may recommend an endometrial biopsy, which can usually be done in the office with minimal discomfort. A D&C (dilation and curettage) procedure, which is usually done in the operating room (often with general anesthesia), may be necessary to complete the evaluation. If endometrial cancer is detected, additional evaluation is carried out, including X-rays, blood tests, and physical examination.

In 75 percent of women with endometrial cancer, the disease is confined to the uterus and can be surgically removed with no recurrence. The surgery includes a total hysterectomy, removal of the ovaries and tubes, and sampling of the lymph nodes in the pelvis and in the area of the aorta. This type of surgery helps determine whether the disease has spread, and if so, how far, which is called *staging*. Alternatives to surgery include radiation and hormonal therapy; however, these are not as effective as surgery. Some women will require these treatments in addition to surgery.

In the United States, fewer than half of women who are diagnosed with endometrial cancer have a gynecologic oncologist complete their initial surgery. This is unfortunate because studies suggest that women treated by this type of specialist are three times more likely to have a comprehensive and adequate surgical staging evaluation.[34] In some cases, such an evaluation allows women to avoid unnecessary postoperative therapy such as pelvic radiation.[35] The vast majority of women with endometrial cancer will be adequately treated by surgery alone. However, as with all cancers, once recovery from surgery or other treatment is complete, regular checkups are wise.

CERVICAL CANCER

DEMOGRAPHICS, RISK FACTORS, AND SCREENING

Cervical cancer is the second most frequent cancer among women worldwide, though much more common in the developing world. According to the American Cancer Society, between 60 and 80 percent of newly diagnosed cervical cancers are found in women who have not had a Pap test in the last five years. In the countries where Pap tests are not available, cervical cancer remains the leading cause of cancer death.

Cervical cancer usually affects women between the ages of 30 and 55, with the mean age of diagnosis being 51.4 years, almost exactly the average age of menopause for women in the United States. More than 20 percent of women who are diagnosed with cervical cancer are over the age of sixty-five, which underscores the importance of postmenopausal women having annual Pap tests if appropriate (see "When to get a Pap," page 274) and yearly gynecologic exams.[36] Women who have had a total hysterectomy, meaning that both the body of the uterus and the cervix were removed, generally require the Pap test only if there was previous treatment for precancerous changes of the cervix or if the surgery itself was done to treat a malignancy.

The most common type of cervical cancer is squamous cell carcinoma, which arises in the thin flat (squamous) cells that line the outer part of the cervix. The remaining 10 to 20 percent of cervical cancers are adenocarcinomas, meaning that they develop from glands that produce mucus in the inner cervical canal.

The major risk factor for cervical cancer is exposure to specific subtypes of the human papillomavirus, or HPV. The virus is sexually transmitted, and most men and women who have had unprotected genital contact have been exposed to it. Most of the time, a woman will clear the virus with her own immune system; only those of us with persistent infections with HPV are at risk. In most cases, HPV does not cause symptoms and may go undetected for years if a woman does not get regular Pap tests. A new screen for HPV, called the HPV test, can be used in combination with the Pap test for women over thirty. Knowing whether you have the HPV virus can help your doctor evaluate your risk of getting cervical cancer and determine how often you may need to be retested. Routine HPV testing is not recommended for younger woman because of the high-positive rate in women who will never have a problem.

Other risk factors for cervical cancer include multiple sexual partners or sexually transmitted infections; suppression of the immune system as a result of HIV, steroids, or medical therapy following an organ transplant; and smoking. You can lower your risk of cervical cancer by practicing safer sex; not smoking; and obtaining regular gynecologic care and Pap tests.

DIAGNOSIS AND TREATMENT

Precancerous changes and cervical cancer confined to the cervix usually do not exhibit symptoms. If the cancer becomes invasive, symptoms may emerge. These include vaginal bleeding after menopause or with vaginal penetration, unusual vaginal discharge, leg pain, or bleeding from the bladder or rectum. If cancer is suspected, colposcopy (an exam of the cervix with binocularlike instruments) followed by a cervical biopsy or a LEEP (loop electrosurgical excision procedure) can be done in the office. (LEEP is a procedure in which an electric wire is used to remove a portion of the cervix.) Alternatively, if needed, a cone biopsy can be done in the operating room.

The prognosis of cervical cancer depends on the stage, which is determined by physical examination together with additional tests that look at the lungs, bladder, and rectum. The five-year survival rate for early-stage cervical cancer is very good, ranging between 80 and 94 per-

WHEN TO GET A PAP

A Pap test involves collecting cells from the surface of the cervix and looking for abnormal cells. This test, along with a pelvic exam, should be done annually starting within three years of beginning sexual activity or no later than the age of twenty-one.[37] After age thirty, the test may be done less often if you have had only normal results in the past. More than 20 percent of newly diagnosed cervical cancers occur in women who are over the age of sixty-five. Therefore, it is important for women to have annual Pap tests until the age of seventy, perhaps longer, depending on risk factors, especially having new sexual partners.

cent. As with all cancer, long-term survival decreases with advanced-stage disease.

Treatment may involve surgery, radiation, chemotherapy, or a combination of these.[38] Depending upon the invasiveness of the cancer, the recommendation may be a simple total hysterectomy, which removes the cervix and uterus, or a radical hysterectomy, which removes the cervix, uterus, surrounding pelvic tissue, part of the upper vagina, and pelvic lymph nodes. In either case, the ovaries may be preserved, since cervical cancer rarely spreads to them. Radiation therapy concurrent with chemotherapy is effective for both radical hysterectomies and early cervical cancers. It is important to discuss the risks, benefits, and long-term effects of these therapies with a gynecologic oncologist.

Following initial treatment, visits to your provider every few months will help identify any recurrence. After a year or so, you can be checked less often.

VAGINAL/VULVAR CANCER

Cancer of the vulva (the external genitals) is the fourth most common gynecologic cancer. It is seen mostly in postmenopausal women and is diagnosed at an average age of sixty-five. Risk factors for developing vulvar cancer include smoking, human papillomavirus, and immunosuppression. In addition, long-standing vulvar dystrophy (one of several skin conditions of the vulva) increases your risk of getting vulvar cancer. If you have lumps or sores on your vulva, especially itchy or painful ones, you may want to request a biopsy. Biopsy is the most important step in diagnosing vulvar cancer and can be done in an office visit.

Treatment for early-stage vulvar cancer involves removing the part of the vulva that is affected and removing the lymph nodes in the groin on one or both sides to evaluate for spread. If two or more lymph nodes are positive for cancer, radiation therapy will likely be needed. If the cancer has spread further to the urethra or rectum, chemotherapy may also be used.

LUNG CANCER

Lung cancer strikes both men and women and is the most frequent cause of cancer death in the United States and in the world. Among women in the United States, lung cancer is second only to breast cancer in frequency, and after menopause the frequency increases, with lung cancer being diagnosed in 1 out of every 123 women aged forty to fifty-nine and 1 in 26 women aged sixty to seventy-nine.[39] The numbers have risen in large part because more women are smoking. About 80 percent of lung cancers in women (90 percent in men) are estimated to be due to tobacco smoking.[40] Prevention strategies have therefore focused on helping people to stop smoking. (For more information, see page 279.) Some nonsmokers develop lung cancer because of exposure to secondhand smoke. The reasons that other nonsmokers develop lung cancer are less clear.

Lung cancer is a highly lethal disease. It is the leading cause of cancer death among women in the United States, accounting for 27 percent of all cancer deaths among U.S. women, as compared to breast cancer, which accounts for 15 percent.[41] Unfortunately, there is still no useful screening test for lung cancer.[42]

At first, I was scared, worried, devastated, wondering whether I was going to live or die. I cried a little bit, worried, prayed a lot. Then—after the surgery—when the doctor told me how small it was, I felt better. Doing fine since then, trying to gain some weight. Feeling good. My life isn't changed too much. I went back to work.

Lung cancer is generally treated with combinations of surgery, radiation, and chemotherapy. Following appropriate therapies for both early- and late-stage lung cancer, women have longer survival rates than men.

COLORECTAL CANCER

Worldwide, colorectal cancer is the third most common cancer in women, and the incidence for women increases considerably around age fifty, making it an important cancer to watch for in the years around menopause.

Colorectal cancer seems to occur more often in regions where meat and animal fat consumption is high and less often where large amounts of fiber are eaten as part of the diet. Other risk factors include being physically inactive, being overweight, or having fat distributed mainly in the middle of your body. If you have one or more close relatives who have colorectal cancer or who had it at an early age, your risk of getting this cancer is higher than average. Overall, colorectal cancer has a good prognosis.

Screening for early detection is often successful in finding precancers and early-stage cancers that can be removed. It is recommended for women and men over age fifty. Screening options include an annual check for blood in the stool, sometimes combined with a flexible sigmoidoscopy, or a full colonoscopy.[43] The sigmoidoscopy and colonoscopy involve procedures by which a specialist uses an instrument to look directly into the colon for cancer or precancerous lesions, called polyps or adenomas. Sigmoidoscopy looks only at the last part of the colon, while colonoscopy looks at the whole colon and is considered the gold standard for diagnosis.

Treatment of colorectal cancer includes combinations of surgery, radiation, and chemotherapy,[44] depending on how widespread the disease is. Proper treatment of early-stage cancer that is confined to the bowel wall and local lymph nodes often leads to long-term survival.

NOTES

1. A. Jemal, T. Murray, E. Ward, A. Samuels, R. C. Tiwari, A. Ghafoor, et al., "Cancer Statistics, 2005," *CA: A Cancer Journal for Clinicians* 55, no. 1 (2005): 10–30.

2. I. E. Smith and M. Dowsett, "Aromatase Inhibitors in Breast Cancer," *New England Journal of Medicine* 348, no. 24 (2003): 2431–42, 2438.

3. Ibid.

4. American Cancer Society, "Breast Cancer Death Rates Dropping," September 22, 2005, accessed at www.cancer.org/docroot/NWS/content/NWS_1_1x_Breast_Cancer_Death_Rat es_Dropping.asp on October 10, 2005.

5. B. N. Polite and O. I. Olopade, "Breast Cancer and Race: A Rising Tide Does Not Lift All Boats Equally," *Perspectives in Biology and Medicine* 48, Supplement 1 (2005): S166–75; see also A. Ghafoor, A. Jemal, E. Ward, V. Cokkinides, R. Smith, and M. Thun, "Trends in Breast Cancer by Race and Ethnicity," *CA: A Cancer Journal for Clinicians* 53, no. 6 (2003): 342–55.

6. M. G. del Carmen, K. S. Hughes, E. Hapern, E. Rafferty, D. Kopans, Y. R. Parsky, A. Sardi, L. Esserman, S. Rust, and J. Michaelson, "Racial Differences in Mammographic Breast Density," *Cancer* 98 (2003): 590–96.

7. National Cancer Institute, "Probability of Breast Cancer in American Women," April 15, 2005, accessed at cis.nci.nih.gov/fact/5_6.htm on October 14, 2005.

8. Y. Yasui and J. D. Potter, "The Shape of Age-Incidence Curves of Female Breast Cancer by Hormone-Receptor Status," *Cancer Causes and Control: CCC* 10, no. 5 (1999): 431–37; see also R. E. Tarone and K. C. Chu, "The Greater Impact of Menopause on ER than ER+ Breast Cancer Incidence: A Possible Explana-

tion," *Cancer Causes and Control: CCC* 13, no. 1 (2002): 7–14.

9. Freddie Bray, Peter McCarron, and D. Maxwell Parkin, "The Changing Global Patterns of Female Breast Cancer Incidence and Mortality," *Breast Cancer Research* 6 (August 2004): 229–39, 230.

10. M. Clemons and P. Goss, "Estrogen and the Risk of Breast Cancer," *New England Journal of Medicine* 344, no. 4 (2001): 276–85.

11. P. G. Toniolo, M. Levitz, A. Zeleniuch-Jacquotte, S. Banerjee, K. L. Koenig, R. E. Shore, et al., "A Prospective Study of Endogenous Estrogens and Breast Cancer in Postmenopausal Women," *Journal of the National Cancer Institute* 87, no. 3 (1995): 190–97; see also S. R. Cummings, J. S. Lee, L. Y. Lui, K. Stone, B. M. Ljung, and J. A. Cauleys, "Sex Hormones, Risk Factors, and Risk of Estrogen Receptor–Positive Breast Cancer in Older Women: A Long-Term Prospective Study," *Cancer Epidemiology, Biomarkers and Prevention: A Publication of the American Association for Cancer Research, Cosponsored by the American Society of Preventive Oncology* 14, no. 5 (2005): 1047–51.

12. J. E. Rossouw, G. L. Anderson, R. L. Prentice, A. Z. La-Croix, C. Kooperberg, M. L. Stefanick, et al., "Risks and Benefits of Estrogen Plus Progestin in Healthy Postmenopausal Women: Principal Results from the Women's Health Initiative Randomized Controlled Trial," *JAMA* 288, no. 3 (2002): 321–33.

13. H. T. Lynch, C. L. Snyder, J. F. Lynch, B. D. Riley, and W. S. Rubinstein, "Hereditary Breast-Ovarian Cancer at the Bedside: Role of the Medical Oncologist," *Journal of Clinical Oncology* 21, no. 4 (2003): 740–53; see also D. M. Parkin, F. Bray, J. Ferlay, and P. Pisani, "Global Cancer Statistics, 2002," *CA: A Cancer Journal for Clinicians* 55, no. 2 (2005): 74–108.

14. P. Lichtenstein, N. V. Holm, P. K. Verkasalo, et al., "Environmental and Heritable Factors in the Causation of Cancer—Analyses of Cohorts of Twins from Sweden, Denmark, and Finland," *New England Journal of Medicine* 343 (2000): 78–83.

15. M. Harvie, A. Howell, R. A. Vierkant, N. Kumar, J. R. Cerhan, L. E. Kelemen, et al., "Association of Gain and Loss of Weight before and after Menopause with Risk of Postmenopausal Breast Cancer in the Iowa Women's Health Study," *Cancer Epidemiology, Biomarkers and Prevention: A Publication of the American Association for Cancer Research, Cosponsored by the American Society of Preventive Oncology* 14, no. 3 (2005): 656–61; see also Z. Huang, S. E. Hankinson, G. A. Colditz, M. J. Stampfer, D. J. Hunter, J. E. Manson, et al., "Dual Effects of Weight and Weight Gain on Breast Cancer Risk," *JAMA* 278, no. 17 (1997): 1407–11.

16. M. Ahlgren, M. Meelbye, J. Wohlfahrt, T. I. Sorensen, "Growth Patterns and the Risk of Breast Cancer in Women," *New England Journal of Medicine* 351 (2004): 1619–23. See also A. Trentham-Dietz, P. A. Newcomb, K. M. Egan, et al., "Weight Change and Risk of Postmenopausal Breast Cancer (United States)," *Cancer Causes Control* 11 (2000): 533–38.

17. C. Byrne, C. Schairer, J. Wolfe, et al., "Mammographic Features and Breast Cancer Risk," *Journal of the National Cancer Institute* 87 (1995): 1622–26; see also N. F. Boyd, J. W. Byng, R. A. Jong, et al., "Quantitative Classification of Mammographic Densities and Breast Cancer Risk: Results from the Canadian National Breast Screening Study," *Journal of the National Cancer Institute* 87 (1995): 670–75; K. Kerlikowsje, J. Shepherd, J. Creasman, et al., "Are Breast Density and Bone Mineral Density Independent Risk Factors for Breast Cancer?" *Journal of the National Cancer Institute* 97 (2005): 368–75.

18. W. Y. Chen, G. A. Colditz, B. Rosner, et al., "Use of Postmenopausal Hormones, Alcohol, and Risk for Invasive Breast Cancer," *Annals of Internal Medicine* 137 (2002): 798–804; see also S. Zhang, D. J. Hunter, S. E. Hankinson, et al., "A Prospective Study of Folate Intake and the Risk of Breast Cancer," *JAMA* 281 (1999): 1632–37.

19. R. A. Smith, V. Cokkinides, and H. J. Eyre, "American Cancer Society Guidelines for the Early Detection of Cancer, 2005," *CA: A Cancer Journal for Clinicians* 55, no. 1 (2005): 31–44; quiz 55–56.

20. Jemal et al., 26.

21. A. J. Alberg et al., "Epidemiology, Prevention, and

Early Detection of Breast Cancer," *Current Opinion in Oncology* 9 (1997): 505–10.

22. Lynch et al.

23. A. Eisen and B. L. Weber, "Prophylactic Mastectomy for Women with BRCA1 and BRCA2 Mutations—Facts and Controversy," *New England Journal of Medicine* 345, no. 3 (2001): 207–8; see also L. J. Pierce, M. Strawderman. S. A. Narod, I. Oliviotto, A. Eisen, L. Dawson, et al., "Effect of Radiotherapy after Breast-Conserving Treatment in Women with Breast Cancer and Germline BRCA1/2 Mutations," *Journal of Clinical Oncology* 18, no. 19 (2000): 3360–69.

24. R. Calderon-Margalit and O. Paltiel, "Prevention of Breast Cancer in Women Who Carry BRCA1 or BRCA2 Mutations: A Critical Review of the Literature," *International Journal of Cancer* 112, no. 3 (2004): 357–64.

25. B. Fisher, J. P. Costantino, D. L. Wickerham, C. K. Redmond, M. Kavanah, W. M. Cronin, et al., "Tamoxifen for Prevention of Breast Cancer: Report of the National Surgical Adjuvant Breast and Bowel Project P-1 Study," *Journal of the National Cancer Institute* 90, no. 18 (1998): 1371–88.

26. National Cancer Institute Press Release, "Initial Results of the Study of Tamoxifen and Raloxifene (STAR) Released: Osteoporosis Drug Raloxifene Shown to Be as Effective as Tamoxifen in Preventing Invasive Breast Cancer," April 17, 2006, accessed at www.cancer.gov/newscenter/pressreleases/STAR resultsApr172006 on April 19, 2006.

27. Jemal et al., 10–30.

28. S. A. Cannistra, "Cancer of the Ovary," *New England Journal of Medicine* 351, no. 24 (2004): 2519–29.

29. The Cancer and Steroid Hormone Study of the Centers for Disease Control and the National Institute of Child Health and Human Development, "The Reduction in Risk of Ovarian Cancer Associated with Oral-Contraceptive Use," *New England Journal of Medicine* 316, no. 11 (1987): 650–55.

30. Cannistra.

31. R. Tozzi and A. Schneider, "Laparoscopic Treatment of Early Ovarian Cancer," *Current Opinion in Obstetrics and Gynecology* 17, no. 4 (2005): 354–58.

32. D. A. Levine and W. J. Hoskins, "Update in the Management of Endometrial Cancer," *Cancer Journal* 8, supplement 1 (2002): S31–40.

33. Smith et al., "American Cancer Society Guidelines."

34. P. Y. Roland, F. J. Kelly, P. Blitzer, M. Curcio, J. W. Orr Jr., "The Benefits of a Gynecologic Oncologist: A Pattern of Care Study for Endometrial Cancer Treatment," *Gynecologic Oncology* 93, no. 1 (2004): 125–30.

35. C. Burke and K. Hickey, "Does Surgical Staging of Clinical Stage I Endometrial Carcinoma Significantly Alter Adjuvant Management?" *Journal of Obstetrics and Gynaecology* 24, no. 3 (2004): 289–91; see also M. M. Juretzka, D. S. Chi, and Y. Sonoda, "Update on Surgical Treatment for Endometrial Cancer," *Expert Review of Anticancer Therapy* 5, no. 1 (2005): 113–21.

36. Smith et al., "American Cancer Society Guidelines."

37. Ibid.

38. W. A. McCreath, E. Salom, and D. S. Chi, "Cervical Cancer: Current Management of Early/Late Disease," *Surgical Oncology Clinics of North America* 14, no. 2 (2005): 249–66.

39. Jemal et al.

40. Centers for Disease Control, "Lung Cancer Questions and Answers," page last reviewed September 16, 2005, accessed at www.cdc.gov/cancer/lung/qa.htm#risk on October 20, 2005.

41. Jemal et al.

42. Smith et al., "American Cancer Society Guidelines."

43. M. Pignone, M. Rich, S. M. Teutsch, A. O. Berg and K. N. Lohr, "Screening for Colorectal Cancer in Adults at Average Risk: A Summary of the Evidence for the U.S. Preventive Services Task Force," *Annals of Internal Medicine* 137, no. 2 (2002): 132–41; see also S. Winawer, R. Fletcher, D. Rex, J. Bond, R. Burt, J. Ferrucci, et al., "Colorectal Cancer Screening and Surveillance: Clinical Guidelines and Rationale—Update Based on New Evidence," *Gastroenterology* 124, no. 2 (2003): 544–60.

44. J. A. Meyerhardt and R. J. Mayer, "Systemic Therapy for Colorectal Cancer," *New England Journal of Medicine* 352, no. 5 (2005): 476–87.

CHAPTER 19

Other Health Concerns

A range of medical conditions can become more pronounced with age and may be of concern to us as we go through the menopause transition. In addition, our use of alcohol and tobacco may create health challenges at this time, inspiring us to seek support and treatment. This chapter covers tobacco, alcohol, type 2 diabetes, migraine headaches, joint health, dry eye and vision changes, hearing loss, gum and dental problems, and thyroid conditions.

TOBACCO

About one in five women between the ages of 45 and 64 smokes (20 percent).[1] However, smoking rates vary dramatically by level of education, race/ethnicity, and other factors. For example, only 7 percent of women with graduate degrees smoke, in contrast to 46 percent of women with GEDs.

Women smoke for many reasons. We may be influenced by advertising that equates smoking with independence, sophistication, and beauty or that plays into the social pressures on us to control our weight. Smoking may help us organize our social relationships, carve out time for ourselves, control our emotions, create an image, and have a source of comfort and dependability in our lives.[2]

I began smoking and drinking in the 1970s as a part of coming out and accepting my identity as a lesbian. At that time we took a lot of health risks in the pursuit of a strong "dyke" image!

We also smoke because we are addicted. The symptoms of addiction can appear within weeks of beginning even occasional smoking, and we may find it difficult to quit. Many obstacles can prevent us from getting the support and treatment we need to stop smoking. These may include being depressed, not having people in our lives who support our desire to quit, or having friends, relatives, and coworkers who smoke. But help is available. For women who smoke, quitting is the single most important thing we can do to protect our own health and the health of those around us.

HEALTH EFFECTS

Smoking has extremely serious consequences for our health. The 2001 U.S. Surgeon General's Report, "Women and Smoking," and a 2004 Surgeon General's report offer the following information on the health effects of smoking for women: [3]

- Nearly 178,000 U.S. women die from smoking-related diseases each year.
- Smokers are twice as likely to have heart attacks and strokes, which are the leading killers of women in the U.S.
- Smoking causes almost 90 percent of all lung cancer deaths in women. It also causes 90 percent of women's deaths from chronic bronchitis and emphysema.
- Smoking also increases a woman's risk of cervical cancer, bladder cancer, head and neck cancer, pancreatic cancer, and kidney cancer. Increased rates of stomach cancer and leukemia also appear to be linked to smok-

ing. [4] Although evidence is not conclusive, scientists are beginning to suggest that there may be a link between breast cancer and smoking (including secondhand smoke).
- Smoking while undergoing treatment for cancer reduces the effectiveness of the treatment, can increase the treatment's adverse effects, causes complications with healing, increases the risk of developing a second malignancy, and decreases the overall survival rate.
- Smokers reach menopause an average of two years earlier than nonsmokers.
- Smoking increases the risk of osteoporosis and bone fractures, ulcers, and cataracts.
- Smoking interferes with healing from surgery.

Quitting smoking *at any age* can reverse the harmful effects of smoking. However, the earlier one stops, the greater the benefit.

Quitting smoking may have particular benefits for women during and after the menopause transition. Smoking increases hot flashes and mood disturbances during the menopause transition and may decrease the benefits of hormone treatment. [5] Smoking also raises our risk of developing many postmenopausal health problems mentioned above, including heart disease, osteoporosis, hip fractures, and difficulties with bone and muscle healing. [6]

As we age we are more likely to require, or elect to undergo, surgery. Quitting smoking prior to surgery is especially important because smoking increases surgical complications and slows wound healing. Smoking also has a negative effect on our quality of life, causing us to feel tired, weak, and out of breath, and reducing our strength, balance, and agility. Smoking increases facial wrinkles, causes skin to be dry and gray, and speeds the process of hair turning gray. [7]

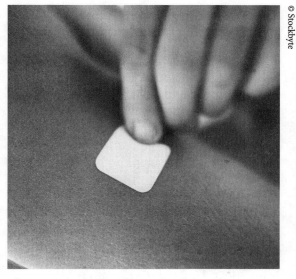

The nicotine patch is one form of assistance that increases your chance of success in quitting smoking.

QUITTING SMOKING

Despite the proven benefits of quitting, women who stop smoking around the time of menopause may find it especially challenging. We may be facing nicotine withdrawal symptoms such as depressed mood at the same time that we are coping with hot flashes or other signs of the menopause transition. We may gain more weight than women who continue to smoke; however, exercise and a healthy diet will help keep weight gain to a minimum.

Right now, I am taking care of my kids and my aging mother, who is ill. Smoking really became my only indulgence—my only time for myself. Now I realize that by using this time to smoke, I wasn't taking care of myself. In quitting smoking, I've started to learn how to say "no" to others and take care of my health first.

All women who smoke can quit, even those who have smoked for many years and those who have previously quit and started again. While nearly three out of every four smokers want to quit, it usually takes several attempts to be successful. Try not to get discouraged by temporary relapses. Focusing on the health benefits and the ways in which being a non-smoker will increase your quality of life can be important in helping you quit and maintain your success.

There are many different and effective ways for women to stop smoking. While many women choose to quit on their own, using a combination of the following methods will increase your odds of success:

- Call telephone "quit lines."
- Use self-help materials and discussion boards available on the Internet.
- Attend clinics, classes, or support groups.
- Seek counseling from health care providers or other trained counselors.
- Avoid secondhand smoke or other places/ triggers for smoking. If you live or work with people who smoke, ask them not to smoke around you.
- Avoid alcohol use, because alcohol and tobacco are often used together, and alcohol use can weaken your resolve not to smoke.
- Take medication, such as nicotine replacement (patch, gum, or lozenge, all available over the counter, or nasal inhaler or spray, available by prescription) or Zyban (a drug used to treat depression that also helps people quit smoking).

The most important thing to know about quitting smoking is that while there is no right or wrong method, using some form of assistance increases the chance of success.[8] Women seem to do best with a combination of methods that includes social support, counseling, and medication. These treatments, which are available through public programs, telephone quit lines, clinics, and hospitals, will double or triple our chances of quitting permanently. It can be helpful to try quitting during a time when you are not feeling overly stressed.

There are many resources to help you stop smoking. Look for them at your workplace, your health care provider's office, community organizations such as the American Lung Association (see www.lungusa.org), and on the Internet. You may be able to find cessation programs for women in your area. A national program called Circle of Friends helps women quit smoking and empowers nonsmokers to support women who choose to quit. Its toll-free telephone number (1-800-243-7000) provides information on how to quit smoking. Its website (www.join-the-circle.org) has information for female smokers and nonsmokers. The National Cancer Institute also provides aid to smokers who want to quit (1-800-4-CANCER or www.smokefree.gov).

Although midlife women are the largest consumers of smoking cessation resources, there are few programs targeted to us. More research is needed to target and tailor cessation programs to the needs of women going through the menopause transition.

ALCOHOL

I can't believe I am at this midpoint in my life still so unable to feel, still needing to drink and smoke to get me through, hating myself for it, feeling so unwell and miserable.

Moderate drinking appears to have beneficial health effects; it can be good for the heart and circulatory system, and probably protects against type 2 diabetes and gallstones. (For more information, see page 183.) But heavy drinking has harmful effects on our health and our lives. Almost 7 percent of U.S. women be-tween forty-five and forty-nine years old and 4 percent between fifty-five and fifty-nine report heavy drinking.[9] Heavy drinking is defined as consuming five or more alcoholic drinks on the same occasion on at least five different days in the past thirty days. The U.S. guideline for moderate drinking by women is to have no more than one drink a day.

HEALTH EFFECTS

Drinking was always part of our life. A glass of wine or two with dinner and maybe more on the weekends. When my husband and I split up and I was suddenly sad and fifty, kids gone, and all alone, a few drinks turned into a bottle of wine every night. I gained thirty pounds in one year, just from drinking! Now I was fat, fifty, and alone.

The short-term effects of alcohol can be pleasurable, but heavy use and abuse can have devastating effects on our bodies:[10]

- Alcohol can diminish motor coordination, judgment, emotional control, and reasoning power, increasing our risk of accidents and injuries and our vulnerability to violence.
- Chronic, heavy drinking can contribute to a wide range of reproductive disorders, including irregular menstrual cycles and early menopause.[11]
- Even average levels of drinking can increase the risk of mouth, esophageal, and liver cancer; major depression; epilepsy; hemorrhagic stroke; cirrhosis of the liver; and other diseases.[12]
- Women develop alcohol-related liver disease after a comparatively shorter period of heavy drinking than do men.[13] Other alcohol-related health risks that are higher for women include hypertension (high blood pressure), particularly for African-American women,

and an increased risk of osteoporosis (thinning of bones), gastric ulcers, and alcoholic hepatitis.[14]

- Some studies have linked alcohol use with increased risk for breast cancer.[15] Postmenopausal women using hormone treatment, which is a known risk factor for breast cancer, and drinking even moderate amounts of alcohol have a higher risk of developing the disease than nondrinkers who take hormone treatment.[16]
- With age, and cumulative alcohol and other drug use, our bodies have more difficulty processing mood-altering substances, increasing the risk of harmful interactions and drug tolerance.[17]

RECOGNIZING A PROBLEM

Addiction to alcohol involves both psychological and physical dependence on the drug. Signs of dependence include having withdrawal symptoms (such as depression, anxiety, irritability, nausea, sweating, and sleeping problems) when we stop using alcohol. Another sign is continuing to drink in spite of the negative effect alcohol has on our life. A third sign is what's called tolerance—the need to drink more and more to achieve the same effect.

FINDING HELP

A serious alcohol problem does not go away overnight, but with time, perseverance, self-care, and lots of support, we can recover our lives. During the menopause transition, we are often ready to look at changes we would like to make in our health and life course, and often women choose this time of life to seek treatment.

Everyone should go to treatment. I feel so lucky to have had the opportunity to spend time thinking

and talking about ME—asking for help and listening to other women's struggles. Some of it makes my choices seem easier and also I feel proud of my accomplishment and have learned to accept my shortcomings. I feel I have the tools to continue my recovery.

SELF-HELP GROUPS

When we face our problems with alcohol, probably the greatest support comes from others who have "been there." There are many self-help groups, with varying approaches, including Alcoholics Anonymous, Women for Sobriety, and 16 Steps for Discovery and Empowerment. Other self-help groups on related topics, such as self-esteem and experience of trauma, can also be helpful in combination with these recovery groups. It's worth putting some effort in to find the right combination of supports in the areas important to you; they can be critical to getting well.

Twelve-step meetings were useful for me. The stories were inspiring and helped to show how well people do who follow the program. I could see the honesty of the speakers once I identified myself as an addict.

MANAGING WITHDRAWAL

For those of us who have been using alcohol or a combination of alcohol and other drugs heavily or for a long time, it may be best to have supervision and support from health care providers when withdrawing. We may need help to relieve withdrawal symptoms and to reestablish sleep patterns, as well as to get treatment for a range of medical problems. A hospital or recovery center can be the best place to get this help. Women with HIV or those who are going through withdrawal from specific drugs, such as opiates and tranquilizers, may need further specialized care. Withdrawal symptoms are temporary; they subside once the body gets used to the absence of the substance, though the desire for the substance may last for a long time.

TYPE 2 DIABETES

Diabetes mellitus is a disease in which the body can't use sugar (glucose) properly. Ninety-five percent of people who have diabetes have type 2 diabetes (which used to be called adult-onset diabetes). Type 2 diabetes occurs when our bodies don't produce enough of the hormone insulin or become resistant to its effects. Insulin helps the body use and store glucose, keeping blood sugar at normal levels.

While type 2 diabetes is treatable, developing diabetes increases our risk for heart attack, stroke, and complications related to poor circulation. Diabetes can damage the kidneys, leading to their failure to filter out waste products. Diabetes also can cause eye problems and may lead to blindness.

DIAGNOSIS

Some people with diabetes develop symptoms that may include frequent urination, excessive thirst, pervasive fatigue, an increase in infections, blurred vision, tingling in hands or feet, and absence of menstrual periods. Many people have no symptoms at all and find out they have diabetes only through testing. One-third of adults with diabetes have type 2 diabetes but don't know it.

Diabetes is diagnosed by measuring blood sugar levels. If they are higher than normal but not yet high enough to indicate full-blown diabetes, you may have what is called prediabetes or glucose intolerance. This means you are more likely to develop diabetes and heart attack or stroke.

WHO GETS TYPE 2 DIABETES?

Women who are overweight and inactive are more likely to develop type 2 diabetes. The risk of developing diabetes can be lowered by keeping weight in control (or losing weight if you are overweight); staying active most days of the week; and eating meals high in fruits, vegetables, and whole-grain foods and low in unhealthy fats.

Other factors associated with diabetes or prediabetes include high blood pressure, low HDL cholesterol and high triglycerides, a family history of diabetes, a history of gestational diabetes (diabetes in pregnancy), giving birth to a baby weighing more than nine pounds, or belonging to an ethnic or minority group at high risk for diabetes (African-American, Asian-American, Latina, Native American, or Pacific Islander).

Age is also a factor. You are more likely to get diabetes as you get older; almost one in five people over age sixty have it. If your weight is normal and you're over age forty-five, a baseline screening test may be appropriate. If you have prediabetes or any of the risk factors mentioned above, you should be checked for type 2 diabetes every one to two years.

DIABETES TREATMENT AND MANAGEMENT

If you have prediabetes, eating healthy, nutritious foods and participating in modest physical activity regularly are recommended. A loss of just ten to fifteen pounds can delay the onset of diabetes or reduce the amount of medication you may need.

If you have type 2 diabetes, its progression can often be controlled by diet and exercise.

Maintaining fitness and a healthy weight will improve your chances of controlling diabetes. Eat properly before working out, because exercise will lower your blood sugar levels. (For more information on exercise, see Chapter 13, "Staying Active"; for more information on a healthy diet, see Chapter 12, "Eating Well.")

If diet and exercise alone do not control the disease, oral medications are usually prescribed. People with type 2 diabetes sometimes need insulin. It is especially important for people with diabetes to reduce other risk factors for a heart attack or stroke, such as high cholesterol and hypertension. (For more information about diabetes and heart health, see Chapter 17, "Heart Health.")

MIGRAINE HEADACHES

Headaches are one of the most common problems for women of all ages. It is thought that the majority of headaches are migraines, experienced by about 20 percent of women and 7 percent of men.[18] Migraines appear to be related to the spasm or contraction of blood vessels, which temporarily decreases blood flow to the brain. During the menopause transition, fluctuating hormones may aggravate existing migraines, cause migraines to recur after a time when they have been absent, or cause migraines for the first time in women without previous headaches. After menopause, about two-thirds of women with migraines will find that our headaches disappear or improve.[19]

Only about half of all migraine sufferers are evaluated, correctly diagnosed, and appropriately treated.[20] Migraines may be underdiagnosed partly because many migraines are not severe and also because the symptoms may not be consistent with what people think of as migraine. This is true for health care providers as well as for the general public. Often mild migraines are misdiagnosed as tension or sinus headaches, because they sometimes accompany or are triggered by tension or sinus symptoms. Also, many of us with migraines find relief with over-the-counter medication, so we do not seek further treatment. New headaches, or headaches that change in type, severity, or frequency, should be evaluated to be sure that there is not a more serious underlying cause.

WHAT IS A MIGRAINE?

Migraines are recurring headache attacks that last between four and seventy-two hours and are accompanied by nausea, vomiting, or sensitivity to light and noise.[21] Migraines often occur mostly on one side, involve a throbbing or pulsating quality, are of moderate or severe intensity (such that they inhibit or prohibit daily activities), and are aggravated by walking up stairs or other similar physical activity.

Migraines can occur with or without *auras,* which are visual or neurological symptoms experienced before the headache.[22] Auras are most often visual, usually consisting of zigzags, dots, or flashing lights across the visual field, or of patches of vision that disappear. These phenomena usually develop gradually over a few minutes, last less than an hour, and then disappear completely. Symptoms that do not completely disappear or that last more than an hour should be evaluated to rule out a more serious cause.

WARNING SYMPTOMS OF MIGRAINES

Common warning symptoms are mood shifts, such as feeling unusually happy or sad; unusual thirst or hunger, including food cravings; drowsiness; increased feelings of stress; fatigue or excessive energy; upset stomach; and increased sensitivity to noise or bright lights. Other signs of impending headaches, which may occur up to a few hours before headache onset, include feelings of facial fullness, nasal stuffiness, and neck discomfort. Menstrual migraines may also be predictable, since many women experience headaches before or during our periods.

I got them for one year in my twenties when I first started using birth control pills. They are back now at menopause with a thirty-year hiatus in between. I get them over my eyes and throughout the top of my head. When they go unrelieved, I sit over the vaporizer or in the bathroom with the shower on.

Headaches can vary in intensity and frequency, even for the same person. Sometimes headaches are mild and easily treated with over-the-counter medication, but at other times they may be more severe. Migraines that are accompanied by a stiff or painful neck may be diagnosed as tension headaches. Nasal congestion or facial discomfort with headache may be interpreted as a sinus headache. Some experts now think that all these headaches may be migraines.[23]

Many people think that migraines always cause severe pain, or that a headache is not a migraine unless there is also an aura (see "What Is a Migraine?" page 285). This means that milder headaches and migraines without aura (which are more common) are often not accurately diagnosed.

TRIGGERS

The most common triggers that stimulate migraines are stress, weather changes, alcohol, changes in dietary or sleep patterns, and hormonal fluctuations, which cause "menstrual migraines" in some women. Other factors, such as caffeine, aged cheese, bright lights, exertion, smoke, and noise, may also be triggers for some people. Triggers can be difficult to identify, as it may be twenty-four to forty-eight hours between the trigger and the headache. Also, a particular factor may trigger a headache at some times but at other times may not. Many women have migraines when we are premenstrual but have them less often at other times.

EARLY WARNING SYMPTOMS

In addition to specific factors that can trigger a migraine, there are also warning symptoms that women are often able to identify as being predictors of an upcoming migraine. For women who can identify these warning symptoms, about half of all migraines may be prevented, if known triggers are then avoided.[24] For example, if a woman knows that feeling a little "down" and needing sunglasses even when the weather is overcast are signs that she may have a migraine within twenty-four hours, she may make a special effort to avoid migraine triggers that day. She might reduce her stress level; perhaps she would skip a glass of wine that night and get a good night's sleep. It is also possible to take medications for migraines early when a headache is predicted, and thus prevent the headache from becoming severe.

I will often start with a very low-grade, what I call prodromal-type [warning] ache. Then, the headache may increase in severity as the day goes on, or I may continue all day with this low-grade ache that is annoying but doesn't require medication. Then, the next day, it may hit full force. When I first started having the migraines, I ignored the ones that started in my neck or affected both sides of my head. I discounted them as tension or sinus headaches and tried to treat them with over-the-counter medications. It was several years later that I actually saw a neurologist who told me they were all *migraines, and I should treat them as such.*

MIGRAINE TREATMENTS

Self-Treatments

The familiar home remedies for migraines include "sleeping the headache off," lying still in a dark room, and avoiding bright lights, noise, and smoky environments. Acupuncture and biofeedback have also been found to be effective for some people.[25] A daily headache diary can help to identify patterns between triggers and headaches. In a diary, you can note such events as the dates of your period, intake of alcohol or other possible food triggers, daily stress level, occurrence and severity of headaches, and effectiveness of particular treatments.

Medications for Acute Treatment and Prevention

Medications for migraines can be thought of as being either for acute treatment of headache pain or for prevention (treatment of the underlying causes of the headaches). Medication for prevention is used daily by women who have very frequent headaches (usually more than two or three per month) or have severe headaches. For mild to moderately severe migraines, over-the-counter medications have been found to be effective. These include *nonsteroidal anti-inflammatory drugs (NSAIDs),* such as aspirin, ibuprofen, and naproxen sodium. Caffeine can also be helpful; however, sometimes too much caffeine can make the headache worse.

Medications for acute treatment are more effective when used early. Earlier treatment also leads to less severe headaches and fewer accompanying symptoms. Sometimes we are reluctant to treat a headache until we are sure it is a migraine, but this often allows the headache to become more severe and makes treatment less effective.

The simplest treatment is high-dose NSAIDs, which are effective for many women. Of all the prescription medications that are used to treat acute headaches, the newest and

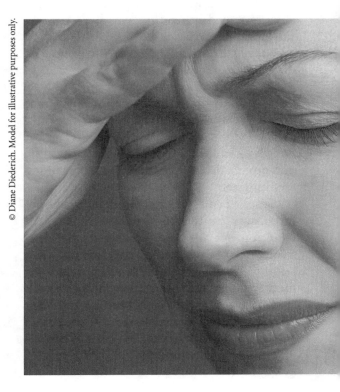

© Diane Diederich. Model for illustrative purposes only.

most widely used is a group of medications called *triptans*. All of these drugs fall into two categories: those that take effect more quickly and wear off more quickly, and those that take longer to take effect but are effective longer. The drugs also vary with regard to adverse effects, and so choice of triptan depends on the individual woman. Triptans can be administered by different routes: for example, sumatriptan may be taken as a pill, by injection, or in a nasal spray. Rizatriptan can be taken as a disintegrating tablet, dissolving in the mouth.

The triptans have been found to be safe and effective in relieving the suffering of many people who have migraines. However, for a woman who has heart disease or who is at high risk for heart disease, triptans may not be the best choice. Evaluation of this risk is especially important for perimenopausal and postmenopausal women, since our risk for heart disease goes up with age. Triptans are not usually prescribed in women over sixty-five, because of this increased risk.

Other treatments for acute migraine pain include the ergotamines, which because of their risks and adverse effects are now used less often than triptans. Also, narcotics are still used, but they should be avoided when possible and used only under careful monitoring, as there is a high risk of dependency. Narcotics are not more effective for migraines than other medications.

Some medications for acute headaches (even over-the-counter drugs) should not be used more than twice a week, since more frequent usage may lead to daily *rebound headaches*.[26] As the rebound headaches become more frequent, they often become more severe. This can lead a person to need medications daily, increasing the frequency and severity of headaches in a vicious circle.

Preventive medications, which can help to avoid or treat migraines and rebound migraines, are usually taken every day. Most preventive medications are safe and can be used at dosage levels that control headaches but have minimal negative effects. Both riboflavin (B2, 400 mg per day) and magnesium (300 mg per day) have been found to be effective preventive nonprescription medications. Both are safe and have few adverse effects, although magnesium may cause diarrhea. Either or both of these medications can be used preventively for migraines, alone or with prescription drugs. Another over-the-counter drug is coenzyme Q10 (150 mg per day), which is also safe and may be effective, although it is more expensive.

A number of prescription medications are effective for preventing migraines. The drugs that are most often used for this purpose are antihypertensives, such as beta-blockers and calcium channel blockers; anticonvulsants; and antidepressants, both tricyclics and selective serotonin reuptake inhibitors (SSRIs). It may take several weeks to several months to tell whether a given medication will improve headaches, and dosage adjustments may be needed during that time. Keeping a headache diary makes it easier to tell if the medication is effective.

I carry my medicine with me everywhere I go. . . . You know, you try not to run out. But sometimes it's gonna happen. . . . It reminds me of carrying tampons so that you don't start your period off someplace. Yes, yes! So, all we have done is traded tampons for pills.

Migraines and Hormones

Many perimenopausal women with migraines use hormone treatment or oral contraceptives without problems. For the individual woman, hormones or oral contraceptives may help migraines or may make them worse. Both hormone treatment and oral contraceptives are less likely to worsen headaches if they are used in low, consistent doses. A woman who has aura with her migraines should consider avoiding oral contraceptives, as having migraine with aura has been found to increase the risk of stroke with oral contraceptives.[27]

Treatment Decisions

The first level of response to migraines includes self-help strategies such as stress management, eating well, exercising regularly, and learning how to avoid your triggers and respond to your warning symptoms. You may want to try over-the-counter medications or, if you need more help, seek acupuncture or consult with your health care provider. If you experience frequent or severe migraines, consulting a neurologist with expertise in managing women's migraines may be beneficial. Migraine treatment is optimal when the woman experiencing the headaches is in an active partnership with her health care provider, keeping diaries for headache patterns and triggers, and tracking which medications helped, how soon they helped, and how effective they were.

Keeping Headaches in Perspective

Women going through the menopause transition often juggle complicated schedules, carrying heavy work responsibilities, managing adolescent children, and caring for aging parents. For many of us, it is not possible to go to bed when we have headaches, although that is where we would rather be. It is necessary to keep going, even when our productivity level is lower and we feel awful. As one woman put it, "If I called in sick every time I had a headache, I would be without a job."

Usually our partners, families, and coworkers are understanding and supportive of our unpredictable, disruptive headaches. However, there is still a common attitude that women use headaches to avoid responsibilities or "give in"

to the headache when we might be able to overcome it. Many of us have internalized this sense that we are responsible for our headaches, even when we know that this is not true.

I sometimes see myself as weak because of this predisposition I have. I don't tell a lot of people about my migraines for fear of sounding like a whiner.

Being able to prevent and treat our headaches effectively, while at the same time continuing to enjoy life in spite of them, is the challenge facing those of us who have migraines. Migraines are rapidly becoming better understood, and more effective medications are being developed. For the individual woman, understanding her headache patterns and finding effective ways to prevent and treat her headaches can make it possible to maintain balance through the menopause transition.

I started having headaches at ten years old. The headaches have been a constant part of my life. If I go a week without a headache, it is great. If I go two weeks without a headache, it is wonderful and very rare. I guess I deal with it like any other disability. I won't stop living and can't afford to miss work.

JOINT HEALTH

With aging, we experience natural wear and tear on muscles and joints. One cause of aches and pains is arthritis, or inflammation of the joints. There are over a hundred different forms of arthritis, some hereditary, some autoimmune, and some aggravated by other conditions. Osteoarthritis, also called degenerative joint disease, is the most common type. It occurs when the cartilage that protects our joints loses its elasticity and wears away. Osteoarthritis can be related to repetitive stress from work, walking, or prior injury to bones and joints. Immune-mediated arthritis diseases (sometimes called inflammatory arthritis) such as rheumatoid arthritis affect a much smaller segment of the population than osteoarthritis and may lead to total body fatigue, stiffness, and swelling.

While arthritis is often diagnosed around the time of menopause, it is not clear if the hormone changes of menopause contribute to it.

DRY EYE AND VISION CHANGES

We experience dry eyes when tear glands cannot make enough tears or produce poor-quality tears. Allergies can also contribute to eye dryness, which can be uncomfortable. Allergies and dry eye increase with age. Certain medications can affect your tear output and cause dry eye. Over-the-counter artificial tears that lubricate the eye are the main treatment for dry eyes.

At age forty, it is important to start getting your eyes examined every one to two years, or more often if you have vision problems, a family history of eye problems, former eye injuries, or diabetes.

As we age, we lose the ability to see close objects or small print clearly. This is a normal process that happens slowly over a lifetime. Some of us find we need reading glasses, or bifocals or progressive lenses, which combine two prescriptions into one pair of glasses. (The upper half of bifocals and progressive lenses corrects distance vision and the bottom half corrects close-up vision.)

HEARING LOSS

Those of us who grew up listening to loud music or who are exposed to loud sounds on the job may find our hearing failing. Cells and nerves in the inner ear are destroyed by continuous or repeated exposure to loud noises.

Hearing loss is rarely painful. The symptoms are usually vague feelings of pressure or fullness in the ears, speech that seems to be muffled or far away, and a ringing sound in the ears that you notice when you are in quiet places. The first sign of a noise-induced hearing loss is failing to hear high-pitched sounds.

To prevent hearing loss, reduce your exposure to loud sounds as much as possible. Develop the habit of wearing earplugs when you know you will be exposed to noise for a long time. Keep television sets, stereos, and headsets low in volume. If you are regularly exposed to loud noise at work or play, you are at risk for hearing loss and should have your hearing tested every year.

GUM AND DENTAL PROBLEMS

Taking care of our teeth and gums by brushing, flossing, and getting regular cleanings and checkups is important in preventing disease and decay (cavities in the teeth).

Gum disease is a chronic infection of the tissues supporting the teeth. Warning signs include gums that bleed easily, are red, swollen, and tender, or have pulled away from the teeth; persistent bad breath or bad taste; permanent teeth that are loose or separating; any change in the way your teeth fit together when you bite; and any change in the fit of partial dentures.

Gum disease begins when the bacteria in plaque (the colorless, sticky material that forms on your teeth) irritate the gums and cause them to swell. In more advanced phases, the disease is known as periodontitis. The bacteria go under the gum line, eventually attacking the tissues and bone around the teeth. This can lead to tooth loss. Treatment may include special cleanings under the gum line and, in more advanced cases, surgery.

Regular checkups can help detect, prevent, and treat cavities, gum disease, and other dental problems. The American Dental Association recommends the following for optimal oral health:[28]

- Brush your teeth twice a day with an ADA-accepted fluoride toothpaste.
- Clean between teeth daily with floss or an interdental cleaner.
- Eat a balanced mix of foods and limit between-meal snacks.
- Visit your dentist regularly for professional cleanings and oral exams.

THYROID CONDITIONS

When I was diagnosed with hypothyroidism, I was put on medication to bring it to normal levels. I was extremely tired and very sluggish. You are so sluggish that you don't retain things well. There is hair loss and brittle nails. Other people experience sweating and weight gain. Doctors treated it by administering a synthetic hormone, putting the thyroid hormone back into my body. Now it is under control. Diagnosing it is the hardest part. Some people don't know it could be your thyroid.

We are more likely to develop thyroid problems as we age. Women also are more likely than men to have thyroid problems. The thyroid gland is located at the base of your neck in front of your trachea (or windpipe). It has two sides and is shaped like a butterfly. It regulates metabolism and can be involved in certain forms of reversible dementia.

If there is not enough thyroid hormone in the bloodstream, the body's metabolism slows down. This is called **hypothyroidism** (underactive thyroid). Symptoms of hypothyroidism include weight gain, hair thinning, weakness,

and mental confusion. In most cases, hypothyroidism is treated with medication that contains thyroid hormone.

If there is too much thyroid hormone, your metabolism speeds up. This is called **hyperthyroidism** (overactive thyroid). Symptoms of hyperthyroidism include tachycardia (fast and sometimes irregular heartbeat), protruding eyes and other eye changes, nervousness, and anxiety. Treatment for hyperthyroidism will lower the amount of thyroid hormone and relieve your symptoms.

Symptoms of thyroid problems are sometimes mistakenly thought to be signs of the menopause transition. Also, changing estrogen levels due to menopause or hormone treatment can complicate the measurement of thyroid hormone levels, making diagnosis of thyroid problems more difficult. If you have symptoms of thyroid disease, learn more about the condition from your health care provider and other sources, and consider being tested.

NOTES

1. Centers for Disease Control and Prevention, "Cigarette Smoking among Adults—United States 2003," *Morbidity & Mortality Weekly Report* 54, no. 20 (2005): 509–13.

2. Greaves, Lorraine, *Smoke Screen: Women's Smoking and Social Control* (Halifax, Canada: Fenwood Publishing, 1996).

3. U.S. Department of Health and Human Services, Centers for Disease Control and Prevention, "The Health Consequences of Smoking: A Report of the Surgeon General" (Rockville, MD, 2004); see also U.S. Department of Health and Human Services, "Women and Smoking: A Report of the Surgeon General" (Rockville, MD, 2001).

4. U.S. Department of Health and Human Services, Centers for Disease Control and Prevention, "The Health Consequences of Smoking."

5. U.S. Department of Health and Human Services, "Women and Smoking."

6. Ibid.

7. Ibid.

8. Fiore M. C., W. C. Bailey, S. J. Cohen, et al., "Treating Tobacco Use and Dependence," U.S. Department of Health and Human Services, Public Health Services (Rockville, MD, 2000).

9. *National Survey on Drug Use and Health,* Office of Applied Statistics, Substance Abuse and Mental Health Services Administration, U.S. Department of Health and Human Services, 2003, accessed at www.oas.samhsa.gov/nhsda.htm on June 15, 2005.

10. National Institute on Alcohol Abuse and Alcoholism, *Alcohol, A Women's Health Issue.* August 2003: Rockville, MD.

11. National Institute on Alcohol Abuse and Alcoholism, "Alcohol and Hormones," *Alcohol Alert* 26 (October 1994); see also Mary Ann Emanuele, Frederick Wezeman, and Nicholas V. Emanuele, "Alcohol's Effects on Female Reproductive Function," *Alcohol Research and Health: The Journal of the National Institute on Alcohol Abuse and Alcoholism* 26, no. 4 (2003): 274–81.

12. Jürgen Rehm, Robin Room, Kathryn Graham, Maristela Monteiro, Gerhard Gmel, and Christopher T. Sempos, "The Relationship of Average Volume of Alcohol Consumption and Patterns of Drinking to Burden of Disease: An Overview," *Addiction* 98, no. 9 (2003): 1209–28.

13. National Institute on Alcohol Abuse and Alcoholism. "Alcoholic Liver Disease," *Alcohol Alert* 64 (January 2005).

14. "Women and Alcohol: An Update," *Alcohol Research & Health: The Journal of the National Institute on Alcohol Abuse and Alcoholism* 26, no. 4 (2002).

15. National Cancer Institute, *Breast Cancer Prevention: Summary of Evidence,* 2005.

16. Petri, Anette Lykke, Anne Tjonneland, Michael Gamborg, Ditte Johansen, Susanne Hoidrup, Thorkild Sorensen, I. A., and Morten Gronbaek, "Alcohol Intake, Type of Beverage, and Risk of Breast Cancer in Pre- and Postmenopausal Women," *Alcoholism: Clinical and Experimental Research* 28, no. 7 (July 2004): 1084–90; see also Dorgan, Joanne F., David J. Baer, Paul S. Albert, Joseph T. Judd, Ellen D. Brown, Donald K. Corle, William S. Campbell, Terryl J. Hartman, Aliya A. Tejpar, Beverly A. Clevidence, Carol A. Giffen, Donald W. Chandler, and Philip R. Taylor, "Serum Hormones and Alcohol–Breast Cancer Association in Postmenopausal Women," *Journal of the National Cancer Institute* 93, no. 9 (2001): 710–16.

17. "Women and Alcohol: An Update," *Alcohol Research & Health: The Journal of the National Institute on Alcohol Abuse and Alcoholism* 26, no. 4 (2002).

18. Richard B. Lipton, Walter F. Stewart, Seymour Diamond, Merle Diamond, and Michael Reed, "Prevalence and Burden of Migraine in the United States: Data from the American Migraine Study II," *Headache* 41, no. 7 (2001): 646–57.

19. Iria Neri, Franco Granella, Rossella Nappi, Gian C. Manzoni, F. Facchinetti, and A. R. Genazzani, "Characteristics of Headache at Menopause: A Clinico-Epidemiologic Study," *Maturitas* 17, no. 1 (1993): 31–37.

20. Richard B. Lipton, Walter F. Stewart, and David Simon, "Medical Consultation for Migraine: Results from the American Migraine Study," *Headache* 38, no. 2 (1998): 87–96.

21. The Headache Classification Committee of the International Headache Society, "Classification and Diagnostic Criteria for Headache Disorders, Cranial Neuralgias, and Facial Pain," *Cephalalgia* 8, supplement 7 (1988): 1–97.

22. Ibid.

23. Roger Cady, Curtis Schreiber, Kathleen Farmer, and Fred Sheftell, "Primary Headaches: A Convergence Hypothesis," *Headache* 42, no. 3 (2002): 204–16.

24. N. J. Giffin, L. Ruggiero, Richard B. Lipton, Stephen D. Silberstein, J. F. Tvedskov, J. Olesen, J. Altman, Peter J. Goadsby, and A. Macrae, "Premonitory Symptoms in Migraine: An Electronic Diary Study," *Neurology* 60, no. 6 (2003): 935–40.

25. William B. Young, Stephen D. Silberstein, and Jeffrey

M. Dayno, "Migraine Treatment," *Seminars in Neurology* 17, no. 4 (1997): 325–33.

26. Stephen D. Silberstein and Dongmei Liu, "Drug Overuse and Rebound Headache," *Current Pain and Headache Reports* 6, no. 3 (2002): 240–47.

27. Stephen D. Silberstein, "Headache and Female Hormones: What You Need to Know," *Current Opinion in Neurology* 14, no. 3 (2001): 323–33.

28. American Academy of Periodontology, "Periodontal Disease," June 11, 2004, accessed at www.perio.org/consumer/2a.html on August 17, 2005.

Knowledge Is Power

CHAPTER 20

The Politics of Women's Health

Our health as we go through the menopause transition depends on many factors, including how our society values postmenopausal women and how we fare in a health care system that focuses more on curing disease and making profit than on maintaining well-being and providing health care for all.

Women's health involves more than physical changes to our bodies and the related medical care we receive. Our health is affected by the social, economic, political, and cultural context of our lives. To enjoy optimum health as we go through the menopause transition, we need supportive living conditions: an unpolluted environment, decent housing, good nutrition, adequate income from honest and satisfying work, retirement security, and access to long-term care and safety. We need policies, programs, and cultural attitudes that recognize the diverse needs of women's lives and supports us through menopause and beyond.

At least 33 million women in the United States will be between forty and fifty-five years old, the average age range when menopause occurs, by the year 2010.[1] A number of younger women who experience early menopause can be added to that large population. We have the political clout to advocate for changes that will support women's health.

I am well aware that I am part of the largest cohort of women going through menopause in the history of our country. I am excited about our potential to feel good and

accepting of ourselves as we age, supporting each other, questioning ageist attitudes and anti-aging marketing pressures and advocating for policies that support us all.

BARRIERS TO GETTING GOOD HEALTH CARE

Access to high-quality health care is an important issue for women. We often coordinate health care for our families and have primary responsibility for medical decisions, and we use the system more than men. Yet women at menopause face many barriers to getting good health care.

MEDICALIZATION AND MARKETING

Menopause, like childbirth, aging, and other biological events and transitions in women's lives, has become medicalized. We are encouraged to see this normal life change as a medical problem requiring medical interventions and chronic use of medications. This view helps convince healthy women that we need a pharmacological fix to cope with menopause, look and feel good, and prevent the diseases of aging. (For more information on medicalization, see page 8.)

DISCRIMINATION AND HEALTH DISPARITIES

Our health is negatively affected by being older women in a culture that values youth. (For more information about ageism and sexism, see page 7.) Disparities due to race, class, and sexual identity also take a toll on our health and life expectancy. Studies show there are racial disparities in the delivery of health care and in health outcomes,[2] and higher income or college degrees do not necessarily protect against health disparities. Black women over fifty-four years old are only half as likely as white women to have a mammogram ordered by a doctor.[3] Women of color have higher mortality rates for conditions such as diabetes, obesity, breast cancer, heart disease, and cerebrovascular disease and get less screening and treatment.[4] Reducing disparities in access to health care and treatment is essential for women of color to stay healthy through the menopause transition and beyond.

Discrimination against lesbian and bisexual women and transgender people, including the presumption that everyone is straight and fits traditional gender norms, profoundly affects quality of life, health, and health care as well. Eliminating such discrimination is crucial to improving health.

LOW INCOME AND LACK OF INSURANCE

Money and status tend to determine who receives good health care. The wealthy are more likely to be healthy and tend to live longer.[5] This is bad news for women, who are disproportionately poor. The highest rates of poverty in the United States are found among single women raising children and women of color. Even those of us who are working full-time often do not earn enough to keep out of poverty.[6] If we are poor, we experience less control over the circumstances of our lives: We may be overworked, inadequately housed, malnourished, sleep-deprived, and stressed, with little energy or time to take the preventive measures needed to maintain our health.

Nearly one in five American women does not have medical insurance.[7] Women are less likely than men to be covered by employer-sponsored insurance, which is the basis of much medical care coverage. Low-income women and women of color are more likely to work in jobs that don't provide this benefit. Midlife women are more likely than men to take time out from work for caregiving, work in low-paid jobs, work part-time and not be eligible for benefits, be unemployed and out of the workforce, or work for companies that don't offer benefits.

I am fifty-five and have been self-employed in a consulting business I started. . . . All my money is going for living expenses and building my business, and I can't afford health insurance. When I have had medical problems, I have gone to the hospital emergency room, which I feel uncomfortable about. I worry all the time that I will have a major medical emergency and not be able to afford treatment. Also, I know I am not getting the screening and annual checkups that I need.

Uninsured and underinsured women are at higher risk for disease than privately insured women and women insured by Medicaid, the federal program that pays for medical care for the poor. The uninsured are three times as likely as the insured to postpone seeking care, not have a good baseline from which to diagnose illness, not get needed care or fill prescriptions, and not follow up on treatment, which raises risk for serious illness, disability, and death.[8]

Women in midlife who develop a serious health problem or chronic condition and are not eligible for Medicare are particularly vulnerable. (Medicare covers people who are over sixty-five or have certain disabilities; for more information, see page 300.) Federal legislation (COBRA, the Consolidated Omnibus Budget Reconciliation Act) allows the unemployed, people on family leave for caregiving, divorced or widowed women, and spouses of retirees the right to stay on their own, their partner's, or their former partner's group plan for eighteen months, but doing so is expensive.

Although [I was] divorced fourteen years ago, my children and I were covered by my ex-husband's medical insurance. A month ago, he lost his job and health insurance. I can't afford it on my limited salary and will not be eligible for benefits on any insurance he gets from a new job.

A philosophy of self-help may be empowering for some, but it puts an unfair burden of blame on individuals for inequities caused by socially created health problems. Having economic security in midlife and retirement, reducing or eliminating the gender gap in wages and benefits, and guaranteeing health care coverage would contribute to better health for all women.

THE U.S. HEALTH CARE SYSTEM

In recent decades, medical care in the United States has shifted increasingly toward being a profit-making industry. This system comprises for-profit medical institutions, pharmaceutical and hospital-supply industries, and insurance/managed care corporations. Corporations now have more control over the delivery of care than doctors or government.[9]

The cost of managing these corporate entities; the administrative expenses of billing and insurance; expenses for scientific research, drug development, and new technologies; protection against litigation; and the profit motive are driving up costs of medical care. Fifteen percent of premiums paid to private insurers goes to funding administrative bureaucracy. The administrative costs of public programs such as Medicare and Medicaid use only 4 percent of premiums paid in.[10]

As a nation, we are facing a health care crisis. The United States spends more on health care than any other industrialized country in the world. In 2003, 15 percent of the U.S. gross domestic product went for health and medical care.[11] This amounted to $5,635 per person per year, about twice the total expenses in health per capita in Sweden, Canada, Japan, or Great Britain.[12] U.S. consumers pay more for services and medications, yet we have shorter, less frequent physician visits and shorter hospital stays than consumers in other countries,[13] and many countries have better health outcomes. The United States lags behind other industrialized countries in life expectancy and in infant mortality rates.[14]

The driving motive in the current health care system is profit, and the need to reduce costs and maximize profits often conflicts with a commitment to providing optimal health care. As for-profit managed care has become more widespread, with more abuses and unfair denials of care, there is a need for more government regulation and for expanded access to health care for all. Lately, doctors have begun to organize in protest against insurance companies' telling them how to practice medicine and limiting what they can do or prescribe. A few doctors are trying to reduce administrative costs and cumbersome paperwork by lowering their fees and not taking insurance. As consumers, we need increasingly to challenge the power of corporate health care management and make the system accountable for our health care needs.

GOVERNMENT INSURANCE: MEDICARE AND MEDICAID

There are two major programs of federal government medical insurance designed to help people in need: Medicare and Medicaid. **Medicare** was established in 1965 under the Social Security Act to provide medical insur-

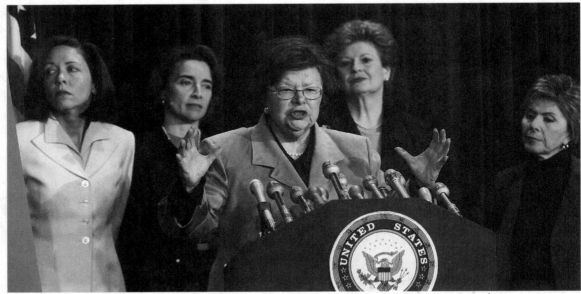

© Associated Press

Senator Barbara Mikulski of Maryland (center) holds a press conference on Capitol Hill in Washington, D.C., in 2005, to discuss proposed Social Security reforms. She is joined by fellow senators (L-R) Maria Cantwell of Washington, Blanche Lambert Lincoln of Arkansas, Debbie Stabenow of Michigan, and Barbara Boxer of California. Without Social Security income, a majority of women over the age of sixty-five would be living in poverty.

ance for people who are sixty-five years old and older and some younger people with disabilities. The other government health insurance program is **Medicaid,** which pays for medical care for poor people.

While these programs provide important coverage, they have limitations, and proposed changes threaten the current benefits. (For more information about Medicare, see "Medicare and Women's Health" at www.ourbodies ourselves.org.)

Medicaid is essential to women's health, since 70 percent of Medicaid beneficiaries are women.[15] This program provides more than 2.5 million women between the ages of forty-five and sixty-four with health care coverage.[16] Yet in half the states, a woman with two children working full-time at minimum wage earns too much to qualify for Medicaid. Cuts in federal shares of the program would mean increased pressure on the states to cover eligible women. States would inevitably reduce services and raise eligibility requirements, and the number of uninsured would go up.

SUPPORTING WOMEN'S HEALTH THROUGH MENOPAUSE AND BEYOND

REFORMING THE HEALTH CARE SYSTEM

With the skyrocketing costs of our medical care, limited medical insurance coverage, disparities in health care services, and discriminating attitudes, our health care system is in crisis and needs reform. The debate centers on whether government should provide universal health insurance for all (called a *single-payer* system); employers should offer insurance as a benefit, with private insurance companies continuing to manage the cost of care through market-based competition; or individuals should be left to choose their own health care and insurance and bear most of the burden of paying for it themselves. Market competition and employer-based health insurance are not more cost-effective than government-funded insurance. The rhetoric of choice in the marketplace masks the reality that many people, including many women at midlife, have no realistic options to pay for health care. The current U.S. system seems to be leading to higher costs, huge discrepancies between rich and poor, and lower-quality health care.[17]

Universal health insurance could lower health care costs.[18] We would no longer have to depend on our work status or our savings for insurance, and we could have continuous access to health care, whether we change jobs, work for small companies, take time off for caregiving, work part-time or at home, or are unemployed. The savings could exceed $200 billion a year, far more than the cost of covering all the uninsured.[19] Although a 2003 poll showed that two-thirds of the public is in favor of the U.S. government guaranteeing medical insurance for all citizens,[20] the power and organization of the medical establishment, the private insurance industry, and drug companies together have thus far successfully opposed reform. Local, state, and federal legislators continue to propose single-payer laws that would be financed like Medicare. Indeed, the Medicare program offers a model that could be expanded into a national health insurance system.

Universal single-payer coverage is probably not going to happen right away, but there are some improvements that could be made right now. Increased coverage could be offered through employer-based insurance, including job-based coverage for part-time workers. Medicaid eligibility requirements could be broadened on the state and federal level to cover women with earnings up to 200 percent of poverty level. Medicare could offer buy-ins for

IMPORTANT GAPS IN KNOWLEDGE
ABOUT THE MENOPAUSE TRANSITION

While scientific understanding of menopause has increased over the years, much remains to be learned. Assessing the knowledge base and identifying important gaps in understanding about the menopause transition were the primary goals of the National Institutes of Health State-of-the-Science (SoS) Conference on Management of Menopause-Related Symptoms, held in March 2005. The conference's independent panel evaluated the risks and benefits of estrogen with or without a progestin as well as other hormonal and nonhormonal strategies for management of short-term symptoms associated with the menopause transition.

The SoS Conference Panel concluded that there was adequate evidence to classify hot flashes, night sweats, vaginal dryness, and sleep disturbances occurring in midlife women as "menopausal" symptoms.[21] Yet it found considerable ambiguity over whether other complaints that are sometimes associated with the menopause transition, such as decreased sexual desire, depression, cognitive difficulties, and urinary problems, are due to menopause and aging changes in ovarian function or are due instead to aging in general. The panel determined that more research is needed to understand when menopausal symptoms appear, why some women suffer greatly from them while others do not, how long menopausal symptoms last and what influences their severity, and how the menopause transition affects subsequent quality of life and healthy aging. More studies on how health problems experienced at midlife are affected by a broad range of biological factors (including but not limited to ovarian aging) and by the socio-cultural environment are also needed.[22]

Although estrogen treatment is highly effective in relieving hot flashes and vaginal dryness associated with the menopause transition, recent studies have shown that certain oral regimens using conjugated equine estrogens increase the risks of cardiovascular disease, stroke, blood clots, breast cancer, and dementia. Therefore, there has been a growing interest in other options: bioidentical hormones, androgens such as testosterone, botanical products (such as phytoestrogens and black cohosh), and other complementary and alternative medicine strategies, such as acupuncture, homeopathy, and exercises (such as paced respiration). However the benefits of such strategies are often minimal or uncertain and/or the risks are poorly understood. Recently, positive preliminary results in managing hot flashes have been reported with nonhormonal pharmaceuticals, including gabapentin and antidepressants (such as venlafaxine and paroxetine). However, the risks of these agents need to be rigorously evaluated in clinical trials. More research on promising behavioral regimens and botanicals as well as new drug development and testing is needed to pinpoint effective strategies and understand adverse effects and safety issues. New customized options to relieve problems associated with the menopause transition and improve women's quality of life will be welcomed by the millions of women experiencing or approaching this milestone.

uninsured women ages fifty-five to sixty-four (13 percent of uninsured women). Hospitals and doctors could accept payments from uninsured patients on a sliding scale adjusted to income. The states could subsidize health insurance plans that would cover basic care, at rates that working people who earn too much to qualify for Medicaid could afford, or the states could set up programs to cover the uninsured.

Women's health care activists have developed a list of features required for health care reform policy to reduce disparities and increase access to all:[23]

Affordability

- Finance health care through government insurance to achieve universal coverage.
- Control costs through streamlined administration, elimination of profits, control over fraud and advertising, and price limits on health-care providers.
- Reduce profits on prescription drugs and focus drug industry research on new treatments instead of profitable copies of existing drugs.

Fair treatment

- Eliminate discrimination against women and all populations confronting geographic, physical, cultural, language, and other barriers to service.

Accountability

- Involve health care users, women, and communities in administration and policy decision making in health care administration and policy making.
- Guarantee provider accountability and the right to sue for grievances.
- Assure confidentiality of medical records.
- Establish our right of ownership over our genetic material and control over who has access to our genetic information.

Comprehensive benefits

- Provide a package responsive to women's needs, including coverage for wellness visits, gynecological/reproductive health, occupa-

tional and environmental health, prescription drugs, mental health, dental care, and long-term care.

Effective planning

- Require consumer participation with ongoing evaluation and planning of the delivery of health services.

Support for public health

- Invest in and recognize public health programs.

High quality of care

- Improve the quality of medical care for all of us.
- Train health professionals in the economic, cultural, psychological, and social (race/gender/age, etc.) determinants of health and effective caregiving for different populations.
- Assess and evaluate medical technology and make results available to the public.
- Provide access to high-quality, unbiased women's health information.

Support for health care workers

- Support education, training, employment, and promotion of professional and other health care workers. Assure advancement of female workers and clinicians who represent diverse communities and provide quality care at all levels.

Social/economic policies

- Direct health institutes to research and implement social and economic policies that improve women's health, including protection of occupational safety and health.

ECONOMIC SECURITY: END GENDER DISCRIMINATION

Since economic status has such a large impact on women's health and access to health care, we need to make sure that every working woman earns a decent wage and acknowledge the diverse work and family patterns in people's lives. Even thirty-five years after the passage of the Equal Pay Act, women are paid 77 percent of what our male counterparts earn, get lower-paying full-time jobs, and have less pension coverage.[24] In 2003, African-American women earned 66 percent of the average of all men's earnings, and Latinas 55 percent.[25] Women are more likely to be part-time or temporary employees with few benefits and no health insurance. Only 53 percent of working Americans can expect to get pensions,[26] and coverage rates are lower for women than men and for part-time workers compared to full-time workers.

Equal pay for equal or equivalent work is the basis for equality in the workplace. The WAGE (Women Are Getting Even) Project, Inc. (www.wageproject.org) is a national nonprofit dedicated to closing the wage gap and ending discrimination against women in the workplace.[27] The Older Women's League, an advocacy group for midlife and older women, promotes legislation to improve women's economic security, including expanding and extending pension coverage to more workers and to part-time and temporary workers, and making it portable from job to job.[28]

FAMILY-FRIENDLY WORKPLACE POLICIES

The challenge of family caregiving in an aging society is a reality for the 76 million baby boomers as we take care of parents, spouses, and relatives and think about long-term care options for ourselves. Medicare covers only a limited amount of home help. Medicaid pays for medical care for women with very low incomes. Most of us rely on the informal help of family members, mostly midlife women. Family caregivers are the backbone of long-term supportive services in the United States. The annual value of this unpaid, sometimes taken-for-granted informal care is estimated at $257 billion![29]

We need affordable, accessible, high-quality, comprehensive long-term care services to support our caregiving work at home, balance caregiving responsibilities with work, and as necessary provide us with paid leave from our jobs to do caregiving. We also need polices, in any health care reform, that address the emotional, financial, and physical challenges caregivers face, as well as the value and importance of this work:

- Increase funding for the National Family Caregiver Support Program. (This program, created in 2001, provides information, support, counseling, respite, and other services to all family caregivers.)
- Guarantee enough paid days of sick leave a year to allow us to care for ourselves or a family member short-term.
- Expand the Family Medical Leave Act to cover more employees and provide paid leave from work to care for chronically ill or disabled family members.*
- Provide a tax credit, tax deduction, or other financial incentives to encourage family caregivers to keep aging relatives at home rather than place them in a nursing home.
- Strengthen Social Security by providing cred-

---

* The Family and Medical Leave Act (1993) requires employers to grant twelve weeks of unpaid leave each year to care for a newborn or adopted child or a seriously ill family member or to recover from one's own serious health condition. It does not cover temporary part-time workers and applies only to companies with more than fifty employees.

its to account for years of contributions lost to homemaking and caregiving.

- Provide comprehensive, affordable, accessible, high-quality services coordinated across home, community, and institutional settings.
- Provide for respite care so that family caregivers can take regular breaks.
- Encourage employers to offer flextime, work-at-home options, job sharing, counseling, dependent care accounts, information and referral to community services, employer-paid services of a care manager, and pension and medical insurance for part-time workers.

RETIREMENT SECURITY

Midlife women need to be assured of a secure retirement. If we don't think about this now, we could be in serious financial trouble later. One-third of recipients of Social Security benefits in the United States are children, widows, and people with disabilities, not retirees. Women make up 58 percent of beneficiaries over age sixty-five and 71 percent of those at age eighty-five,[30] and Social Security is the major source of retirement income for most, despite increased participation of women in the workforce.

Women need the program more than men because women make up 70 percent of the people who live in poverty. We also, on average, are out of the workforce longer to care for children or aging parents and have less money in pension income, savings, and private accounts than men. We tend to live longer than men and, in old age, are more likely to run out of resources and be alone. Without the guaranteed income, 52 percent of white women, 61 percent of Latinas, and 65 percent of African-American women would be poor at age sixty-five and older.[31]

The economic and social realities of women's lives must be factored into the current debate about ways of preserving the long-term solvency of the Social Security Trust Fund, given the increasing numbers of people approaching retirement and the dwindling number of younger workers. The Trustees' 2002 annual report estimated that in 2041 the Trust

SOCIAL SECURITY REFORM

Social Security must always provide equitable coverage for those who are eligible. We need to strengthen the current program for caregivers, widows, divorced women, and same-sex partners.

For caregivers: Give credits for unpaid caregiving, and expand spousal disability benefits to adults caring for a disabled spouse.

For widows: Increase widows' benefits to 75 percent of couples' combined benefits.

For divorced spouses: Reduce how long a divorced spouse has to have been married to qualify for benefits, increase divorced spouse's benefit from 50 to 75 percent of former spouse's benefit.

For disabled widows: Benefits should be increased.

For same-sex partners: Make Social Security benefits available to same-sex couples and our families.

Since women are a majority of those who depend on Social Security for lifetime benefits, we have a special stake in preserving this universal social insurance program.

Fund will be exhausted. There are many ways to close the gap and keep the program solvent, but privatization—diverting payroll taxes into individually owned private accounts—would shift the collective risk and gain onto the individual and would not improve Trust Fund solvency. Privatization would undermine women's economic security. There are many reasons it will not work for women: It requires more risk; it doesn't insure us against unexpected events; it is tied to stock market volatility; it will speed up the insolvency of the Trust Fund;[32] and it may lead to benefit cuts.

CONCLUSION

With supportive policies and programs, we can improve the health, well-being, and financial and social status of women through menopause and beyond. The more that women going through the menopause transition give voice to our experiences and advocate for reform, the more we become a force for social change now and for future generations.

NOTES

1. U.S. Census Bureau, State Interim Population Projections by Age and Sex 2004–2030 based on the 2000 census, accessed at www.censusgov/population/www/projections/projectionssagesex.html on July 5, 2005.

2. Apryl Clark, Claire Fong, and Martha Roman, "Health Disparities among U.S. Women of Color: An Overview," Jacobs Institute of Women's Health, from the Margaret E. Mahoney Annual Symposium Health Disparities among Women of Color, April 16, 2002, accessed at www.jiwh.org on October 23, 2005.

3. Margaret Cruikshank, *Learning to Be Old: Gender, Culture and Aging* (Lanham, MD: Rowman & Littlefield Publishers, Inc., 2003), 98.

4. Clark et al.

5. Janny Scott, "Life at the Top of America Isn't Just Better, It's Longer," *New York Times,* May 16, 2005.

6. U.S. Census Bureau, "Income, Poverty and Health Insurance Coverage in the United States: 2003," Table 3, accessed at census.gov/prod/2004pubs/p60-226.pdf on July 5, 2005.

7. Jacobs Institute on Women's Health, transcript from briefing, "A New Year: A Dialogue on Women's Health," Anne Kaspar, January 24, 2005, 7, accessed at www.jiwh.org on October 23, 2005.

8. Kaiser Commission on Medicaid and the Uninsured, "The Uninsured: A Primer: Key Facts About Americans Without Health Insurance," January 2006, accessed at www.kff.org/uninsured/upload/7451.pdf on March 15, 2006.

9. David Himmelstein, M.D., and Steffie Woolhandler, M.D., "Why the U.S. Needs a Single Payer System," June 29, 1995, Physicians for a National Health Program, accessed at www.pnhp.org on October 20, 2005.

10. Paul Krugman, "Passing the Buck," *New York Times,* April 22, 2005.

11. Organisation of Economic Co-Operation and Development, "Health Data 2005," accessed at www.oecd.org/els/health on October 23, 2005.

12. Ibid.

13. Gerard F. Anderson, Uwe E. Reinhardt, Paeter S. Hussey, and Varduhi Petrosyan, "It's the Prices, Stupid: Why the United States Is So Different from Other Countries," *Health Affairs: The Policy Journal of the Health Sphere* 22, no. 3. (May/June 2003): 89–105.

14. Organisation of Economic Co-operation and Development.

15. Jacobs Institute on Women's Health, "A New Year," 11.

16. Cynthia B. Costello and Vanessa R. Wright, "Improving the Health of Midlife Women: Policy Options for the 21st Century," report by the Women's Research and Education Institute, May 2001.

17. NIH State-of-the-Science Panel, "National Institutes of Health State-of-the-Science Conference Statement: Management of Menopause-Related Symptoms." *Annals of Internal Medicine* 142 (2005): 1003.

18. Sherry Sherman, Heather Miller, Lata Nerurkar, and Isaac Schiff, "Research Opportunities for Reducing the Burden of Menopause-Related Symptoms." *American Journal of Medicine* (in press).

19. Gerard F. Anderson, Peter S. Hussey, Bianca K. Frogner, and Hugh R. Waters, "Health Spending in the United States and the Rest of the World," *Health Affairs* 24, no. 4 (July/August 2005): 912.

20. Kenneth E. Thorpe, "Impacts of Health Care Reform: Projections of Costs and Savings," National Coalition on Health Care, 2005.

21. Paul Krugman, "One Nation, Uninsured," *New York Times,* June 13, 2005.

22. Pew Research Center for the People and the Press, "Bush Approval Slips—Fix Economy, Say Voters," August 2003, accessed at http://people-press.org/reports/pdf/190.pdf on January 17, 2006.

23. Boston Women's Health Book Collective, *Our Bodies, Ourselves: A New Edition for a New Era* (New York: Simon & Schuster, 2005), 728–29.

24. Evelyn Murphy and E. J. Graff, "Why Women Are Still Paid Less than Men," *Boston Globe,* October 9, 2005.

25. National Women's Law Center, Fact Sheet, "The Paycheck Fairness Act: Helping to Close the Wage Gap for Women," 2005, accessed at www.pay-equity.org/PDFs/PaycheckFairnessAct_April2005.pdf on January 17, 2006.

26. OWL: The Voice of Midlife and Older Women, "Social Security Privatization: A False Promise for Women," Mother's Day Report 2002, accessed at http://massowl.com/issues.htm on January 17, 2006.

27. Evelyn Murphy, with E. J. Graff, "Mind the Wage Gap," *Ms.* (fall 2005): 46–49.

28. OWL: The Voice of Midlife and Older Women, "The State of Older Women in America," OWL Report 2001.

29. Peter S. Arno, *Economic Value of Informal Caregiving,* Annual Meeting of the American Association of Geriatric Psychiatry, Orlando, FL, February 24, 2002; see also Peter S. Arno, Carol Levine, and Margaret M. Memmott, "The Economic Value of Informal Caregiving," *Health Affairs* 18, no. 2 (March/April 1999): 182–88.

30. OWL: The Voice of Midlife and Older Women, "Social Security Privatization."

31. Ibid.

32. Ibid.

CHAPTER 21

Finding Our Power, Organizing for Change

Finding my power? I am still searching for it . . . but it gets a little easier every day . . . What is power? To me, it means having control of my life in large areas and small, living my values as they change and develop, reflecting on life, and seeking balance, harmony, and wholeness, making my own decisions, even when I flail and fail occasionally, and determining the direction and purpose of my life.

Despite many advances, we still live in a society where a woman's worth is partially determined by her sexual attractiveness and her ability to have children. The loss of our reproductive capabilities, other physical changes, and ageist attitudes in society and ourselves can make some of us feel old, powerless, and unsupported as we experience menopause. Many women are also dealing with additional pressures, such as chronic health conditions, financial insecurity, and caring for children as well as aging parents.

Yet many of us find that this stage of life offers an opportunity to reassess our lives and to experience positive growth. Even if we face events that we would never have chosen, such as the loss of a job or a life partner, our experience may give us confidence and wisdom to deal with such challenges, and our heightened awareness of our mortality may bring us an appreciation of time. While much of our lives is now behind us, we still have room to grow.

Women my age (baby boomers) made opportunities previous generations didn't have. So we don't really want to talk about something that is "our mothers' issue." We don't see [menopause] as "the change," just a change like a lot of others. We may be changing what we do, but we aren't stopping the doing. Sometimes, though, you need false sorts of benchmarks to get yourself reorganized toward some purpose. In the past, I have never left a job without having a job to go to, but I left a twenty-year job. I wasn't learning and didn't want to mark time. Menopause did play a part in tipping me over the edge.

BUILDING COMMUNITY

During the change itself, I suffered so much, physically, mentally, and emotionally, that it was definitely not empowering—just the opposite! . . . If I had more happy and proud older women to hang out with and chat with, I would feel better.

Because menopause can sometimes be a frustrating and isolating experience, it is important that we build good emotional support systems for ourselves. By joining or forming support groups with other women, such as friends, family, colleagues, neighbors, and other community members, we can share our ideas, dreams, goals, and fears as well as get affirmation from each other on a regular basis. As a fifty-eight-year-old Mexican-American woman said, in Spanish, women going through menopause need friends:

People around them who can help tell them where they're going or where to look . . . a network of women to talk to them. Women networking is probably going to be the best piece of

treatment that you can have [for menopause], and saying, It is okay. It's gonna pass.

Women's groups and friendships of all kinds can support us while we embrace the changes and challenges of our lives. Traversing this midlife passage is often easier if we can talk with other women and share our experiences. Women who are older than we are can help us learn more about what to expect as we age, and we can offer similar knowledge to women younger than ourselves. "Do ask, do tell" should perhaps be our watchwords, so that we can break the silence about menopause and aging and replace it with solid information and wisdom based on experience.

You can look for groups to join by checking the community activities announcements in your local newspaper or searching on the Internet. Hospitals, community centers, religious institutions, and other groups often have support groups. If you have difficulty finding an existing group you're comfortable with, consider creating your own. A great source to consult is *The Support Group Sourcebook: What They Are, How You Can Find One, and How They Can Help You* by Linda Klein.[1] A women's group need not be focused on talking about menopause; in their book, *Girls' Night Out: Celebrating Women's Groups across America*, Tamara Kreinin and Barbara Camens chronicle a range of women's groups that offer shared interests as well as emotional support and a good bit of fun in the bargain.[2]

More people are turning to the Internet for information, advice, and support. Through e-mail discussion lists, message boards, websites, and blogs (online postings, also called web logs, that are often updated daily), we can communicate and connect with people beyond our local communities. Many Internet companies, such as Yahoo (www.yahoo.com) and

Topica (www.topica.com), provide free services that allow users to create and manage e-mail lists and groups. Also, Internet service providers often provide users with space to create their own websites and blogs. For those of us who do not have access to the Internet in our homes, public libraries and community centers often offer free access.

New initiatives recognizing midlife as a time of social contribution and engagement are cropping up throughout the United States. Civic Ventures (www.civicventures.org), an organization committed to transforming aging into a source of social and individual renewal, has created two. They are Experience Corps, a national program that involves midlife and older adults in vital community service, and Next Chapter (Life Options), an initiative to develop centers in communities nationwide that will offer life-planning programs, learning opportunities, and peer and community connections.

MAKING HEALTHY DECISIONS

I say what I want to more often now.

Many women find that the menopause transition is an impetus to make healthy changes in our lives. At this time, we may feel more confident than ever before. Yet many of us are still learning how best to take care of ourselves.

My daughter turned fifteen the year I went through menopause. It was the year from hell. . . . What I had to learn was to be kinder to myself.

My plan (when I thought about menopause) was to eat a little more soy and ignore the whole thing. And here I am a public health person. But then I found it would take a little more than that!

The menopausal transition inspires many of us to make more time for our health. Eating a nutritious diet and reducing or managing stress can help us feel better and provide other health benefits. Regular physical exams help us to keep in touch with our bodies, assure that our health care practitioners have a good baseline from which to diagnose ailments, and sometimes identify problems early enough that they are treatable. Taking care of ourselves helps put our minds and bodies at ease.

It is sometimes possible not just to maintain but to improve our physical strength. Exercise is important, and not just for physical health or appearance.

It is wonderful for the head: You're happier and have a better outlook. Forty-five minutes on a treadmill and I feel different.

When I learned to lift weights at fifty, I gained a new sense of physical strength and psychological power at a time when women often begin to feel invisible. And it has practical benefits, too, when I need to heave a suitcase into an airplane overhead bin unassisted or carry a grandchild in my arms.

Even the simplest of exercises can yield many health benefits, and a gym is not necessary. Byllye Avery, founder of the Black Women's Health Imperative, started the Walking for Wellness program in 1990 to encourage women to walk to improve our health and spiritual well-being. Over the years, more than 10,000 women in twenty-five cities across the country have made the pledge to take daily group walks with their friends, families, and neighbors.[3]

IMPLEMENTING OUR PLANS

It may feel easy to make big plans for changing our lives, but taking the necessary day-to-day steps to implement our good intentions is often a challenge. Assessing our priorities can help us make changes. Try asking yourself what you want to do and learn in the next year, five years, and ten years, and then take action on your answers.

I made a values reassessment at midlife. . . . I had spent a lot of years making money, and now I wanted to be with a socially responsible company. The skills I had developed in the business world applied to nonprofits, too. I joined a not-for-profit organization where I feel that I can make a difference. A bonus to making this change was the freedom of making decisions for one reason alone—what is the best for the organization and its mission. . . . I realized I was not willing to compromise, and if it didn't have that social responsibility, I was not willing to go there.

Whether implementing our plans means making major career changes or taking incremental steps, such as eating more fruits and vegetables, the process of choosing and doing supports our continuing growth. One success builds upon the next. Perhaps more important, even when our plans do not result in success as we have defined it, we can learn from that experience, too.

I was forty years old before the idea of my having any power at all to determine anything at all occurred to me. For the first eighteen years, I responded to my parents' power; for the next twenty-two, I responded to a husband's power. Little by little over the years, I came to realize that I was a marionette, my limbs jerking to whatever strings someone else pulled. Then one fateful day, I cut those strings, fled from a life of privilege but quiet desperation, financially broke, but swelling with my own power to direct my life for the first time. I entered my forties and began the most productive, satisfying period of my life.

ORGANIZING FOR SOCIAL CHANGE

With so many of us now entering midlife, our potential to influence the culture is immense. But to realize that power, we must come together to support each other and advocate on our own behalf. Women at midlife and in old age are not only more likely to register to vote, we vote in higher numbers than our younger counterparts.[4] We can use this civic consciousness to advocate for programs and policies that support our health and the health of our communities.

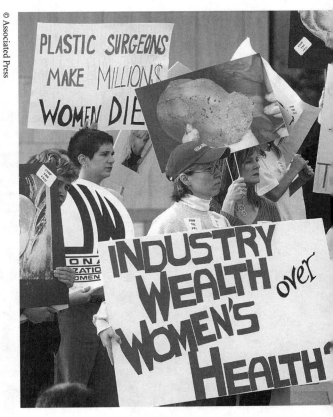

© Associated Press

Women rally outside the Health and Human Services Department in Washington, D.C., against the approval of silicone gel breast implants.

TAKING POLITICAL ACTION

If you are interested in becoming politically active, a good place to start is to become more informed. While all social, economic, and political issues affect women going through the menopause transition, some issues—such as ageism, Social Security, pension reform, health care reform, caregiving, and long-term care—are especially relevant to our lives. You can begin to learn more by following the news, reading reports and fact sheets produced by research and advocacy groups, or talking with people in your communities. (For more information, see Chapter 20, "The Politics of Women's Health.")

You may want to become more active within your community. You can start by joining a community health organization or a local chapter of an existing national organization, such as the Older Women's League (OWL). If you are already a member of an advocacy organization such as AARP, Gray Panthers, the National Latina Institute for Reproductive Health, the National Asian Women's Health Organization, or the Black Women's Health Imperative, encourage it to focus on the issues of midlife women if it does not already.

If a chapter of a national group doesn't already exist in your local community, think about starting one yourself with the help of friends and colleagues. You may even consider starting your own advocacy group. According to the Midwest Academy, which trains grass-

ACTION STEPS

There are many ways to influence politics and the public's opinions on social and political issues that you care about. Whether you are acting as a representative of a group or involved as a private citizen, here are a few actions to consider:[5]

- Contact local, state, and federal elected officials and their staff through phone calls, letters, faxes, and e-mails. Joining the action network of an organization you trust can make these activities easy, and your voice will be multiplied by those of other members.
- Schedule meetings with your elected representatives and participate in lobby days set up by an organization.
- Write letters to editors or op-ed pieces for your local newspaper.
- Pitch story ideas to journalists of your local newspaper.
- Create and distribute your own newsletter or set up a blog.
- Sponsor town hall meetings, public educational campaigns, rallies, and other public events.
- Conduct press conferences and other media activities.

To learn how to do these activities and to see examples, consult *The One-Hour Activist* (2004) by Christopher Kush; the civic education guides published by the League of Women Voters (www.lwv.org/elibrary, or 202-429-1965); and *The Community Action Kit* by SIECUS (Sexuality Information and Education Council of the United States) at www.communityactionkit.org. (You may also reach SIECUS at 212-819-9770 or 202-265-2405.)[6]

roots organizers,[7] the following five strategies are important to consider when taking on a political issue:

- Define your issue.
- Set achievable short-term and long-term goals, such as changing a specific state or federal law or electing a political candidate who supports your issue.
- Get support from the community, such as individual voters, community leaders, and civic and religious organizations.
- Build coalitions with organizational and individual allies.
- Define your opponents.

Another important organizing strategy is to decide what tactics you will use to achieve your goals. (Consider some of the actions listed on page 312.)

If you are not satisfied with the performance of your local, state, or federal elected representatives, consider running for political office yourself. Women still make up only a small percentage of elected officials in the United States at all levels of government.[8] Our voices are sorely needed. Groups like EMILY's List (www.emilyslist.org, or 202-326-1400) and the National Women's Political Caucus (www. nwpc.org, or 202-785-1100) provide training and give advice to women running for office.

EXAMPLES OF GRASSROOTS ORGANIZING

While many national, state, and community groups focus on the reproductive health needs of women in their childbearing years, few groups specifically focus on women who are transitioning through menopause, which makes it even more important for us to advocate on our own behalf. The idea of becoming more politically active can be intimidating, es-

pecially if we are new to it or have other issues to deal with in our lives. Sometimes, we just need a small spark of inspiration to get us going. Here are a few examples of groups of women who have successfully organized.

OWL: Older Women's League
In 1980, Tish Sommers and Laurie Shields gathered a group of friends and acquaintances around a kitchen table in Oakland, California, to talk about the lack of attention paid to issues that affect women over the age of forty. That night, they laid the foundation for a new grassroots organization that would become the "voice of midlife and older women." In October of that year, the Older Women's League, or OWL, was officially launched at the White House Mini-Conference on Older Women in Des Moines, Iowa, with over 300 women serving as charter members.

Over twenty-five years later, OWL is still the only national organization dedicated solely to the issues that affect women at midlife and in old age. It now has sixty chapters in twenty-seven states and the District of Columbia and a membership network of 15,000. The organization, now based in Washington, D.C., publishes reports and advocates for laws in the U.S. Congress and state legislatures on a wide range of issues, including Social Security, pension reform, health care, prescription drugs, Medicare, caregiving, long-term care, housing, and mental health.[9] To learn more about OWL and its activities, visit www.national-owl.org or call 1-800-825-3695.

Planned Parenthood's *Promotora* Programs
Concerned that many Latinas in the Los Angeles area were not taking advantage of its services, Planned Parenthood Los Angeles developed the *Promotoras Communitarias* Training Program in 1991. The program was

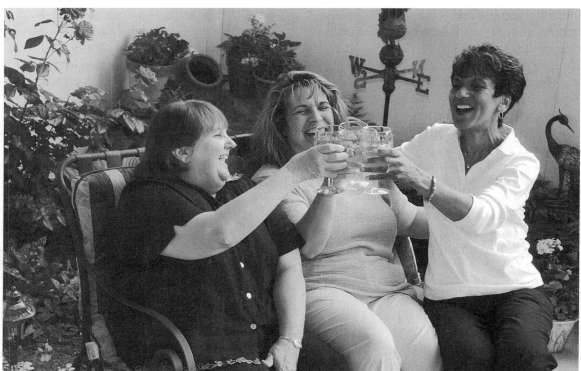

inspired by similar programs run by clinics in Mexico and other parts of Latin America and had been pioneered in the United States by Planned Parenthood of Central and Northern Arizona.

Promotoras are women who work as lay health educators within their local communities. After undergoing a lengthy training process, they provide information in group presentations and in one-on-one sessions on a wide range of reproductive health issues, including birth control, abortion, sexuality, anatomy, breast cancer, and domestic violence, as well as menopause.

The program has provided vital health information and support to women and their families. It also has been vital in developing leadership skills and providing economic support to the trainers, many of whom had not previously worked outside the home or finished high school.

To learn more about *promotora* programs, visit the website of the Planned Parenthood Federation of America at www.plannedparenthood.org or call 1-800-230-7526, or visit the website of Our Bodies Ourselves at www.ourbodiesourselves.org.

The HERS Foundation

Nora Coffey, who had a hysterectomy at age thirty-six, has made it her life's mission to end "the conspiracy of silence" on unnecessary hysterectomies. In 1982, Coffey founded the Hysterectomy and Educational Resources and Services (HERS) Foundation. She recalls the inspiration for her own activism:

Doctors told me I was the only woman who experienced post-hysterectomy problems. To find out if that was true, I took out a small, two-line classified ad in Ms. magazine that said, "Author writing book about hysterectomy would like response to confidential questionnaire." I was unprepared for the 425 responses from women who filled out my forty-five-page questionnaire. Each one validated my own experience. For the first time, I knew I was not the only one.

Based in Bala Cynwyd, Pennsylvania, HERS has provided health consumer information and counseling services to more than 700,000 women in the United States and abroad. In March 2004, the organization began a yearlong, fifty-two-city demonstration to raise the public's awareness about unnecessary hysterectomies. In conjunction with the campaign, HERS sponsored the production of the play *Un Becoming* in several of the cities. The play confronts the complex physical and emotional issues surrounding hysterectomies. To learn more about HERS and the play, go to www.hersfoundation.com or call 1-888-750-4377.

The National Council of Negro Women, Inc.

Founded in 1935 by renowned educator and political activist Mary McLeod Bethune, the National Council of Negro Women, Inc. (NCNW) advocates for African-American women, our families, and our communities. It has more than 200 affiliated chapters and organizations in thirty-four states that reach out to a network of over 4 million women.

After learning that many African-American women at midlife are not sufficiently prepared for old age, NCNW launched a public educational initiative called "Tomorrow Begins Today: African American Women As We Age" in 2005. The purpose of the campaign is to provide advice on aging, financial planning,

healthy living, and emotional well-being to African-American women between the ages of thirty-five and fifty-nine. It publishes an inspirational book, sponsors community forums in several cities, and supports ongoing activities in local communities.

Ultimately, NCNW wants to change the way in which we think about midlife and aging to help ensure that it is not an isolating and frightening process for women. To learn more about the organization and the Tomorrow Begins Today initiative, visit its website at www.ncnw.org or call 202-737-0120.

MOVING FORWARD

Menopause offers an opportunity for us to reassess our lives, support one another in making healthy individual choices, and work together for broader social changes. We may well learn that we don't have to *find* our power after all: It is right there in our hands if we can but see it. Each of us has much we can contribute to our families, our communities, and the world. Suzanne Braun Levine, author of *Inventing the Rest of Our Lives,* calls this part of life "second adulthood" and says it has two components: making peace with the reality of midlife and taking charge of our own futures.[10] We are not alone in this process. Together, we can find ways to share our knowledge with other women; affirm our creative power, our passions, and our compassion; and even live our wildest dreams during this journey.

Yes, there were night sweats and discomfort. Yes, there were times when . . . I chaired meetings with increasingly soggy tissues in the hand mopping my face—periods when my exultant power surges turned into electrifying hot flashes. But medication and time soon alleviated these discomforts, and the last ten years or so have been the greatest "period" of my life. It is the period that I feel—outside of bringing three beloved children into the world—that I have made and continue to make my strongest contribution to the lives of other people, as teacher, writer, lecturer, and counselor. I continue to direct my own life, and that direction is outward toward making life better physically, mentally, and spiritually for others.

NOTES

1. Linda A. Klein, *The Support Group Sourcebook: What They Are, How You Can Find One, and How They Can Help You* (New York: John Wiley & Sons, 2000).

2. Tamara Kreinin and Barbara Camens, *Girls' Night Out: Celebrating Women's Groups across America* (New York: Crown Publishing, 2002).

3. Julie Flaherty, "Preaching the Merits of a Multistep Program," *New York Times,* June 13, 1999, Section 15, p. 3; see also Beatrice Mutamedi, "Walking the Walk: The Best Exercise," WebMD Health, November 20, 2000, accessed at my.webmd.com/content/article/12/1689_51173.htm on September 20, 2005.

4. United States Census Bureau, "Table A-1. Reported Voting and Registration by Race, Hispanic Origin, Sex, and Age Groups: November 1964 to 2004," Current Population Survey, 2005, accessed at www.census.gov/population/www/socdemo/voting.html on April 21, 2005.

5. Gloria Feldt, *The War on Choice: The Right-Wing Attack on Women's Rights and How to Fight Back* (New York: Bantam Books, 2004); MoveOn.org, *MoveOn's 50 Ways to Love Your Country: How to Find Your Political Voice and Become a Catalyst for Change* (Maui, HI: Inner Ocean Publishing, 2004).

6. Christopher Kush, *The One-Hour Activist: The 15 Most Powerful Actions You Can Take to Fight for the Issues and Candidates You Care About* (San Francisco, CA: Jossey-Bass, 2004).

7. Kimberly Bobo, Jackie Kendall, and Steve Max, *Organizing for Social Change: The Midwest Academy Manual for Activists,* 2nd ed. (Washington, DC: Seven Locks Press, 2001).

8. Center for American Women and Politics at the Eagleton Institute of Politics, Rutgers University at New Brunswick, "Women in Elective Office 2005," fact sheet, April 2005.

9. Older Women's League, "About Us," fact sheet, accessed at www.owl-national.org/about/index.html on May 30, 2005.

10. Suzanne Braun Levine, *Inventing the Rest of Our Lives: Women in Second Adulthood* (New York: Viking, 2005).

Resources

The list below includes resources on menopause and on women's health advocacy. For a more extensive list of resources on women's health, visit the Our Bodies Ourselves website at www.ourbodiesourselves.org.

GENERAL

Books

Barbach, Lonnie. *The Pause: Positive Approaches to Perimenopause and Menopause.* 2nd ed. New York: The Penguin Group, 2000.

Boston Women's Health Book Collective. *Our Bodies, Ourselves: A New Edition for a New Era.* New York: Simon & Schuster, 2005.

Doress-Worters, Paula B., and Diana Laskin Siegal in cooperation with the Boston Women's Health Book Collective. *The New Ourselves, Growing Older.* New York: Simon & Schuster, 1994.

Greer, Germaine. *The Change: Women, Aging, and the Menopause.* Ballantine Books, 1993.

Gullette, Margaret Meganroth. *Aged by Culture.* Chicago: University of Chicago Press, 2004.

Kagan, Leslee, Bruce Kessel, and Herbert Benson. *Mind over Menopause: The Complete Mind/Body Approach to Coping with Menopause.* New York: Free Press, 2004.

Love, Susan M. *Dr. Susan Love's Menopause and Hormone Book.* New York: Three Rivers Press, 2003.

National Women's Health Network. *The Truth about Hormone Replacement Therapy: How to Break Free from the Medical Myths of Menopause.* Roseville, CA: Prima Publishing, 2002.

North American Menopause Society. *Menopause Guidebook.* Cleveland, OH: North American Menopause Society, 2003.

Ojeda, Linda. *Menopause without Medicine.* Alameda, CA: Hunter House Publishers, 2003.

O'Leary Cobb, Janine. *Understanding Menopause.* Toronto: Key Porter Books Limited, 2001.

Seaman, Barbara. *The Greatest Experiment Ever Performed on Women: Exploding the Estrogen Myth.* New York: Hyperion, 2003.

Stewart, Elizabeth Gunther, and Paula Spencer. *The V Book: A Doctor's Guide to Complete Vulvovaginal Health.* New York: Bantam Books, 2002.

Topp, Elizabeth, and Dr. Carol Livoti. *Vaginas: An Owner's Manual.* New York: Thunder's Mouth Press, 2004.

Weed, Susun. *New Menopausal Years: The Wise Woman Way.* Woodstock, NY: Ash Tree Publishing, 2002.

Periodicals

A Friend Indeed
Newsletter for Women in Menopause and Midlife
PO Box 260, Pembina, ND 58271-0260
294-989-8029
or
The Winnipeg Women's Health Clinic
Main Floor, 419 Graham Ave., Winnipeg, Manitoba CANADA R3C 0M3
www.afriendindeed.ca

The Women's Health Activist
The National Women's Health Network
514 Tenth Street NW, Suite 400, Washington, DC 20004
www.womenshealthnetwork.org

Organizations

American Menopause Foundation
350 Fifth Avenue, Suite 2822, New York, NY 10118

212-714-2398
www.americanmenopause.org

National Women's Health Information Center, Menopause & Hormone Therapy
8270 Willow Oaks Corporate Drive, Fairfax, VA 22031
1-800-994-WOMAN or 1-888-220-5446 (for hearing impaired)
www.4woman.gov/menopause/index2.htm

National Women's Health Network
514 Tenth Street NW, Suite 400, Washington, DC 20004
202-347-1140 or 202-628-7814 (for health information)
nwhn@nwhn.org
www.nwhn.org

North American Menopause Society (NAMS)
PO Box 94527, Cleveland, OH 44101
440-442-7550
info@menopause.org
www.menopause.org

SUDDEN AND EARLY MENOPAUSE

Books

Banerd, Karin. *Menopause Before 40: Coping with Premature Ovarian Failure.* New Bern, NC: Trafford Publishing, 2004.

DeAngelo, Debbie. *Sudden Menopause: Restoring Health and Emotional Well-Being.* Alameda, CA: Hunter House Publishers, 2001.

Elson, Jean. *Am I Still a Woman? Hysterectomy and Gender Identity.* Philadelphia, PA: Temple University Press, 2004.

Icon Health Publications. *Premature Menopause: A Medical Dictionary, Bibliography, and Annotated Research Guide to Internet References.* San Diego, CA: Icon Health Publications, 2004.

North American Menopause Society. *Early Menopause Guidebook.* Cleveland, OH: North American Menopause Society, 2003.

Vliet, Elizabeth Lee. *It's My Ovaries, Stupid!* New York: Simon & Schuster, 2003.

Organizations

Hysterectomy Educational Resources and Services (HERS) Foundation

422 Bryn Mawr Avenue, Bala Cynwyd, PA 19004

888-750-HERS

www.hersfoundation.org

The International Premature Ovarian Failure Association (IPOFA)

PO Box 23643, Alexandria, VA 22304

support line: 703-913-4787

www.pofsupport.org

RESOLVE: The National Infertility Association

7910 Woodmont Avenue, Suite 1350, Bethesda, MD 20814

301-652-8585, helpline: 888-623-0744

www.resolve.org

WOMEN'S HEALTH ADVOCACY

Books

Abramson, John. *Overdosed America: The Broken Promise of American Medicine.* New York: HarperCollins, 2004.

Agnew, Vijay, ed. *Women's Health, Women's Rights: Perspectives on Global Health Issues.* Toronto: Centre for Feminist Research (CFR), 2003.

Baumgardner, Jennifer and Amy Richards. *Grassroots: A Field Guide for Feminist Activism.* New York: Farrar, Straus and Giroux, 2005.

Bobo, Kimberly, Jackie Kendall, and Steve Max. *Organizing for Social Change: The Midwest Academy Manual for Activists.* 2nd ed. Washington, DC: Seven Locks Press, 2001.

Klein, Linda A. *The Support Group Sourcebook: What They Are, How You Can Find One, and How They Can Help You.* New York: John Wiley & Sons, 2000.

Krieger, Nancy, ed. *Embodying Inequality: Epidemiologic Perspectives.* Amityville, NY: Baywood Publishing Company, 2004.

MoveOn.org. *MoveOn's 50 Ways to Love Your Country: How to Find Your Political Voice and Become a Catalyst for Change.* Maui, HI: Inner Ocean Publishing, 2004.

Pogrebin, Letty Cottin. *Getting over Getting Older: An Intimate Journey.* New York: Berkley Publishing Group, 1997.

Sered, Susan, and Rushika Fernandopulle, *Uninsured in America: Life and Death in the Land of Opportunity.* Berkeley: University of California Press, 2005.

Worcester, Nancy, and Mariamne H. Whatley, eds. *Women's Health: Readings on Social, Economic, and Political Issues.* 4th ed. Dubuque, IA: Kendall/Hunt Publishing, 2004.

Organizations

Black Women's Health Imperative (formerly National Black Women's Health Project)

600 Pennsylvania Ave. SE, #310, Washington, DC 20003

202-548-4000

www.BlackWomensHealth.org

Breast Cancer Action

55 New Montgomery, Suite 323, San Francisco, CA 94105

877-2STOPBC (toll-free)

www.bcaction.org

Canadian Women's Health Network

419 Graham Avenue, Suite 203, Winnipeg, Manitoba Canada R3C 0M3

888-818-9172
www.cwhn.ca/indexeng.html

Center for Medical Consumers
239 Thompson Street, New York, NY 10012
212-674-7105
www.medicalconsumers.org

The Feminist Majority
1600 Wilson Boulevard, Suite 801, Arlington, VA 22209
703-522-2214
www.feminist.org

Gray Panthers
1612 K Street NW, Suite 300, Washington, DC 20006
800-280-5362 or 202-737-6637
www.graypanthers.org

The League of Women Voters
1730 M Street NW, Suite 1000, Washington, DC 20036-4508
202-429-1965
www.lwv.org

National Asian Women's Health Organization
One Embarcadero Center, Suite 500, San Francisco, CA 94111
415-773-2838
www.nawho.org/index.html

National Council of Negro Women, Inc.
African American Women as We Age Campaign

633 Pennsylvania Ave. NW, Washington, DC 20004
202-737-0120
www.ncnw.org

National Organization for Women
1100 H Street NW, 3rd floor, Washington, DC 20005
202-628-8NOW
www.now.org

National Women's Law Center
11 Dupont Circle NW, Suite 800, Washington, DC 20036
202-588-5180
www.nwlc.org

OWL: Older Women's League, The Voice of Midlife and Older Women
1750 New York Avenue NW, Suite 350, Washington, DC 20006
202-783-6686 or 800-825-3695
www.owl-national.org

SisterSong Women of Color Reproductive Health Collective
PO Box 311020, Atlanta, GA 31131
404-344-9629
www.sistersong.net

Universal Health Care Action Network
2800 Euclid Avenue, Suite 520, Cleveland, OH 44115
216-241-8422 or 800-634-4442
www.uhcan.org

Authorship and Acknowledgments

THE PRODUCTION TEAM

Editor: Heather Stephenson
Editorial Advisors: Judy Norsigian, Marcie Richardson, and Kiki Zeldes
Graphics Editor: Sarai Walker
Interns: Adrianne Ortega, Heather Town, and Amie Vaccaro

SPECIAL THANKS TO:

Other Our Bodies Ourselves staff and consultants: Jessica Halverson, Elana Hayasaka, Sally Whelan, Zobeida Bonilla, Pam McCarthy, and Marianne McPherson
At Simon & Schuster: Doris Cooper, Sara Schapiro, Cherise Davis, Meghan Stevenson, Ellen Silberman, Chris Lloreda, Debbie Model, Marcia Burch, Sue Fleming, Mark Gompertz, and Trish Todd
Our Bodies Ourselves board members (2005): Shahira Ahmed, Elizabeth Daake-Kelly, Sally Deane (past chair), Vilunya Diskin, Nancy Forsyth, Ileana Jimenez Garcia, Teresa Harrison, Neda Joury-Penders, Mary (Bebe) Poor, Penelope Riseborough, Patricia Roche, Bonnie Shepard (co-chair), Donna Soodalter-Toman, Amanda Buck Varella (co-chair), and Rachel A. Wilson
Our Bodies Ourselves advisory board members: Marjorie Agosin, Hortensia Amaro, Byllye Avery, Joan Bavaria, Teresa Heinz, Cathy Inglese, Paula Johnson, Wanda Jones, Florence Ladd, Susan M. Love, Meizhu Lui, Ngina Lythcott, Evelyn Murphy, Cynthia Pearson, Vivian Pinn, Ellen Poss, Joan Rachlin, Allan Rosenfield, Isaac Schiff, and Gloria Steinem
Founders of the Boston Women's Health Book Collective: Ruth Bell-Alexander, Pamela Berger, Paula Doress-Worters, Joan Ditzion, Vilunya Diskin, Paula

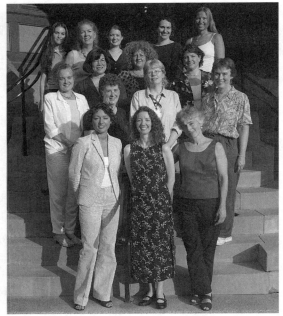

Some members of the board and staff of Our Bodies Our-seves: Front row, left to right: Teresa Harrison, Heather Stephenson, Judy Norsigian. Second row: Sally Whelan, Kiki Zeldes, Patricia Roche, Bonnie Shepard. Third row: Sally Deane, Donna Soodalter-Toman, Rachel A. Wilson. Back row: Amie Vaccaro, Penelope Riseborough, Amanda Buck Varella, Neda Joury-Penders, and Jessica Halverson.

Doress-Worters, Nancy Miriam Hawley, Elizabeth MacMahon-Herrera, Pamela Morgan, Judy Norsigian, Jane Pincus, Esther Rome (1945–1995), Wendy C. Sanford, Norma Swenson, and Sally Whelan

AUTHORSHIP AND ACKNOWLEDGMENTS BY CHAPTER

Approaching Menopause
Chapter 1: Understanding Our Menopause Experiences

By Josephine Etowa, Barbara Keddy, Janice Acton, Vicki Meyer (medicalization and the role of hormones), and Margaret Lock ("Is Menopause the Same around the Globe?").

Thanks for help to Zobeido Bonilla, Joan Ditzion, Paula Doress-Worters, Anna Freixas, Malkah Notman, Edith Silvas, and Susan Sered.

Chapter 2: Making Health Care Decisions

By Judith Costlow and Mara Taub, with Susan Sered; John Abramson and Barbara Seaman ("Can We Trust the Evidence in Evidence-Based Medicine?"); Katy Backes Kozhimannil and Marianne McPherson ("Understanding Research Results"); and Susan Green Cooksey ("Group Visits").

Thanks for help to Karen Carlson, Kay Dickersin, and Elaine Rosenblatt.

A Transition and Its Challenges
Chapter 3: What's Happening in Our Bodies

By Nancy Fugate Woods and Ellen Sullivan Mitchell.

Thanks for help to Stacie Geller, Patricia Rackowski, Nancy Reame, and Diana Siegal.

Chapter 4: Sudden and Early Menopause

By Jean Elson with Patricia Noone.

Thanks for help to Nora Coffey, Debbie DeAngelo, and Wendy Garling.

Chapter 5: Hot Flashes, Night Sweats, and Sleep Disturbances

By June Rogers.

Thanks for help to Janine O'Leary Cobb, Leilani Doty, Joel Lexchin, and Margaret Moloney.

Chapter 6: Vulvovaginal Health

By Rebecca Kightlinger, with Shannon Berning ("Vaginal Health after Vaginoplasty").

Thanks for help to William M. Burke, Jane Goto, Rebecca Kightlinger, Eric Leach, Susan Levenstein, Esther Morris, Elizabeth Stewart, and Moonhawk River Stone.

Chapter 7: Hormone Treatment

By Amy Allina and Kristen Suthers, with Shannon Berning and Moonhawk River Stone ("Hormones and Transgender Health").

Thanks for help to the National Women's Health Network, Becky Alison, Kay Dickersin, Patricia Dougherty, Stacie Geller, Elizabeth Mandell, JoAnn Pinkerton, Elizabeth Plourde, Lynn Rosenberg, Ben Singer, and Jessica Xavier.

Changing Selves, Changing Relationships
Chapter 8: Body Image

By Patti Owen-Smith, with Diana Zuckerman (breast implants).

Thanks for help to Margaret Morganroth Gullette, Christina Roache, and Deborah Sullivan.

Chapter 9: Sexuality

By Lenore Pomerance with Wendy Wolfson (birth control and unexpected pregnancy).

Thanks for help to Adrienne Asch, Barbara Boston, Liz Coolidge, Suzanne Folger, Sandra Leiblum, Susan Levenstein, Phyllis Mansfield, Maurizio Macaluso, Gina Ogden, Nancy Reame, Jeanne Shaw, Victoria Wright, and all the women who generously shared their stories.

Chapter 10: Family Life and the Workplace

By Joan Ditzion and Nancy London ("Becoming a Mother").

Thanks for help to Nada Stotland, Anita Taylor, and Trish Wilson.

Taking Care of Ourselves
Chapter 11: Emotional Well-Being and Stress Management

By Kristin DeJohn and Leslee Kagan, with Joan Ditzion.

Thanks for help to Nada Stotland, Anita Taylor, and Trish Wilson.

Chapter 12: Eating Well

By Ellen Barlow.

Thanks for help to Marion Nestle and Elaine Rosenblatt.

Chapter 13: Staying Active

By Ellen Barlow and Miriam Nelson.

Thanks for help to Diane Dahm, Mickie Randazza, and Maria Skinner.

Health Concerns
Chapter 14: Uterine and Bladder Health

By Susan Green Cooksey (uterine health) and Carolyn Sampselle (bladder health).

Thanks for help to Dianne Bailey, Kate Beadle, Jeanette Brown, George Flesh, Janis Luft, Aldie Rol, and Nanette Santoro.

Chapter 15: Memory and Mood

By Jeanne Leventhal Alexander, based on earlier work by Jeanne Leventhal Alexander, Lorraine Dennerstein, Nancy Fugate Woods, Victor Henderson, and Krista Kotz.

Thanks for help to Vivien Burt, Janet Currie, Leilani Doty, Anne Rochon Ford, Joel Lexchin, Donna Stewart, and Nada Stotland.

Chapter 16: Bone Health

By Charlea Massion.

Thanks for help to John Abramson, Amy Allina, Ellen Barlow, Adriane Fugh-Berman, Bonnie Hillsberg, Betsy McClung, Michael McClung, Cindy Pearson, and the National Women's Health Network.

Chapter 17: Heart Health

By Judith Hsia and Ginny Levin, with John Abramson ("Questioning the Role of Cholesterol") and Aggie Casey ("Stress and the Heart").

Thanks for help to Warren Bell, Beatrice Golomb, and Vicki Meyer.

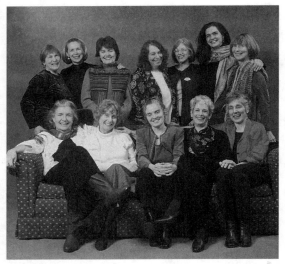

© Jörg Meyer

Founders of the Boston Women's Health Book Collective. Front row, seated left to right: Norma Swenson, Pamela Berger, Sally Whelan, Nancy Miriam Hawley, Judy Norsigian. Back row, left to right: Jane Pincus, Pamela Morgan, Vilunya Diskin, Joan Ditzion, Paula Doress-Worters, Elizabeth MacMahon-Herrera, Wendy C. Sanford. Not pictured: Ruth Bell-Alexander and Esther Rome (deceased).

Chapter 18: Cancers

By Barbara Brenner, William Burke, Barbara Dunn, Angela Kueck, and Jennifer Rhode, with Wendy Garling.

Thanks for help to Sheldon Cherry, Wanda Davis, Marcela Del Carmen, Margaret Moloney, and Ellen Richmond.

Chapter 19: Other Medical Concerns

By Margaret Moloney (headache), Amy Lazev (smoking), Nancy Poole (alcohol), Lenore Riddell (alcohol), and Wendy Wolfson (all others).

Thanks for help to Victoria Almquist, Michelle Bloch, Elisabeth Broderick, and Martha Katz.

Knowledge Is Power
Chapter 20: The Politics of Women's Health

By Joan Ditzion, with Sherry Sherman ("Important Gaps in Knowledge about the Menopause Transition").

Thanks for help to Jacqueline Lapidus, Ruth Palombo, Susan Sered, and Ellen Shaffer.

Chapter 21: Finding Our Power, Organizing for Change

By Gloria Feldt and Kimala Price.

Thanks for help to Nancy Becker, Eileen Breslin, Ceil Cleveland, Vickie Costa, Vanesa Cullins, Joan Ditzion, Wendy Garling, Tamara Kreinin, Friedrike Merck, Sandy Owen, Joyce Roche, Susan Roll, Ema Rosero, Edith Silvas, and Jean Woody.

About the Contributors

OUR BODIES OURSELVES STAFF

Judy Norsigian is executive director of Our Bodies Ourselves. A cofounder of the Boston Women's Health Book Collective and coauthor of all Simon & Schuster editions of *Our Bodies, Ourselves,* she is a renowned speaker and writer on women's health.

Heather Stephenson is a program manager for Our Bodies Ourselves. She was the managing editor of the 2005 edition of *Our Bodies, Ourselves.*

Sarai Walker is a former associate editor at Our Bodies Ourselves and served as the graphics editor for the 2005 edition of *Our Bodies, Ourselves.* She is currently earning her doctorate in English literature and writing a novel.

Kiki Zeldes is the website manager for Our Bodies Ourselves, where she has worked since 1997. She was part of the editorial team for the 2005 edition of *Our Bodies, Ourselves* and developed its companion website.

CONTRIBUTORS

John Abramson, M.D., is the author of *Overdosed America* and a clinical instructor at Harvard Medical School. He practiced family medicine in Hamilton, Massachusetts, for twenty years, and served as chairman of the Department of Family Practice at Lahey Clinic.

Janice Acton is a writer, researcher, and adult educator. Over the past thirty years, she has worked with community-based health, women's, solidarity, and peer network organizations. She is a partner in Tides Turning Consulting and lives in Halifax, Nova Scotia.

Jeanne L. Alexander, M.D., is the director of the Northern California Kaiser Permanente Medical Group Psychiatry Women's Health Program, an adjunct assistant clinical professor of psychiatry, Stanford University, and founder of a 501(c)3 nonprofit, Alexander Foundation for Women's Health (www.afwh.org).

Amy Allina is program director of the National Women's Health Network, a nonprofit organization based in Washington, D.C. She is also an author of *The Truth about Hormone Replacement Therapy: How to Break Free from the Medical Myths of Menopause.*

Ellen Barlow is a freelance writer specializing in health and medicine. Formerly a writer/editor at Harvard Medical School, she is coauthor of a book on diabetes and women and contributed to the original *Ourselves, Growing Older,* among numerous other publications.

Shannon Berning is an editor for Alyson Books, the oldest publisher of books by, for, and about lesbians, gay men, bisexuals, and transgender people. She wrote the "Relationships with Women" chapter for the 2005 edition of *Our Bodies, Ourselves.*

Barbara Brenner is executive director of Breast Cancer Action (www.bcaction.org), a national grassroots education and advocacy organization. Since first diagnosed with breast cancer at age forty-one, in 1993, she has led activists in challenging the status quo in breast cancer.

William Burke, M.D., received bachelor and medical degrees from Columbia University. He completed his residency in obstetrics and gyne-

cology at Columbia Presbyterian Medical Center and a fellowship in gynecologic oncology at the University of Michigan, where he now teaches.

Aggie Casey, M.S., R.N., is the director and clinical nurse specialist for the Cardiac Wellness Program of the Mind/Body Medical Institute. She is also a researcher and an associate in medicine at Harvard Medical School.

Susan Green Cooksey, Ph.D., is a nurse practitioner and researcher with Kaiser Permanente Northwest. A certified menopause clinician and a lead practitioner at the Portland site for the Women's Health Initiative, she has completed research on women's menopause experiences.

Judith Costlow has been facilitating menopause workshops since 1977. She is a founding member of the Santa Fe Health Education Project, coauthor of *Menopause: A Self-Care Manual,* and a health education specialist for the state of New Mexico.

Kristin DeJohn, an award-winning writer and television producer, has been honored by the American Medical Association and by American Women in Radio and Television. She began researching women's midlife experiences as primary writer for the book *Mind over Menopause.*

Joan Ditzion is a founder of the Boston Women's Health Book Collective and a coauthor of all editions of *Our Bodies, Ourselves.* A geriatric social worker and educator, she appreciates the love and support of her husband and two sons.

Barbara K. Dunn has a Ph.D. in genetics from the University of Wisconsin and an M.D. from

Georgetown University. She also trained at the National Cancer Institute in medical oncology. Her focus is on breast cancer chemoprevention and genetics.

Jean Elson, Ph.D., M.A., M.Ed., is the author of the book *Am I Still a Woman? Hysterectomy and Gender Identity,* as well as several academic and popular articles. She teaches sociology at the University of New Hampshire.

Josephine Etowa, Ph.D., R.N., is a professor of nursing at Dalhousie University. Her nursing career spans international, multicultural, community development, and women's health issues. She is a founding member and past chair of the Health Association of African Canadians.

Gloria Feldt capped thirty years at Planned Parenthood by serving as president and CEO of Planned Parenthood Federation of America from 1996 to 2005. She is the author of *The War on Choice* and *Behind Every Choice Is a Story.*

Wendy Garling, M.A., is a writer and editor specializing in health care and women's issues. She earned her master's in Sanskrit at the University of California at Berkeley and teaches at the Women's Well in Concord, Massachusetts, www.womenswell.org.

Margaret Morganroth Gullette is the author of *Aged by Culture,* which the *Christian Science Monitor* named a Noteworthy Book of 2004, and of the prizewinning *Declining to Decline.* She is a resident scholar in the Women's Studies Research Center at Brandeis University.

Judith Hsia, M.D., is a professor of medicine in the Division of Cardiology at George Washington University and a principal investigator for the Women's Health Initiative.

Leslee Kagan, M.S., N.P., is a nurse practitioner and director of the Mind/Body Medical Institute's Menopause and Infertility Programs. An associate in medicine at Harvard Medical School, she coauthored *Mind over Menopause: The Complete Mind/Body Approach to Coping with Menopause.*

Barbara Keddy is a retired professor of nursing and women's studies at Dalhousie University in Halifax, Nova Scotia, Canada.

Rebecca Kightlinger, D.O., is an assistant professor at the University of Virginia and a board-certified obstetrician gynecologist in practice at the University of Virginia Midlife Health Center. She has a special interest in vulvar disease.

Katy Backes Kozhimannil is a researcher and advocate whose work focuses primarily on program and policy evaluation in sexual, reproductive, and maternal health care. She is pursuing a doctorate in health policy at Harvard University.

Angela Kueck, M.D., received a bachelor's degree from Notre Dame. She attended medical school and completed her residency in obstetrics and gynecology at Georgetown University. She is currently a fellow in gynecologic oncology at the University of Michigan.

Amy Lazev, Ph.D., is a faculty member in the Psychosocial and Behavioral Medicine Program, part of the Division of Population Science at the Fox Chase Cancer Center. She is a clinical psychologist and specializes in behavioral medicine and smoking cessation.

Ginny Levin, M.P.H., is a health educator and research coordinator of disease prevention clinical trials for women at George Washington University. She worked on PEPI, HERS, and

WHI, three large clinical trials of hormone use in postmenopausal women.

Margaret Lock is a professor of medical anthropology in the Department of Social Studies of Medicine at McGill University. Her books include *Encounters with Aging: Mythologies of Menopause in Japan and North America.* Her writing has earned numerous awards.

Nancy London, M.S.W., was a coauthor of the original version of *Our Bodies, Ourselves* and is the author of *Hot Flashes, Warm Bottles: First-Time Mothers over Forty.* She runs support groups for older first-time mothers. For information, see www.mothersoverforty.com.

Charlea T. Massion, M.D., has been a board-certified family physician and women's health specialist since 1981. She is an adviser to the American College of Women's Health Physicians and a coauthor of *The Truth about Hormone Replacement Therapy.*

Marianne McPherson, M.S., is a doctoral student in social policy at Brandeis University's Heller School and an Our Bodies Ourselves program consultant. Her research interests concern gender, reproductive health, and menstruation. She thanks her family and friends for their support.

Vicki Meyer earned a doctorate in community health at Texas Woman's University. She is the founder of the International Organization to Reclaim Menopause (www.inorm.org) and is an adjunct professor at the University of South Florida, where she teaches women's studies.

Ellen Sullivan Mitchell, R.N., Ph.D., is an associate professor at the University of Washington School of Nursing. She is currently responsible for a large, long-term research study about women's health during midlife, focusing on the menopausal transition and early postmenopause.

Margaret F. (Peggy) Moloney is an associate professor and nurse practitioner at Georgia State University. She has migraine headaches, and she conducts research into perimenopausal women's experiences of migraines. In the 1970s, she learned about women's health from *Our Bodies, Ourselves.*

Miriam E. Nelson, Ph.D., is an associate professor at the Friedman School of Nutrition Science and Policy at Tufts University. She is the author of the best-selling *Strong Women* book series and founder of Strongwomen.com.

Patricia Noone is a Ph.D. student in sociology at the University of New Hampshire. She is involved in research on women, the family, and medical sociology.

Patti Owen-Smith, Ph.D., is a professor of psychology and women's studies at Oxford College of Emory University. She has conducted award-winning research on homeless women and is the recipient of numerous honors for her teaching.

Lenore M. Pomerance, M.S.W., is a psychotherapist in Washington, D.C., specializing in midlife and menopause issues. Through her Menopause Counseling Center, www.menopausecounseling.com, she holds periodic workshops on healthy emotions and aging. Family, work, and masters competitive rowing are her passions.

Nancy Poole works as a provincial research consultant on women's substance use with BC Women's Hospital in Vancouver, and with the British Columbia Centre of Excellence for

Women's Health on research related to women's substance use and associated health issues.

Kimala Price, Ph.D., is an assistant professor of women's studies at San Diego State University. Formerly a post-doc at Ibis Reproductive Health in Cambridge, Massachusetts, she holds a doctorate in political science from the University of Michigan.

Jennifer Rhode, M.D., received her bachelor's degree from Auburn University. She attended the University of Alabama for medical school and completed her residency at Keesler Medical Center. She is a fellow in gynecologic oncology at the University of Michigan.

Marcie K. Richardson, M.D., is codirector of the Harvard Vanguard Menopause Consultation Service, an adviser to the Harvard Woman's Health Watch, and a trustee of the North American Menopause Society. She has two sons who know a lot about menopause.

Lenore Riddell, R.N., M.S.N., is an advanced practice nurse (women's health) in Vancouver, BC, Canada. Lenore is very active in giving presentations and workshops on reproductive health and general women's health concerns in Vancouver and other communities in British Columbia.

June Rogers is the editor of *A Friend Indeed,* a North American health newsletter for women in menopause and midlife (www.afriendin deed.ca). She is the recipient of the Margaret Mead Journalism Award from the American Medical Writers Association, among other awards.

Carolyn M. Sampselle, Ph.D., R.N.C., F.A.A.N., is a professor of nursing and associate dean for research at the University of Michigan School of Nursing. Her research on behavioral prevention of incontinence won recognition from the National Association for Continence in 2002.

Barbara Seaman is the author of *The Doctor's Case against the Pill, The Greatest Experiment Ever Performed on Women: Exploding the Estrogen Myth,* and other books on women's health. She cofounded the National Women's Health Network in 1975.

Susan Sered is author of *Uninsured in America: Life and Death in the Land of Opportunity.* A medical anthropologist, she is senior research associate at Suffolk University's Center for Women's Health and Human Rights.

Sherry Sherman, Ph.D., is program director of Clinical Aging and Reproductive Hormone Research in the Geriatrics and Clinical Gerontology Program, National Institute on Aging, NIH, DHHS. She is program officer of the NIH Study of Women's Health Across the Nation.

Moonhawk River Stone, M.S., is a psychotherapist in private practice specializing in working with transgender people. He is himself an out transsexual man who is an activist, educator, and writer in the transgender community.

Kristen Suthers, Ph.D., M.P.H., is the Menopause and Aging Program specialist at the National Women's Health Network. Originally a social scientist in gerontology, she now devotes her career to advocating for social justice in scientific research and women's health.

Mara Taub has been facilitating menopause workshops as a member of the Santa Fe Health Education Project since 1980. She is also a founding member and the editor of the free, national Coalition for Prisoners' Rights Newsletter, begun in 1976.

Wendy Wolfson writes about the effects of innovations in science, medicine, and technology on society for national and international publications. She has been a radio commentator and online columnist. She holds degrees from Bryn Mawr College and Boston University.

Nancy Woods, Ph.D., is dean of the School of Nursing and professor of family and child nursing at the University of Washington. She has led thirty years of research in women's health, the menstrual cycle, and the menopausal transition.

Diana Zuckerman, Ph.D., is president of the National Research Center for Women & Families, a nonprofit research and advocacy organization in Washington, D.C. She is trained in psychology and epidemiology, and is widely quoted on health policy and safety issues.

Disclosures

Our Bodies Ourselves is a nonprofit group committed to providing fair and accurate health information. In the interest of maintaining its independence, Our Bodies Ourselves does not accept any funding from pharmaceutical companies. All contributors who wrote sections of this book were asked to disclose any financial interest or other relationship since January 1, 2000, with any manufacturers of products or providers of services that they have discussed in the book. That information is listed below.

John Abramson serves as an expert consultant to plaintiffs' attorneys on a number of cases involving the drug industry, including litigation regarding the marketing of Lipitor to women and people over 65 who don't have heart disease or diabetes.

Gloria Feldt is the former president of Planned Parenthood Federation of America.

Judith Hsia receives research support from Pfizer, AstraZeneca, KOS, and Novartis, and is on the speaker's bureaus of Pfizer, AstraZeneca, and Sankyo.

Miriam Nelson serves on the board of directors and is a consultant to LLuminari, Inc., a lifestyle and health media corporation that markets the "Strong Women" brand. She is also a consultant to Mission Pharmacal, makers of citracal, where she assists with public relations, and serves on McDonald Corporation's Global Advisory Council. She has been a consultant to Stonyfield Farm.

Marcie Richardson is a consultant for Procter & Gamble Pharmaceuticals, serving as a member of its advisory board on female sexual dysfunction, and for Tufts Health Plan and Harvard Pilgrim Health Care, serving on physicians' advisory committees for each of them. She is also a consultant to LLuminari, Inc. The Harvard Vanguard Menopause Consultation Service that she directs has received unrestricted educational grant support from Alliance for Better Bone Health, Barr Laboratories Inc., Eli Lilly and Company, and Solvay Pharmaceuticals, Inc.

Carolyn Sampselle serves as an advisory board member for the National Association for Continence. She also serves on a Cognimed committee that focuses on educating health care providers about stress urinary incontinence.

Index

intercourse, painful, 47, 92, 93, 95, 106, 139, 148, 153
Internet, 309–10
intersex condition, 94
intestinal malabsorption, 238
intimacy, 154–55
introitus, 92, *92*, 93
in-vitro fertilization, 158
irbesartan (Avapro), 260
iron deficiencies, 85
iron supplements, 85
irritability, 192, 221, 229
ischemic cardiomyopathy, 256
isoflavones, 182
itching, vaginal, 91, 92, 107
IUDs, 145, 210

Japan, 12, 235, 300
Japanese-Americans, 13, 49, 54
  early menopause among, 61
  hot flashes among, 76
jobs, 15
job sharing, 305
jogging, 196, 199, 236
Johnson, Virginia, 148
joints, 194
 health of, 279, 289–90
  pains in, 51, 63, 105
junk food, 181, 185, 190

kale, 184
Kegel, Arnold, 215
Kegel exercises, 213, 215
Kensington Ladies' Erotica Society, 144
kidney cancer, 184, 280
kidney disease, 235
kidney failure, restless leg syndrome and, 85
kidneys, 47, 255, 257, 259
kidney stones, 238
Kilbourne, Jean, 131
Klein, Linda, 309
knee exercises, 201
knee problems, 196
Kreinin, Tamara, 309
Kush, Christopher, 312
K-Y lubricant, 93

labia, lesions of, 209
labia majora, 92, *92*
labia minora, 92, *92,* 95
laboratory tests, 35
language, medical, 21
language barriers, 32
laparoscope, 211, 212
laparoscopic surgery, 272
Latinas, 12–13
  diabetes and, 284
  early menopause among, 61
  earnings of, 304
  hot flashes among, 76
  Social Security and, 305
  see also Hispanic-Americans
legumes, *179,* 184, 250
leiomyomas, 208
lentils, 111
lesbians, 29, 32, 142, 152–53, 280, 298
Lescol (fluvastatin), 252
letrozole, 266
lettuce, dark green, 184
leukemia, 76, 280
Levine, Suzanne Braun, 315
Lexapro, 228
libido, 67, 147, 148, 152, 155
lichen sclerosus, 91, 94–95
lichen simplex chronicus, 91, 96
licorice root, 80
lidocaine, topical (Xylocaine), 97
life expectancy, 300
Life of My Breasts (Bosch), 269
Lincoln, Blanche Lambert, *300*
lipid metabolism, 52
lipids, 53
Lipitor (atorvastatin), 252, 260
lipoproteins, 53
liposuction, 131
lisinopril, 260
liver disease, 100, 109, 235, 238, 282
living wills, 161
locally grown food, 180, 185
long-term care, 297, 304, 312, 313
long-term memory, 222–23
loop electrosurgical excisions procedure (LEEP), 274

Lopid (gemfibrozil), 254
Loppie, Charlotte, 14
Lopressor (metoprolol), 260
losartan (Cozaar), 260
lovastatin (Mevacor), 252, 260
low-density lipoprotein (LDL) cholesterol, 53, 182, 247, 252, 253, 254
low-fat diets, 183
low-impact aerobics, 251
low self-esteem, 127
lubricants, 93, 139, 140, 143, 154
Lubrin, 93
lumpectomy, 269
Lunesta (eszopiclone), 86
lung cancer, 264, 275–76, 280
lung disease, 152
lungs, 197
Lupron, 60, 66
lupus, 62
luteinizing hormone, 64
Luvox, 228
lymph nodes, 269, 275, 276

mackerel, 237
macular degeneration, 179
magnesium, 288
magnesium supplements, 85
magnetic resonance angiography, 259
magnets, 78, 259
male-to-female (MTF) transgender, 116
mammograms, 265, 267–68, 269, 298
managed care, 29, 299–300, 301
margarine, 180
Massachusetts Women's Health Study, 6, 52, 54
massage, 83
massage therapy, 70
mastectomy, 269, 269–70, *269* reconstruction after, 129, *269,* 270
Masters, William, 148
masturbation, 139, 153
Mavik (trandolapril), 260

selective estrogen receptor
  modifiers (SERM), 113, 242
Selective Extrasynaptic GABA
  Agonists (gaboxadol), 86
selective serotonin reuptake
  inhibitors (SSRIs), 228, 288
self-confidence, 194
self-esteem 127, 189
self-hatred, 126
self-nurture, 134
sentinel node biopsy (SNB), 269
serotonin, 224
serotonin and norepinephrine
  reuptake inhibitors (SNRI),
  81
serotonin receptors, 229
serum cholesterol, 53
Serzone, 152
set points, 75
sex, 3
  genitally-centered, 143
  see also sexuality
sex hormone-binding globulin
  (SHBG), 47–48, 49
sexism, x, 6, 7–8, 15, 170, 298
sex reassignment surgery, 94
sexual attractiveness, 308
sexual concerns, 50–51
sexual desire, 63, 67, 110–11
  medicalization of, 148–52
sexuality, ix, 51, 138–56, 302
  changing relationships and,
    140–43
  early menopause and, 67
  expressions of, 143–45
  illness, disability and, 152–54
  strategies and approaches to,
    154–56
sexually transmitted infections
  (STIs), 32, 146–47, 149, 209,
  274
sexual orientation, 11, 298
sexual pleasure, 90
sexual problems, 228
sexual response cycle, 148
shark, 182
Shields, Laurie, 313
short-term memory, 222

sick leave, 304
side effects, 21
silicone gel breast implants, 129
Silk-E moisturizer, 93
simvastatin (Zocor), 252, 260
Sinequan (doxipin), 86, 228
Single energy X-ray
  absorptiometry, 243
single-payer system, 301
sinus headaches, 285, 286
16 Steps for Discovery and
  Empowerment, 283
skin, 63, 132, 134, 280
skin cancer, 238, 264
skin patches, for hormone
  treatment, 109
sleep, 170, 172
  exercise and, 194, 196
  improvement of, 83
  memory and, 222, 224, 226
  relaxation and, 172
  schedules, 82
  warm milk and, 185
sleep apnea, 82, 83, 84–85
sleep deprivation, 298
sleep-disordered breathing, 84
sleep disturbances, 74, 82–86, 105,
  106, 192, 302
  depression and, 227, 229, 230,
    231
  see also insomnia
sleep hygiene, 83, 84
sleep medications, 85–86
sleep patterns, migraines and,
  286
smoke, migraines and, 286, 287
smoking, 13, 42, 53, 76, 83, 85,
  210, 253
  as addiction, 280
  bladder health and, 216
  and cardiovascular disease, 247,
    247, 250, 251
  cervical cancer and, 274
  depression and, 230
  early menopause and, 62
  hot flashes and, 76–77
  lung cancer and, 275
  osteoporosis and, 235, 237

quitting of, 6, 15, 19, 76–77,
  182, 225, 281–82
  and skin health, 132
  uterine prolapse and, 213
  and vulvar cancer, 275
  wrinkles and, 134
snacks, 180, 181, 186
soaps, 97, 132
social change, 170, 176, 311–15
social connections, 167, 175–76,
  226, 247, 248, 281, 309–10
social isolation, 247, 248
social policies, 303
Social Security, 300, 304–6, 312,
  313
Social Security Act, 300–301
social workers, hospital, 31
society:
  body image and, 128–30
  and postmenopausal women,
    297
sodas, 181
sodium, 251
Sommers, Tish, 313
Sonata (zaleplon), 86
sonohysterogram, 210
soy, 11, 79–80, 80, 111, 180, 182,
  184–85
soy milk, 237
soy oil, 179
speculum, 211
spicy foods, 77, 114, 185
spinach, 179
spine, curvature of, 235
spirituality, 13, 169, 170, 172,
  173–74
sports drinks, 181
spotting, 45, 208, 209, 210
sprue, 238
squamous cell carcinoma, 274
squats, 199–200, 199
Stabenow, Debbie, 300
Stages or Reproductive Aging
  Workshop (STRAW), 43
staging, 273
stair climbing, 236
stamina, 196
statins, 82, 252–54, 260

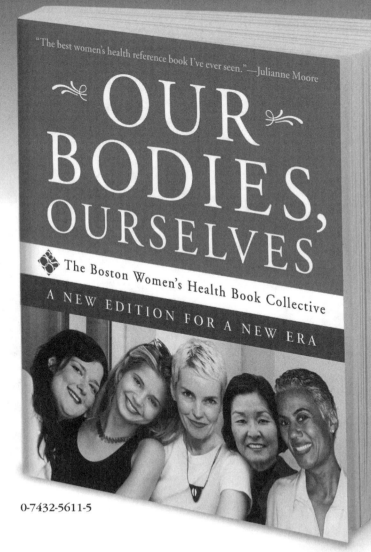
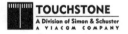